second edition

INTRODUCTION TO
HEALTH EDUCATION
AND
HEALTH PROMOTION

Bruce G. Simons-Morton, Ed.D., M.P.H.
National Institute of Child Health and Human Development
National Institutes of Health

Walter H. Greene, Ed.D.
Temple University

Nell H. Gottlieb, Ph.D.
University of Texas at Austin

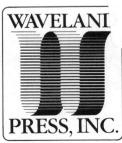

WAVELAND
PRESS, INC.
Prospect Heights, Illinois

To our students and colleagues and

To Denise—BS-M
To Francie—WHG
To Paul and Erin—NHG

For information about this book, write or call:
Waveland Press, Inc.
P.O. Box 400
Prospect Heights, Illinois 60070
(847) 634-0081

Photo Credits: Pages 1, 243, 375, Nora Byrne; pages 119, 316, 317, 319, 320,
Bruce G. Simons-Morton.

Contents

Foreword

Health education is both a process and a profession. As a process, several professional groups as well as layworkers use educational and other interventions to help individuals or groups make changes in behavior or conditions of living to promote health and prevent disease. Health education specialists are professionals who have unique training to plan, implement, and evaluate programs that include educational and related interventions. The revised edition of *Introduction to Health Education and Health Promotion* addresses the methods involved in the process of health education as well as the professional grounding that supports the knowledge and skills necessary to function as a professional health educator. *Introduction to Health Education and Health Promotion, 2/E* provides the scientific basis for conceptualizing and designing health education programs as well as for the art of working with individuals and groups to make programs effective within the context and realities of delivering programs that are relevant and practical.

The first edition of this text was very well received by health education faculty and practitioners and has become one of the standard texts in the field. This revised edition retains the general chapter structure but the content has been significantly updated and expanded. In the 10 years since the first edition was published, the field of health education has grown and matured, resulting in the expansion of conceptual models for program development, improvements in the application of behavioral and social science theory, increasing evidence to show that interventions can be effective, and greater acceptance of health education and promotion as central strategies for the prevention of disease and health problems. The authors have done an excellent job of assessing and capturing the recent developments in health education and integrating them into the knowledge base and skills addressed by the individual chapters. The result is comprehensive, up-to-date coverage of health education and health promotion program development, implementation, and evaluation.

As a survey text, *Introduction to Health Education and Health Promotion, 2/E* cannot provide in-depth coverage of all of the knowledge and skills needed to practice health education. For the advanced student, specialized texts and published research and practice literature are necessary to develop the competencies necessary to carry out the full range of practice activities. However, this text provides an excellent foundation for the beginning student to conceptualize the field and to be socialized into the profession of health education.

The authors of the second edition have extensive experience in teaching health education students in the environments of schools of education, schools of public health, allied health sciences, and medical school. In addition, they have been extensively involved in research and demonstration projects that require them to practice health education and promotion. Thus, the authors speak from a voice of experience not only in the academics of health education but also in the actual planning, implementing and evaluating of programs. They have tested their conceptualizations for health education practice in the real world of community, school, worksite, and patient education programs. The authors are leaders in the field through their work in professional health education organizations and through their research and development projects published in the research and practice literature.

Introduction to Health Education and Health Promotion, 2/E represents current state-of-the-art practice guidelines and conceptual foundations for health education and promotion. The book is highly appropriate for use as a text for undergraduate and graduate education majors in health education as well as for other health professional training that includes roles and responsibilities related to health education and promotion. Professionals involved in planning and providing health education programs will also find the text very useful to update knowledge and to serve as a guide for developing new programs.

Guy S. Parcel, Ph.D.
Professor and Director
Center for Health Promotion Research and Development
University of Texas, Houston Health Science Center

Preface

Many significant changes have taken place in the world and within the profession of health education since the first edition of this text was published in 1984. This has made the task of revising both challenging and exciting.

The cold war, which provided the backdrop for the entire adult life of most Americans, has given way to a "cold peace" in which the specter of a nuclear holocaust has receded, only to be replaced by numerous, small-scale international conflicts and heightened global economic competition. Within our own borders, America suffers from a growing epidemic of domestic violence and seemingly unsolvable social problems such as unintended pregnancies, substance abuse, hopelessness, poverty, and crime. Health and social problems are now recognized as being highly interconnected. Relatedly, many chronic health problems have proven themselves largely to be the product of lifestyle, modifiable only through changes in the environment and the social norms of the population.

Rising concerns over the national deficit and run-away medical costs, combined with general disenchantment with government-funded programs, have led to rigorous cost cutting by private business and government agencies. Therefore, no matter what setting health educators work in they are constrained by economic realities. Consequently, some health education programs have struggled to maintain their funding. Generally, however, prevention has come to be viewed as the cost-efficient path to containing medical care costs, making health education a growth field. This trend is expected to continue in future years as the evidence accumulates that prevention efforts are frequently more cost effective than enforcement or curative approaches. The emphasis on prevention has been crystallized by *Healthy People 2000*, which provides national health goals for the nation's major health problems and target populations. National health insurance and other federal initiatives also are a considerable force for prevention.

In keeping with the modern understanding of the multidimensional causes of health and disease, the mission of health education has expanded considerably in recent years. Health education was once seen as mainly information oriented. Today, health education is the core profession responsible for health promotion in school, worksite, clinical, and community settings. Health education was once seen as being oriented exclusively toward the individual, whereas today it is in the forefront of the movement toward multilevel intervention approaches targeting individuals, groups, organizations, and communities.

Education remains the essential process by which healthful changes are facilitated, but in the modern practice of health education the targets of that education are just as likely to be decision makers, support persons, or health professionals as the groups whose health and health behavior are of primary interest. A range of theories has been identified that is particularly useful in guiding health education interventions. In addition, effective educational methods have been developed for use in various settings with various populations. While many professions are concerned with health and education in some way, health education has established itself as the one profession whose primary and exclusive mission is health promotion.

In keeping with new challenges, the profession of health education has continued to develop rapidly and favorably. Credentialing of health education specialists is a thing of the present. Opportunities for continuing education have increased substantially and improved greatly in recent years. Employment opportunities for capable health educators continue to expand.

The authors have retained much of the same chapter structure of the first edition, with a few notable exceptions. Part I contains an expanded discussion in Chapter 4 of the relationship between health education and health promotion. Part II contains updated and expanded sections on needs assessment, planning, and intervention approaches. In Part III we have greatly expanded the discussion of cognitive theories and methods and added a chapter on organizational change. Part IV now includes a chapter on practice settings. Moreover, all chapters have been revised to reflect the modern practice of health education. Recognizing that many students begin their study of health education at the graduate level, the general tone and style of the book has been modified in an effort to appeal to both upper level and graduate students. The profession and its practitioners are diverse and wide ranging. It is difficult, if not impossible, to describe the essential foundations of the profession and to characterize the profession without leaving out some important perspectives and activities. We have attempted, however, to provide a comprehensive introductory text that is nevertheless practical and readable.

PART I

HEALTH EDUCATION AND PROMOTION

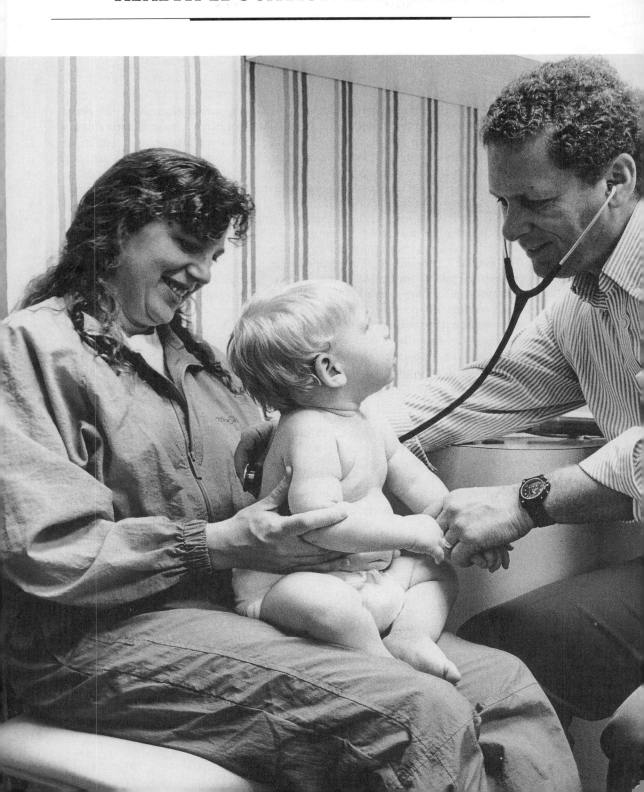

H ealth is a quality vitally important to living satisfaction. As an idealized concept it virtually defies definition. Somewhat like beauty, its true nature exists in the mind, if not the eye, of the beholder. However, in the more practical world of public policy, health professionals have come to rely on an array of relatively precise indicators, such as life expectancy, infant mortality, and freedom from disability, that are used to assess year-to-year progress or to compare the health status of various population groups.

Both the vast historical experience of humankind and the explosive growth of knowledge in the current century have revealed many complex physical, cultural, economic, and political factors that directly or indirectly determine the level of health of any given population. Consequently, a variety of health professions and organizations have been established to assist individuals and communities in their pursuit of better health. These typically well-regarded and well-intentioned professionals often vary in their degree of training and competence; they sometimes aid and complement, and sometimes hamper and duplicate one another's activities.

Health education in the United States was conceived and nurtured as part of the early development of the public schools and public health organizations. In its original form, it focused on the single task of disseminating health information. More recently, health educators have embraced the broader concept of health promotion. Health promotion is a set of processes that can be employed to change the conditions that affect health. Health education is the profession principally devoted to employing such processes to foster healthful behavior and, thus, health itself. Accordingly, health educators are now concerned with the full gamut of personal and environmental factors that affect health behavior. Moreover, they seek positive changes in those factors within the workplace, the community, and the realm of public policy.

Health Status

Many years ago someone questioned the late, great Louis Armstrong about the true meaning and essence of jazz. "How can I tell if the music I hear is really jazz?" The old performer thought a moment and then replied, "If you have to ask, you'll never know." What he probably meant by this cryptic reply was that jazz was essentially an aesthetic concept— something to experience rather than to define, to feel rather than to know. Mere words could not convey its meaning. And such is the case with many significant things in our lives.

Introduction

The term "health" certainly represents a broader and more complex entity than does "jazz," yet health professionals are seldom put in Louis Armstrong's position. Outside of college classrooms the question "Just what is health anyway?" is seldom asked. Most people assume that they know what health is. They are far more likely to ask, "Just what is heart disease anyway?" "What is cancer? Arthritis? Schizophrenia? AIDS?" Although most of us place a high value on health, we tend to think of it as an absence of certain disease conditions rather than a condition unto itself. We support, with very little objection, the annual expenditure of millions of federal tax dollars for research on disease and we contribute millions more via charitable donations. Then, more grudgingly, we spend billions on the treatment of disease. It is logical enough to mount a vigorous fight against these potent enemies, yet we should also give significant attention to the desired quality at the opposite end of the continuum. Within this chapter we seek to provide a balanced approach by first examining the sometimes frustrating and sometimes fascinating efforts to formulate a more positive definition of health and then presenting an assessment of our society's current health status and future outlook.

Defining Health

We live in a society that places great importance on the fight against disease. Themes involving serious illness or injury provide dramatic content to popular soap operas, films, and novels; the people who help the sick and the injured— physicians, nurses, paramedics, and so on—are, for the most part, highly respected. We may occasionally accuse them of greed, neglect, or inattention to our problems but seldom do we challenge their competence. This fascination has helped fuel the growth of a massive health care industry with revenues projected to exceed one trillion dollars in 1994, an amount more than triple the annual budget for national defense.

Our tendency is to think of health simply as the absence of disease. This view has become a *de facto* definition that is generally unspoken and unwritten, yet is reflected in most health-related actions. As such, it has generated a number of problems. Conceptually, it puts us in the awkward position of drawing a sharp focus on that which we wish to avoid (disease) while leaving that which everyone desires (health) very fuzzily described. On a practical level, such an outlook exerts strong influences on both individual health actions and social policies. Nearly 97 percent of America's "health" dollars are spent on facilities, equipment, supplies, and services used to treat disease, leaving little more than 3 percent for all local, state, and federal public health departments and agencies (National Center for Health Statistics, 1993).

The Need for Definition

Definitions are often of little importance, particularly when they remain safely concealed in dictionaries and textbooks. But sometimes they impact directly on an underlying idea or concept with far reaching effects. For example, early in this century a few progressive health professionals fostered the idea that good health involves normal emotional responses and stable, rational behavior and that certain disturbances of mood or behavior (as in anxiety, neuroses, and schizophrenia) are illnesses and thereby merit treatment. Many victims of these maladies who had previously been regarded as "nuts" or criminals now are recognized as ill persons in need of treatment.

As a result, psychiatry has been established as a medical specialty and clinical psychology has emerged as a new field. A small trickle of public funds has grown into a respectable stream of support and this has nourished a new industry complete with hospitals, clinics, psychiatric technicians, and a host of other support personnel, not to mention an important new market for the drug companies. Granted, some efforts are more successful than others; however, for better or worse, a basic change in the concepts of health and disease has had a dramatic impact on people's lives.

The persistent, negative concept of health (i.e., the absence of disease) that has been held by most members of the general public and too many members of the health profession is giving way to a more positive, constructive view of health. This redefinition of health has been a necessary step in establishing the philosophical basis needed for shifting society's priorities from after-the-fact treatment to disease prevention and health promotion.

Difficulty of the Task

"Jazz is beautiful—but what is beauty?" "Love is vital—but what is love?" Most people get by with their implicit, unexamined concepts of such basic entities;

but health professionals need clear perceptions of what they seek to promote. Daniel Callahan, while director of the Institute of Society, Ethics and the Life Sciences, warned that "like most other very general concepts—'peace,' 'justice,' 'freedom'—that of 'health' poses enormous difficulties of definition." He also noted that "oddly enough, for all the debates about 'health,' few attempts have ever been made to give the term some substance; it seems to be taken for granted that everyone knows what is being talked about" (Callahan, 1977:25–26).

The issue of scope soon arises in any serious consideration of health as a concept. What does it include? What is excluded? Michael Dolfman reviewed the changes that have occurred in the generally accepted meaning of the term over the years and concluded that it has, in effect, traveled full circle from a very general term to a very narrow one, then back to a broad interpretation (Dolfman, 1973:491–497). The word "health" first appeared in the English language in approximately A.D. 1000 as a means of referring to the quality of soundness and wholeness in a very broad sense. As its usage is traced in the literature of the period, it soon became apparent that physical prowess, wit, intelligence, and spiritual salvation were included as an aspect of one's wholeness. But, apparently during the 1800s, as modern science entered an "adolescent" phase accompanied by great faith in its physical explanations for human phenomena, the meaning of health gradually shed many of its intellectual and spiritual connotations; by the beginning of the present century it meant little more than the absence of physical illness.

Modern Definitions

Fortunately, a broadening of the concept of health began in the twentieth century as the fields of psychology and sociology attained respectability and contributed to broader and more positive views. The eventual result of this trend was the formulation of the World Health Organization's widely accepted definition.

The WHO Definition: A Broad and Positive View

In 1946 the newly established World Health Organization (WHO) included a twenty-word statement in its constitution which identified three dimensions of health:

> Health is a state of complete physical, mental, and social well-being and not merely the absence of disease or infirmity. (WHO, 1947)

Since its publication the reaction among health professionals to this definition has varied considerably. A few have expressed serious concern. Daniel Callahan, for example stated:

> It is a dangerous definition, and it desperately needs replacement by something more modest. Its emphasis on "complete physical, mental, and social well-being"

puts both medicine and society in the untenable position of being required to attain unattainable goals. There is no reason to think that medicine can, for instance, make more than a modest contribution to "complete social well-being." (Callahan, 1977:26)

Others have ignored it or given it lip service without actually acting on its implications. For the most part, however, the WHO definition has been praised and used as a tool for innovative change. It definitely merits a closer look by those seeking to enter any health profession.

Physical and Mental Well-Being

Although there is broad agreement regarding the inclusion of the physical and mental dimensions in the WHO definition, one may still question the extent of the acceptance of the mental component. It seems clear, for example, that the acceptance of mental or emotional problems is much more certain when something "physical" is involved either as a causative factor or as a symptom. If the harassed businesswoman, for instance, develops a peptic ulcer big enough to reveal itself on an X-ray, she will generally receive more sympathy and more thorough treatment than if her symptoms were expressed in insomnia and its resultant fatigue. For years the many thousands of people who suffer from chronic fatigue syndrome have had difficulty finding physicians who would treat their complaints seriously; this situation is much improved now that there appears to be evidence of a physical cause. Similarly, the schoolchild whose behavioral problems result from brain damage incurred during birth may be regarded more sympathetically than if his or her behavior resulted from long-term interpersonal conflicts. Regrettably, this tendency to regard only physical symptoms as indicative of "real illness" is not restricted to the lay public. Many sophisticated health professionals define health in holistic terms when in the lecture hall, but tend to think in physical terms when in the clinic.

Social Well-Being

As Callahan (1977) implied, the social dimension appears as the most ambiguous member of the triad and thus remains open to individual interpretation. One possible way of viewing social health is to take the position that to be healthy one must make a positive contribution to one's family and community. The parent who does a responsible job of parenting is viewed as socially healthy; the abusive parent is deemed socially ill. The bank clerk who chairs the United Fund drive exhibits social health, whereas his colleague who embezzles the bank's funds exhibits social illness. One's social health status, according to this scheme, is measured not in terms of personal feelings of well-being, but in terms of one's affect on the well-being of others. The neurotic do-gooder therefore moves up a notch or two whereas the happy, well-adjusted criminal, if such exists, is downgraded. This may be what is meant by social well-being, but if it is, one finds very little commentary or clarification in the professional literature.

A more common view holds that social health is characterized by the ability to establish and maintain good interpersonal relationships, to develop a warm circle of friends, to "connect" with other people, to receive and express affection. These are undoubtedly important qualities but they pose a difficult question: do they represent a discrete dimension of their own or are they simply important aspects of mental health? Granted that the human personality is developed, nourished, and sustained in a social context; however, this social context is more an external determinant of health rather than a dimension of health itself. Ware (1981:621), following an extensive review of literature, expresses a similar view:

> A model of health status that defines social factors (along with others such as life events) as external but related to an individual's health status explains empirical results better than one that includes social factors as an integral component of individual health.

Patrick and Bergner (1990:166) express a similar view stating that "health status should be distinguished from the social, familial, and behavioral factors and processes that influence it. . . ." It may be argued that social maladjustment or deprivation, for instance, becomes a problem as it is reflected in reduced mental health. Good social interaction thus becomes analogous to good nutrition; the proper types and amounts, free of pathological contaminants, contribute to good health. According to this view social interaction becomes a means for achieving health rather than a part of health itself.

This alternative view that social interaction is a means of gaining health rather than a part of health itself suggests the possibility that the concept of "social health" could be more properly applied to the surrounding society rather than to the individual. The individual's prospects for physical and mental well-being are enhanced by a "healthy" social environment that provides such essentials as education, opportunity, security, and employment.

Spiritual Well-Being

The inclusion of a spiritual dimension in the concept of health is very common among health professionals. Howard Hoyman, for example, states emphatically, "For us to ignore man's psychospiritual nature in developing our model of health would be to deal with a caricature of man—with modern man dehumanized" (1975:511). Despite this popularity the framers of the WHO definition chose to ignore the issue completely. In view of the potential pitfalls, this omission was probably deliberate rather than accidental.

The validity of the spiritual dimension of health is dependent not only upon one's belief in the existence of spiritual forces, but one's beliefs concerning the particular nature and manner of functioning of these forces. The situation is further complicated by the tendency for writers to hopelessly entangle spiritual with psychological concerns (note Hoyman's use of the term "psychospiritual"). For example, it is relatively easy to demonstrate the health benefits that occur to many devout people who regularly pray; in addition to these persons achieving peace of mind, their blood pressure may ease and their digestion may improve.

But while some would argue that prayer in these instances evoked intervention of metaphysical forces, others would interpret these events merely as an example of autosuggestion involving a placebo effect. Perhaps the framers of the WHO definition were wise to sidestep such questions. Probably the best resolution of this issue is to recognize and respect the comfort that many receive from their spiritual beliefs and practices while focusing one's professional activities on the more secular dimensions. This view is presented in figure 1.1.

Figure 1.1

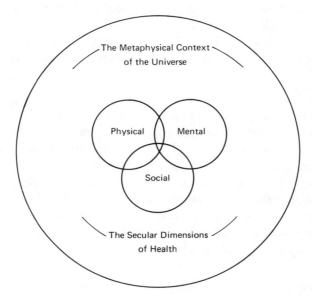

The three dimensions of the WHO definition lend themselves to scientific investigation; however, they exist within a spiritual context which is viewed in highly individual ways.

Holistic Health

As noted, it is difficult to develop a precise list of health factors to which most people will agree. Physical and mental? Physical, mental, and social? Physical, mental, emotional, and social? And dare we add spiritual? Many health professionals say that such lists should not be attempted. They view health as a tightly integrated **gestalt**, a term that refers to the development of a unique entity with an existence of its own, as opposed to a loose collection of components. According to this view, the process of identifying dimensions causes one to lose sight of the whole and so creates an invalid conception. This danger may exist; however, to recognize the dimensions of a certain thing is not the same as reducing it to its separate components. Moreover, it is difficult to nourish and sustain something if we are unable to categorize the things that are needed. Growing children need nutritious food. They need love and praise. They need intellectual stimulation. They need friends. They need faith. The goal is an integrated whole, but the needs are specific and require study and analysis.

The Dynamics of Health: Sharpening the Criteria

How do we determine the presence of health? What is the impact of health on a person's life on a day-to-day basis? What do healthy people do or experience better than unhealthy people? Such questions concern the dynamics of health and may address themselves to its real meaning better than those of dimension. They very quickly lead into a discussion of health criteria. If you have red, itchy eyes; a runny nose; and a dusky red, blotchy rash on your skin, you probably have measles. But how do you know when you have health?

Subjective Feelings

Milton Terris identifies two major aspects of health: ". . . one subjective and the other objective. The subjective aspect relates to feeling well, the objective aspect to ability to function" (Terris, 1975:1038). The quality of "feeling well" as a criterion for health is not only very straightforward but unique in the potential control it gives to the individual over his or her own health. Although obviously influenced by a variety of external stimuli, feelings themselves originate within the mind of the individual; according to this view, perceptions become more important to health than the reality of one's circumstances. Thus many severely disabled people can be ranked very highly according to this criterion, whereas many "clinically healthy" types who happen to become severely depressed or suicidal would be ranked near the bottom.

Ability to Function

Terris's second major criterion, ability to function, seems to have obvious validity and universal acceptance; however, opinions vary on what functions are most important and what standards of competence are associated with health. Many clinical examinations of functional ability, for example, are focused on the minimal requirements for independent living, such as feeding oneself, getting dressed, and bathroom chores. At the other extreme are those advocates of ideal health, such as Halbert Dunn. He felt that the term "health" had been distorted by such minimal concepts beyond any hope of clarification. He decided to use, instead, the term "high-level wellness." He defined it as follows:

> Wellness, in the sense here used, signifies something quite different from good health. Good health can exist as a relatively passive state of freedom from illness in which the individual is at peace with his environment . . . High-level wellness for the individual is defined as an integrated method of functioning which is oriented toward maximizing the potential of which the individual is capable within the environment where he is functioning. (Dunn, 1977:9)

Dunn's basic criterion is thus a method of functioning that permits maximum productivity within the limits of one's inherent potential. The authors generally endorse this positive view but differ with Dunn's limited concept of good health; if health is a "complete state of physical, mental, and social well-being," it would seem to be very similar to "wellness." Both conditions would enable an individual to make maximum progress toward his or her life goals and thus are very compatible with another positive view, that of psychologist Abraham Maslow who defines his concept of self-actualization as "the full use and exploitation of talents, capacities, potentialities, etc." (Maslow, 1970:150).

Both Dunn and Maslow describe people who have succeeded in life in terms of their own particular potential. Health is not success, but that which permits success. This very indirect and subjective approach poses a challenging task for those people seeking valid criteria for ideal health. One must first identify successful people, which is not easy, then identify the particular personal qualities that facilitated this success. This type of thinking goes far beyond the traditional, safe concept of health as a simple state of normality and freedom from disease.

Ability to Adjust or Adapt

René Dubos, who has written extensively on this topic, provides a definition of health that reflects his professional training as a microbiologist:

> The states of health or disease are the expressions of the success or failure experienced by the organism in its efforts to respond adaptively to environmental challenges. (1965:xvii)

The key to this definition lies in the words "respond adaptively to environmental challenges." Dubos uses the term "environmental challenges" to mean virtually any threat to the individual's well-being. The privations of a wartime prison camp provide a prime example of an environment containing many such challenges. Here the prisoner may have to endure unsanitary conditions; an improper diet and insufficient food; prolonged exposure to excessive heat or cold; a lack of exercise or excessive physical labor; emotional stress, including fear of execution or torture; loneliness and boredom; and a variety of similar stresses. The ability to endure and survive such challenges requires a type of physical and emotional toughness that is difficult to assess without putting the individual to the actual test. Many well-documented cases exist of "hale and hardy" types who soon developed pneumonia, dysentery, or other infections which eventually resulted in their death; others seemed to "give up" emotionally—they lost interest in food and over a period of weeks simply shriveled up and died. Still others who appeared to be less well-endowed physically have, in similar circumstances, shaken off the infections, thrived on a sparse diet, coped with the emotional stress, found companionship with both prisonmates and prisonkeeper, and otherwise "adapted" and survived.

Although essential to health, the quality of "adaptability" provides only a partial answer in our search for a positive definition. The human organism has learned to adapt quite well to daily exposure to microorganisms and, given sufficient time, could learn to handle a variety of exotic chemicals just as well. But in this case it is probably better to eliminate the chemicals; in other words, to master the environment rather than adapt to it. However, the concept of adaptability does introduce a useful time perspective into our view of health. According to Dubos, to be truly healthy one must not only be functioning well at the moment but must also possess the capacity to resist future threats. The child whose bloodstream contains antibodies against tetanus, pertussis, polio, and a variety of other infections, presumably as a result of immunizations, thus receives a higher health rating than one who is not similarly protected, even though both may be disease-free at the time of assessment. Likewise, the person with good skills for coping with emotional stress is considered healthier than one lacking these skills, even though neither is currently experiencing any significant problems.

Terris addresses a closely related issue when he emphasizes the difference between **illness** and **disease**. He defines disease as the underlying defect or malfunction within the organism, whereas illness is the visible presentation of symptoms that make a person feel distressed. As he points out:

> Disease may occur without illness. Health and illness are mutually exclusive, but health and disease are not. . . . Since health and disease may coexist, one cannot construct a continuum to show their relationship. (1975:1037)

The distinction between disease and illness seems interesting and useful; however, many health professionals might quarrel with the conclusion that health and disease may coexist. If we say that a person is in a high state of health because that person feels good and performs well, for example, and then we find that the individual dropped dead of a massive heart attack the following day, perhaps we didn't know enough in the first place.

Directions and Ambivalence

In which direction should you look as you search for health? Do you look forward toward an idealized concept of complete physical, mental, and social well-being? Or do you look backward toward disease and attempt to move away from illness in its various forms? Clearly, health professionals are for the most part disease oriented; however, this fact in itself is not a problem. Illness and its prevention should receive the bulk of professional attention. Few people advocate shifting resources to the task of helping "healthy" people move on to high-level wellness at the expense of helping those who are ill to get well or helping "healthy" individuals avoid illness. The problem is that our disease orientation has led to a misguided strategy in how to best carry on the struggle. Guy Steuart makes this clear:

> Firstly, . . . although many of us quote the WHO definition with such conviction, we remain strangely untroubled that so much curative and preventive action in the health field still consists of a fragmentary disease-by-disease approach, with considerable emphasis on the physical, somewhat less on the mental, and to a negligible extent on the social. . . .

Secondly, the term "merely the absence of disease" seems to imply this would constitute a mean, unworthy goal in itself. When we take the state of health of the world's populations today, we would after all be doing exceedingly well if we were able to achieve even a "near" absence of disease. (1969:428)

Steuart thus sees nothing wrong with a health care establishment that single-mindedly studies, treats, and prevents disease; his concern is with the fragmentary, after-the-fact, disease-by-disease approach that currently absorbs so much of the nation's resources. He implies that broad health promotional activities such as providing nutritional support, prenatal care, and training in child rearing to low-income families would effectively combat many potential disease conditions at a much lower cost.

Measuring Health

Efforts to both control disease and enhance health represent the pursuit of an ideal. Regardless of how hard we try to treat or prevent disease, everyone eventually dies; and regardless of how hard we work to enhance health, no one has achieved a "state of complete physical, mental, and social well-being." Consequently, we are never satisfied; resources are always short; there is never time and money enough to do everything we would like to do for health. We are thus forced to make choices, and this brings us to the task of measuring health to determine such things as (1) which groups of people are most in need of help, (2) which diseases are most troublesome, and (3) which methods of control are most promising.

As noted in the previous section, the task of defining and establishing criteria for positive health is difficult yet worthwhile because it provides guidelines for our efforts to attain such a desirable state either for individuals or for our society. Perhaps some day in the future it may be appropriate to direct the bulk of professional attention to the task of helping people move from the "normal" to the "ideal" end of the health-illness continuum. However, in the current stage of the struggle—with so much disease and premature mortality occurring in the world—health professionals generally find it more efficient to measure health progress with such admittedly negative indicators as the reduction of the incidence of disease or the lowering of death rates.

Over the years the various public agencies responsible for health and safety have developed an elaborate system for compiling statistics on births, deaths, disease, and accidents. When used properly, such data can help insure that decisions as to which health-care bill to support and which programs to fund are made in a fair and efficient manner. Although statistics can be abused and misinterpreted, they provide a much better guide than the press releases of well-funded lobbyists or highly vocal interest groups.

The Traditional Indices

Throughout the health field certain traditional indices of health status are commonly used for such tasks as making comparisons between different geographic areas or different periods of time, pinpointing areas of need, and setting future goals. The categories into which these indices fall are mortality, life expectancy, morbidity, and disability. Definitions are provided in table 1.1.

Table 1.1 Definitions of Common Health Indices

Index	Definition
Mortality Rates	
Crude Mortality Rate (per 1,000)	$\dfrac{\text{Number of deaths during a specified year}}{\text{Number of persons in the population at the middle of the same year}} \times 1{,}000$
Infant Mortality Rate (per 1,000)	$\dfrac{\text{Number of infant deaths (0–1 years) in a year}}{\text{Number of live births in the same year}} \times 1{,}000$
Cause-specific mortality rate (per 100,000)	$\dfrac{\text{Number of deaths due to a specific cause during a specified year}}{\text{Number of persons in the population at the middle of the same year}} \times 100{,}000$
Life Expectancy	
	Average number of years of life remaining
Morbidity Rates	
Disease Incidence Rate (per 1,000)	$\dfrac{\text{Number of new cases of a specific disease during a specified year}}{\text{Population at risk for the disease during the same year}} \times 1{,}000$
Disease Prevalence Rate (per 1,000)	$\dfrac{\text{Number of existing cases of a specific disease at one time}}{\text{Number of persons in the population at the same point in time}} \times 1{,}000$

Mortality Rates

One way to keep track of deaths is to simply count how many occurred in a specified time period, such as one year, and compute totals for various groups and/or causes. Totals have their usefulness but make it difficult to compare populations of varying sizes. Generally it is helpful to change the total number of deaths to a rate by dividing it by the number of people in the population you are studying; the inscrutable decimal fraction that results is quickly improved by multiplying it by a large number, usually 1,000 or 100,000, to yield something like the current 8.6 per 1,000 for the United States. This example would be termed a **crude** rate because it has not been adjusted for any differences between the ages of the current population and any other group to which it might be compared.

Mortality rates may be computed for specific populations, such as particular states or cities; racial groups such as black, white, or Asian; or age groups such as 25 to 34 years. The particular cause of death may also be dealt with separately (e.g., heart disease or cancer) to form **cause-specific rates.** Rates for specific age groups are termed **age-specific rates,** such as the current 117 per 100,000 for ages 15 to 24 years. The **infant mortality rate** is a rather special age-specific rate which represents the number of deaths occurring among persons in their first year of life, divided by the number of live births, and multiplied by 1,000; it is used as a rather sensitive indicator for comparing the health status of countries or of the major racial or ethnic groups within them.

Mortality rates may be statistically adjusted for the proportion of young versus old people in a population. Such **age-adjusted** rates are exceedingly useful indicators when comparisons are made between either the mortality rates of (1) different communities, regions, or nations or (2) different historical periods of a particular population group. If unadjusted mortality rates were used to compare deaths from heart disease between Sweden and Egypt, for example, we would find a much lower rate in Egypt because of its higher birth rate and consequently much younger population. Also, if we attempted to compare the relative progress these countries were making to prevent such deaths, it would be necessary to statistically adjust the rates of these two nations to show what they would be if they had identical proportions of young and old within their respective populations.

Morbidity Rates

A number of different statistics are used in the quantification of disease. **Disease incidence** refers to the number of new cases of a disease that occur in a given time period divided by the population at risk for that disease during that time period. Such rates are commonly expressed as number of cases per year for each 1,000 or 100,000 persons and are particularly useful when discussing such acute conditions as the infectious diseases which tend to be of relatively short duration. **Disease prevalence** refers to the number of cases that are present in a given population at any point in time divided by the size of the population. These rates also are based on either 1,000 or 100,000 of the population and are most useful when discussing chronic conditions such as diabetes or arthritis which tend to accumulate because of their longer duration.

Disability Measures

As the health establishment slowly expands its mission beyond the reduction of mortality to include the restoration and maintenance of functional ability, disability measures are becoming more important. A variety of disability measures exist. The most common are **restricted activity days**, wherein a person cuts down on his or her usual activities because of an illness or injury, and **bed-disability days** wherein a person stays in bed for more than half of the normal waking hours for similar reasons. Other measures are **work-loss days** and **school-loss days**. One obvious threat to the accuracy of such measures is their dependence on personal assessment. They also are vulnerable to possible distortion due to changes in sick leave policies, disability insurance rules, and other such incentives or disincentives to judging oneself to be either temporarily or permanently disabled.

Life Expectancy

As perhaps the only positive measure of health among the traditional indicators, **life expectancy** is defined as the average number of years of life remaining. Life expectancy figures have a close and obvious relationship to mortality rates. They must be specified for a given age (e.g., life expectancy at birth, life expectancy at age 65, and so on). Note also that the commonly used life expectancy at birth figure is most heavily affected by deaths among the young. If, for example, one member of a pair of twins dies a few hours after birth and the other lives to an age of 90, their average life expectancy would be 45 years. This explains why some primitive societies have many elderly members even though the average life expectancy might be very low.

Modern Innovations

The recent emphasis on more positive health indices has prompted efforts to quantify many desirable features of life that were formerly reported in purely subjective terms. Although used less frequently than the traditional measures, these modern innovations are gradually gaining in popularity.

Years of Healthy Life

During the current century the average life span in the United States has been extended from 47 to 75 years, a notable accomplishment. However, critics often say that the mere extension of life expectancy does not indicate health progress when the added years are spent in an infirm or severely disabled state. One response to this view has been the development of a formula, based on the current rates of disability among various age groups, for the estimate of the **years of**

healthy life one might expect for any given age. In 1990, for example, a child at birth could look forward to approximately 75 years of life divided into 64 healthy years and 11 dysfunctional years (National Center for Health Statistics, 1993). There is surprisingly little known about the possible increase in disability as a result of longer life spans (Verbrugge, 1989). The advent of this new statistical tool should help answer this important question.

Quality Adjusted Life Years

We may all prefer to be fully functioning during all our years and yet realize that life can still be worth living even with a few disabilities. An elderly Mark Twain once exclaimed that "old age is not so bad when you consider the alternative." This point of view has led to a variation on the "years of healthy life" measure in which each remaining year of life is "weighted" by a figure based on the dysfunction typically experienced by persons of that age. A proposed use of this measure is to compare the relative cost per quality adjusted year of life saved by various health promotion campaigns (Patrick and Bergner, 1990).

Self-Assessment of Health

If one wants to know how healthy people are, why not ask them? Strangely enough, this direct approach was ignored by those surveying health until 1976, when it was added as a routine question to the National Center for Health Statistics annual survey. The subject is asked, "Compared with other persons your age, would you say your health is excellent, very good, good, or fair or poor?" This simple device has proved to be perhaps the best single indicator of general health status (Fingerhut, Wilson, and Feldman, 1980:3). In 1991 for example, 39.7 percent of the population placed themselves in the "excellent" category whereas 9.3 percent said they were in "fair or poor" health (National Center for Health Statistics, 1993). Although they are asked to compare themselves with others in their age group, people still tend to rate themselves lower as they move into the older categories.

Health Risk Appraisal

Unlike the other indices discussed in this section, health risk appraisal is a process rather than a single measure. It involves the simultaneous assessment of the major risk factors to which an individual or community may be exposed in regard to specific health threats. In one of its simplest forms, a **health habit questionnaire** is used to elicit information concerning various behaviors that put a person at risk of developing heart disease or various forms of cancer and subsequently to identify the particular factors that appear most in need of change. This process thus goes beyond the measurement of health status to measure the factors that affect health.

Beery and others (1986) describe three essential elements of health risk appraisal:

1. An assessment of personal health habits and risk factors based on questionnaire responses provided by the client or patient. This may be supplemented by biomedical measurements such as height, weight, blood pressure, urinalysis, blood chemistry, and fitness level, etc.

2. A quantitative *estimation* of qualitative assessment of the individual's future risk of death and/or other adverse outcomes from several specific causes.

3. The provision of *educational messages and/or counseling* about ways in which changes in one or more personal risk factors might alter the risk of disease or death.

Although people have probably always sought to estimate their risk of encountering various adverse health conditions, the formal process of risk assessment has made great strides since the late 1970s when it became apparent that research into the causes of many disease conditions, unintentional injuries, and other threats to health had progressed to the point where risks could be quantified with reasonable accuracy. Through the use of sophisticated statistical techniques, many types of health risk appraisal have been refined and made available in the form of computer software that can be periodically updated as new research results appear. This newly emerging technology lies at the heart of modern efforts to prevent disease and promote health (DeFriese and Fielding, 1990).

Using Health Indices

The various indices described here are commonly expressed in the form of health statistics. Members of the lay public are often confused by the complexities of statistical data or deceived by its manipulation by those with political motives. However, trained health professionals, particularly those in public health, view health statistics as a vital tool in their efforts to assess progress, determine priorities, and evaluate specific programs. Here are a few things to keep in mind when using health statistics:

- To paraphrase an old saying, "liars figure but figures don't lie." Statistics can be used to achieve a fair, even-handed assessment of a health issue; the alternative is anecdotal evidence, another useful tool, but one that is subject to far more misuse. The anecdote takes its most infamous form as the 30-second TV spot wherein whichever cause has the most heart-rending story receives public support.

- Keep in mind that each individual case (datum) that contributes to a particular health statistic represents a person with hopes, aspirations, feelings, and usually a cadre of relatives and loved ones. Statistics should not be divorced from their human context. If there were 53,000 motor vehicle deaths in 1980 and only 49,000 in 1988, for example, public health workers see these figures and think of 4,000 fewer phone calls or visits by police officers telling of the death of one's son, daughter, wife, father, or whomever. Truly, "statistics are people with the tears wiped off."

- Although generated by real events, these underlying events themselves must be evaluated. Death from a stroke at 85 years of age may need to be viewed differently than the death of an 18-year-old in an auto accident. Statistics are exceedingly useful "measures" but measures require "evaluation" in a broader context.

- There are many considerations that arise when attempting to use health statistics as a measure of progress; one of the most important of these is the selection of a proper base line or frame of reference. For example, compared with the situation in 1900, progress appears outstanding; however, compared with 1980, progress looks much less impressive. Compared to the rest of the world, which is predominated by nations much poorer than ourselves, our health status measures look good; however, when we restrict our comparison to nations of comparable wealth, the numbers are disappointing.

The Nation's Health

The proper interpretation of current health trends requires a brief historical review of progress made during the twentieth century. In 1900 most of the people in the United States lived in small towns or on farms. Despite the development of urban manufacturing centers, farming was still the dominant occupation. This rural life of the past, often romanticized in the media, looks much less attractive when viewed more objectively.

The "Good Old Days"?

Whether one labored on a farm or in a factory, debilitating 12- to 14-hour workdays were the rule for adults and for many children who were frequently pressed into service at an early age. Income levels were low and food prices were relatively high; the family diet was often meager and monotonous. The average 10-year-old, for example, was approximately 10 centimeters (4 inches) shorter than his or her modern counterpart (Terris, 1975). Common childhood diseases such as measles, whooping cough, and diphtheria frequently struck and took a heavy toll because of the undernourished and generally run-down condition of much of the young population. After the threat of childhood diseases was past, young adults were still susceptible to the two leading causes of death of the time, tuberculosis, and the lethal combination of influenza and pneumonia. Surprisingly enough, accidents caused even more death and disability within the working population than in our current, highly mechanized society. This higher toll probably resulted from the lack of safety regulations and effective trauma care. Women were often subject to the hazards of factory work plus the added risk of frequent childbearing. Despite high mortality rates among children, family size was large because births more than offset deaths. Obstetrical care was primitive or nonexistent, putting both mother and child at risk. Childbed (puerperal) fever was common and helped raise maternal mortality rates to significant levels. As for the infants, more than 80 of every 1,000 died in their first year of life, usually from intestinal infections. This is more than eight times the current rate.

Table 1.2 Mortality and Longevity Comparisons: 1900 versus 1992*

1900		1992	
Ten Leading Causes of Death:			
Tuberculosis	185	Heart Disease	283
Pneumonia & influenza	184	Cancer	204
Heart Disease	153	Cerebrovascular disease	56
Diarrhea & enteritis	115	Chronic obstructive respiratory disease	36
Cerebrovascular disease	106	Unintentional injuries	34
Nephritis & nephrosis	84	Pneumonia & influenza	30
Unintentional injuries	79	Diabetes mellitus	20
Cancer	68	HIV/AIDS	13
Diphtheria	33	Suicide	12
Typhoid fever	27	Homicide and legal intervention	10
All causes	1622	All causes	853
Infant mortality	77**		9
Life expectancy at birth:			
Male	46	Male	72
Female	48	Female	79
Both sexes	47	Both sexes	76

* (per 100,000 population)
** Earliest available data is for 1920–24.

Source: National Center for Health Statistics. *Health, United States, 1993*, Hyattsville, MD: Public Health Service, 1994.

A Century of Progress

It is well known that when current levels of health are compared with those existing during the relatively primitive conditions of the early 1900s, the progress appears spectacular. Less well known, however, is the fact that this progress has continued at a relatively steady, although slower, pace into the 1990s. A brief review of selected indices as provided by the National Center for Health Statistics (1993) will illustrate this point.

Life Expectancy

Since 1900 life expectancy at birth has risen quite steadily from 47 years to 68 years in 1950, 71 in 1970, and to 75 years in 1990. And contrary to popular opinion, the bulk of the improvement is the result of saving the lives of infants, children, and young adults rather than prolonging the life of the elderly with feeding tubes and ventilators. Since 1980 the National Center for Health Statistics has compiled data on years of life lost below age 65 and recorded a 12 percent reduction between 1980 and 1990. This increase in longevity has not resulted in increased disability or infirmity. The percentage of people over age 65 with significant limitation of their activities caused by chronic conditions actually declined slightly from 39 percent in 1986 to 38 percent in 1991. Also, the proportion of people within the total population whose self-assessments placed their own health in the lowest category, "fair or poor," declined slightly from 10.7 percent in 1983 to 9.3 percent in 1990. Thus, life expectancy continues to increase with no apparent increase in disability or infirmity.

Infant Mortality

A very large part of the increase in the average life span is explained by the steady progress in saving the lives of infants during their first year of life. Between 1950 and 1990 infants deaths were reduced to less than one-third their former level; from 29 to 9 per 1,000 live births. However, as will be discussed later, this apparently solid achievement looks poor when compared to what other countries have accomplished and the composite total masks large differences among our various population groups.

Heart Disease and Stroke

The increased life span of modern Americans also is explained in part by the near spectacular reduction in mortality from two closely related conditions, coronary heart disease and cerebrovascular disease (stroke). Both conditions result from the deterioration of the arteries and thus have similar causes. During the 1950s and 1960s it was relatively common for people to die from heart disease in their 40s and 50s. Such events have since been reduced by almost one-half. On an age-adjusted basis, deaths from heart disease were reduced by half from 307 to 152 per 100,000 between 1950 and 1990. The fact that we have an older population and a stronger effort at public education tends to make the threat of heart disease highly visible while masking the tremendous progress that has been made. During the same time period, deaths from stroke were reduced to less than one-third of their former level from 89 to 28 deaths per 100,000.

Cancer

Far less encouraging is the progress against cancer which has seen an increase from 125 to 135 deaths per 100,000 between 1950 and 1990 despite major efforts at control. This increase, however, can be explained in large part by added deaths from respiratory cancer (primarily of the lung). When this category is excluded, all other categories combined show a modest decline from 112 to 94. Some comfort may be provided by the fact that most deaths from respiratory cancer, which account for approximately 40 percent of the total, are attributable to cigarette smoking which, at this writing, is on the decline.

Motor Vehicle Accidents

The death rate from auto accidents declined from 23 to 19 per 100,000 between 1950 and 1990. This modest improvement actually represents good progress when the large per capita increase in miles driven is considered. But despite this progress, more than 40,000 people die each year (41,462 in 1991) and a disproportionate number of these deaths occur among younger people. This fact, together with the ready availability of many under-utilized safety items and prevention strategies in the form of seat belts, air bags, safer car design, better law enforcement, and other such remedies, make this a high priority area for further improvement.

A Modern Lesson

By any fair analysis, health in America is getting better. When today's population is compared with any other historical period we see improvement. People are living longer and more productive lives than ever before. Significant progress is being made in combating virtually all the major sources of death and disability. Surprisingly, such optimistic assessments are not widely publicized for fear of creating complacency and a consequent reduction in public support for the persistent, and expensive, efforts needed for further progress. However, the main lesson to be learned from progress is that health programs and related efforts are effective. The tools exist. We do not have to await the invention of new technology; rather, we need to make optimal use of the means at hand. And most important, modern progress notwithstanding, there is still far too much death, disability, and other detractors from the quality of life, along with gross inequities among population groups.

Serious Concerns

One can argue that, as a society, we are already making a good effort at health improvement and that, after all, there is a limit to the resources that can be allocated to this effort. Although there is some truth to this argument, close examination reveals two major problems: (1) we are not using our resources very efficiently; too much goes for medical treatment and too little for prevention, and (2) we are applying these resources unevenly across various population groups. The young are neglected in favor of the old; minorities receive far less attention than whites; males receive more than females; rich more than poor. In the first instance we are unwise, in the second unjust. Let's consider a few of the more troublesome health issues.

Infant Mortality

Among public health workers, infant mortality is regarded as the single best indicator of a particular society's health status. It serves as a sensitive barometer because it is affected by several health factors. Low rates are dependent on good maternal nutrition, protection from toxic substances, protection from infections, and access to medical care. Throughout the twentieth century America's infant mortality rate declined to 9.2 deaths per 1,000 live births by 1990. This looks good until we compare it with 1989 data showing rates of 7.5 for Denmark, 7.34 for Switzerland, and 5.77 for Sweden. And, within the United States, we find major differences among population groups—the 1990 rate was 7.7 for whites and 17.0 for blacks.

Suicide and Homicide

The suicide rate has edged upward in recent years despite significant prevention efforts affecting all age groups. Within particular societies, homicide rates traditionally vary according to the proportion of younger males within the population. Consequently the crude or unadjusted rate within the United States rose as our "baby boom" population grew older—from 5.3 per 100,000 in 1950 to a peak of 10.7 in 1980. Although it eased a bit to 9.0 by 1988 it increased sharply to 10.0 in 1990. Again we pale in comparison with other modern countries and there are huge disparities within our own population: the 138.3 rate for black males 25–35 years of age for 1990 is nearly nine times the 15.4 rate of their white cohorts. The issues surrounding the excessive death rate for black males are complex; but simply stated, many in this group appear to be paying the price of being young, male, and poor while living in an urban environment.

HIV/AIDS

During 1992, 33,875 persons died of HIV/AIDS. The accumulated total deaths from this disease since it was identified is now approximately 195,226, when the incomplete data for 1993 are included. Thus far, special population groups have borne the brunt of the devastation—approximately 60 percent of the deaths occurred among men who had homosexual contact and 21 percent among men or women who used drugs intravenously. This condition merits high priority on a number of counts. It is invariably fatal. At this writing there is no effective treatment currently available; the prognosis is grim for the more than 100,000 victims under treatment and the more than one million persons already exposed who have not yet developed the disease. Although the pace of new cases has slowed from the annual doubling of the early 1980s, it is still growing rapidly and it is making a slow but relentless incursion into the ranks of the heterosexual population. It has also changed the thinking of health professionals who had hoped that the conquest of polio in the 1950s had extinguished the last major threat in the infectious disease category. One wonders what new pathogen may evolve or enter the human population from some hidden reservoir.

Alcohol and Drug Abuse

In terms of mortality, alcohol kills young people through fetal alcohol syndrome and increased auto fatalities while attacking older persons through liver cirrhosis and its contribution to homicides and suicides. Perhaps more devastating, however, is the long-term disability caused by alcoholism. The abuse of other drugs, such as cocaine and heroin, is now a major factor in the spread of HIV infection, in addition to its traditional role of producing dependency.

These are but a few examples of largely preventable conditions that continue to diminish our quality of life, weaken the productivity of our workforce, and raise the costs of medical care. Many other such examples come easily to mind: unwanted pregnancies, particularly among teenagers; family disorganization and divorce; and the plight of the homeless.

Goals for the Future

As this brief overview has shown, health progress has proceeded at a more or less steady rate throughout the twentieth century. However, any comfort we might derive from this progress has been tempered by the fact that much more could be done, that we are far from making the optimal effort, and that every year thousands of our citizens die before their time or live lives diminished by crippling disabilities. Finally, the fact that makes this general situation truly unacceptable is that it is largely unnecessary; most of our health woes are preventable through use of materials and procedures that are well known and moderate in cost. Such measures as improved diets, less use of toxic substances, regular prenatal care, routine screening exams, seat belts, condoms, exercise, and so on quickly return benefits in reduced medical expenses and improved quality of life far beyond the cost of their implementation.

Public health professionals have been aware of this situation for many years; however, their efforts to marshal public opinion have largely been met with indifference. Yet, during the past twenty years two developments occurred that make such a task easier. First, information as to the distribution, magnitude, and apparent causes of disease has become more readily available and more accurate. The apparatus for recording, compiling, and analyzing health statistics is much improved as is the conduct of epidemiological research into causes and risk factors. Second, the public health establishment has become much more adept at publicizing health risks and needed responses. These two factors are best illustrated by two prominent initiatives spearheaded by the United States Public Health Service. Among other things, these initiatives were designed to effect a major change in national priorities from an overwhelming emphasis on treatment to a more preventive orientation.

The Surgeon General's 1979 Report

In 1979 the U.S. Public Health Service (USPHS) published a landmark report entitled *Healthy People: The Surgeon General's Report on Health Promotion and Disease Prevention.* The purpose of this progressive document was "to encourage a second public health revolution in the history of the United States" (USDHHS, 1979:vii). Simply stated, this revolution sought to shift the nation's priorities from treatment-oriented, after-the-fact medicine to an emphasis on the prevention of disease and disability. The report provided (1) a thorough analysis of the nation's current health status, (2) an appraisal of trends over the past several years, and (3) specific goals in the form of priority tasks for the decade of the 1980s.

Goals

This report reviewed the substantial progress made since the turn of the century and identified the outstanding health problems that were preventable by use of current technology. Then, as now, several other nations were doing better in infant mortality, life expectancy, circulatory disease, and cancer. The death rate for one age group, 15–24 year olds, was actually increasing largely because of auto accidents among the white population and homicides among black males. The nation's health care costs were increasing at an unacceptable rate, consuming 9.3 percent of our gross domestic product in 1980. All of these concerns appeared related to a disproportionate emphasis on treatment rather than prevention. The report culminated in a relatively simple set of goals for the 1980s organized by age groups as follows:

- To reduce infant mortality by 35 percent to fewer than 9 deaths per 1,000 live births.
- To foster optimal childhood development and reduce deaths among children aged 1 to 14 years by 20 percent to fewer than 34 per 100,000.
- To improve the health habits of adolescents and young adults and reduce deaths by 20 percent to fewer than 93 per 100,000.
- To reduce deaths among people aged 25 to 64 by at least 25 percent to fewer than 400 per 100,000.
- To reduce the average annual number of days of restriction due to acute and chronic conditions by 20 percent to fewer than 30 days per year for people aged 65 and older.

Results

This report and its accompanying *1990 Objectives for the Nation* (USDHHS, 1980) served to focus resources in the public and private sectors on common, high priority tasks. The objectives were organized into categories of primary prevention, health promotion, health protection, and health services. The notable success of this major effort is shown in table 1.3.

Although not all the goals were met, it was apparent that the "goals" approach did indeed provide a useful stimulus to health promotion efforts and a more efficient allocation of resources. Consequently, a second, more ambitious attempt was mounted for the 1990s.

Table 1.3 Progress Toward 1990 Life Stage Goals

Life stage	1980 Status	1990 Target	1990 Status
Deaths per 1,000 Live Births			
Infants (under 1 year)	12.6	9	9.1
Deaths per 100,000 Population			
Children (1-14 years)	38.5	34	30.1
Adolescents/Young Adults (15-24 years)	115.4	93	104.1
Adults (25-64 years)	529.9	400	400.4
Restricted Activity Days per Person			
Older Adults (65 years and over)	36.5	30	31.4
Bed Disability Days per Person			
Older Adults	13.8	12	13.6

Source: National Center for Health Statistics. *Health, United States, 1991.* Hyattsville, MD: Public Health Service, 1992.

Healthy People 2000

Several important forces converged during the late 1980s to set the stage for the massive effort which was eventually entitled *Healthy People 2000* (USDHHS, 1990). Positive motivation for such a project was provided by the aforementioned success of the previous goal-setting project, whereas a negative force was exerted by the continued rise in health care costs. Fortunately, this call for action came at a time when the tools for such an effort were undergoing rapid improvement. The process of descriptive epidemiology, i.e. the measurement and assessment of the importance of various forms of disease and mortality, was becoming increasingly effective as a guide to setting priorities among the various adverse conditions vying for attention. Meanwhile the closely related field of health risk appraisal, which focuses on the causes of such conditions and the subsequent vulnerability of individuals and groups, had reached a level of development that enabled it to target specific behaviors or environmental conditions most in need of change.

The success of the previous goals project also provided added encouragement and useful experience for the difficult task of mobilizing and guiding the actions of the nation's health organizations as they undertook the massive effort needed to realize the *Healthy People 2000* goals. Consequently, "the process for formulating the year 2000 objectives has placed greater emphasis on public and professional participation" (McGinnis, 1990:245). The U.S. Public Health Service, which led the planning effort, heard testimony from more than 750 persons and organizations before drafting its year 2000 goals. These were subsequently reviewed and revised before publication in an effort that ultimately involved at least 10,000 people. The many participants brought a vast amount of expertise to the goals-setting process and, perhaps more importantly, these people returned to their parent organizations with a sense of commitment toward the goals they had helped establish.

In addition to motivation there must be guidance; therefore, a manual entitled *Healthy Communities 2000: Model Standards* (USDHHS, 1991b) was prepared to help direct state and local efforts. Finally, specific federal health agencies, such as the Centers for Disease Control and the Food and Drug Administration, were designated as lead organizations for the efforts in specific areas of health promotion.

Goals

This report was modeled on the previous 1990 objectives; it was more comprehensive than its predecessor and gave increased attention to secondary prevention, i.e., finding and treating disease in its early stages. In another similarity to the first report, the goals for *Healthy People 2000* were not restricted to reductions in death and disability but also addressed the underlying factors that affect health status, such as health habits and the availability of health services. Its targets or expected outcomes were expressed in a two-tiered arrangement of broad general goals and more specific objectives (USDHHS, 1990:4). The three broad goals were:

1. Increase the span of healthy life for Americans.
2. Reduce health disparities among Americans.
3. Achieve access to preventive services for all Americans.

Objectives

The list of specific objectives extends for approximately 35 pages and addresses 22 priority areas which are organized into four categories; a summary appears in table 1.4.

Implications

The content and structure of the *Healthy People 2000* report illustrate several important concepts in regard to society's general effort to improve health,

Table 1.4 *Healthy People 2000* Priority Areas

Health Promotion

1. Physical Activity and Fitness
2. Nutrition
3. Tobacco
4. Alcohol and Drugs
5. Family Planning
6. Mental Health and Mental Disorders
7. Violent and Abusive Behavior
8. Educational and Community-Based Programs

Health Protection

9. Unintentional Injuries
10. Occupational Safety and Health
11. Environmental Health
12. Food and Drug Safety
13. Oral Health

Preventive Services

14. Maternal and Infant Health
15. Heart Disease and Stroke
16. Cancer
17. Diabetes and Chronic Disabling Conditions
18. HIV Infection
19. Sexually Transmitted Diseases
20. Immunization and Infectious Diseases
21. Clinical Preventive Services

Surveillance and Data Systems

22. Surveillance and Data Systems

Source: USDHHS. *Healthy People 2000: National Health Promotion and Disease Prevention Objectives.* Washington, DC: USDHHS (PHS), 1990.

particularly in regard to the question of "which factors are most important in the determination of health ?" Emphasis is placed on **health promotion** activities that relate to personal health behavior or life-style choices such as exercise, food selection, and avoidance of alcohol and drugs. These measures are largely dependent upon the knowledge and will of the individual citizen. **Health protection** efforts refer mainly to regulatory measures that are designed to make the overall environment safer. Examples include workplace safety rules, improved crash worthiness of automobiles, and the purity of food and drug items. These measures are generally dependent upon legislation and enforcement with the individual's role being relatively passive except for the important task of supporting their initial adoption. Preventive services require both societal and personal action; society must insure that the services are available and the consumer must make proper use of them. These include such things as prenatal care, immunizations, and mammograms. Finally, the inclusion of a specific objective regarding the recording and reporting of information related to health and disease demonstrates the importance placed on actual data for monitoring progress and making decisions as to which actions are effective.

One disappointment to many health professionals was the notable lack of attention to broader improvements in the social environment such as measures to attack poverty or reduce unemployment; as will be discussed in later chapters, such problems are highly related to health status. On balance, however, the *Healthy People 2000* initiative represents the largest and most clearly defined commitment to the improvement of health conditions thus far taken in the nation's history.

Summary

Within this chapter the authors have reviewed both the philosophical bases of health as presented by various writers from several different fields and the more action-oriented efforts of modern-day health professionals as they have sought to assess health status and trends in order to properly set priorities for the improvement of health within our society. This information was presented in support of six broad concepts that will undergo further development throughout the balance of this book.

1. Health is a complex quality with physical, mental, and social dimensions. Individuals with high levels of health tend to feel good, function close to their potential, and cope effectively with various forms of adversity. Its large subjective component has led to measurement problems and a historic tendency to rely on mortality and morbidity statistics as indices of health progress. But despite the difficulties in definition and measurement, health has been highly valued and pursued throughout history.

2. Although progress in the improvement of health has been uneven, it has shown a steady upward trend during the twentieth century with longer life expectancies, less disability, and reduced infant mortality occurring from decade to decade. Despite this improvement our society still compares unfavorably with progress in other industrialized countries and with reasonable estimates of what is technically possible. Moreover, the wide disparities among our major population groups—such as between the white majority and the various ethnic and racial minority groups, and between our lower and higher income groups—are unacceptable.

3. The most effective strategies for health improvement emphasize the promotion of health and the prevention of disease rather than the treatment of illness. Despite the considerable evidence in support of this generalization, such factors as the natural compassion and sense of urgency for those acutely ill, public ignorance concerning the dynamics of health, and the inherently short-term outlook of legislatures and other governmental bodies have led to a disproportionate emphasis on treatment as opposed to prevention.

4. Personal health behavior or life-style factors in the form of food selection, exercise habits, substance use or abuse, use of contraceptives, and so forth are the single most important factor influencing health progress. Problems within this category account for an estimated 50 percent of preventable mortality and disability. Personal health behavior is dependent in large part on (1) the knowledge and motivational state of individuals and (2) their access to the resources needed to act on their motivations. Both categories provide implications for health education.

5. Preventive health services such as mammograms, hypertension screening, prenatal care, and immunizations are also important; their effective utilization is dependent on the active participation of the individual. Here again, there is an important role for health education in disseminating information, developing knowledge, and changing attitudes.

6. Health progress is often dependent upon knowledgeable and well-motivated political action. When it comes to protecting the environment, providing pure foods and drugs, constructing safe automobiles, and similar activities the individual is dependent on proper legislation and effective law enforcement. In this realm the health educator often has a role in alerting people to the issues, informing them, and generally getting them involved in the political process.

Chapter 2

Health Determinants

Risks to good health come in various guises. Some are biological, and many of these are inherited. Others result from individual behavior. Still others arise from the environment in which individuals find themselves. Environmental influences on health include the physical environment and socioeconomic conditions, with the family an important part of the socioeconomic environment. Because risks often work in concert to produce a particular disease, and synergistic action can multiply risk enormously, controlling risk is rarely a simple matter.

—Vicki Kalmer, *Healthy People*, (USDHHS, 1979)

Introduction

As Kalmer suggests, the sheer complexity and comprehensiveness of the general field of health presents a serious challenge to its practitioners. Virtually every aspect of human existence either affects, or is affected by, health. This fact is particularly troublesome to health educators, whose principal mission is the improvement of health related behavior. Given that virtually all behavior is somehow related to health, how can they hope to define the proper scope of their activities? If a community experiences an abnormally high suicide rate, health education along with other health services would appear to have a legitimate helping role; but, what if the problem is a high homicide rate? Or perhaps international conflicts? Currently, it seems that every newly industrialized nation seeking to emerge from the Third World aspires to develop an arsenal of atomic weapons. This is not a healthy situation; but, can health professionals address this problem without the risk of being told to "mind their own business"? Few things show a higher relationship to one's health than the ability to find and hold a job with decent working conditions that yields a living wage; yet as health educators, we must often wait until unemployment leads to alcoholism, mental illness, or spousal abuse before being asked to intervene. Although this restricted view of the health educator's role too often prevails, support is developing for a broader function—one that will mandate involvement with the broader social issues that form the root causes of many health problems (Minkler, 1989).

Overview of Health Determinants

Perhaps the best response to this complex situation is to review the broad array of factors that affect health, organize them into logical categories, and seek some reasonably clear understanding of the whole in order to be better equipped to prevent problems. What is needed is what Terris (1975) has described as an "epidemiology of health," an inquiry into its causes and the reasons for its distribution in various degrees among different population groups. Because of the scope and complexity of individual determininants of health, it is impossible to measure their relative contribution with any great precision; however, it is possible to make reasonable estimates for the formulation of effective public policy and good individual decisions among health professionals.

Several writers, including Dubos (1959), LaLone (1974), McKeown (1978) and, more recently, Last and Wallace (1991) have addressed the topic of health determinants. One result of their examination has been the organization of the many determinants into four broad categories, namely: (1) genetics, (2) environment, (3) health care, and (4) personal behavior. This chapter follows this scheme except it divides the environment into physical and social categories in order to give closer attention to differences in their respective mechanisms and dynamics. Given this modification our categories may be described as follows:

- Genetics—Much of one's body size and configuration, special abilities, disease resistance, and general robustness may be attributable to genetic factors. In some cases, lives are dominated by some specific genetic disease or defect.

- Physical Environment—Temperature, humidity, altitude, noise level, the presence or absence of various pollutants, and exposure to natural and/or artificial radiation all affect health to varying degrees.

- Social Environment—The vast network of customs, mores, and laws, as well as the activities of social, commercial, and governmental organizations determine political and economic circumstances that profoundly affect the quality of each person's life.

- Health Care—The quality, availability, and proper use of medical, dental, and other health services can have important effects.

- Personal Behavior—The choices each person makes in regard to nutrition, exercise, rest, substance use, sexual behavior, and other life-style factors exert a powerful influence on health.

Before considering the differences among these categories it is useful to note a number of important commonalties. The various categories overlap; they are not discrete and mutually exclusive. If an expectant mother, for example, decides to cancel a needed appointment for prenatal care because she feels she cannot afford to miss a half day's wages, it may be difficult to identify the factor mainly responsible for this event. Is this primarily a personal decision, as the woman forsakes medical care for added income? Is it a problem with the social environment which may not have provided her with the opportunity to qualify for a better paying job or may not have insisted on a more generous sick leave policy on the part of the employer? Or should we blame the health care system for not being available after working hours?

At the risk of displaying a professional bias, the authors attribute much of this overlap to the pervasive effects of personal behavior, whose elements are typically involved in every other category. The individual with a genetic tendency toward high cholesterol levels must be knowledgeable and motivated enough to note his or her family history of heart disease, get tested, and then take steps to offset this risk factor. Physicians offering preventive health services must wait until a patient decides to make an appointment and then hope that any instructions are followed. The quality of both the physical and social environments is dependent on the actions of individual citizens who often may choose to honor or ignore the various laws and recommendations designed to safeguard these environments. Within every category, time, money, and other resources are needed if there are to be improvements. Consequently, there are political and economic restraints on health programs of all types. This means that health professionals must set priorities and allocate limited resources to areas that will accomplish the most good while garnering increased levels of support.

Genetic Determinants

Health-conscious people generally show considerable interest in their possible exposure to chemicals whether they be in the form of pollutants, food additives, pharmaceuticals, or other sources. But often overlooked is the fact that each of the several million cells in the human body contains approximately 100,000 separate genes, each of which contains information for the production of a specific chemical component for incorporation into the structure of the cell, regulation of its functioning, or perhaps for release into the bloodstream so that it may exert its influence elsewhere. Enzymes, antibodies, blood components, and every other aspect of our physiological functioning is either controlled or significantly influenced by genetic action. Although genetic makeup is established at conception, gene functioning affects every moment of our lives.

The implications provided by genetic factors are so profound and pervasive as to make analysis difficult. However, the task may be simplified somewhat by dividing it into two broad categories: (1) the broad general effects of multifactorial conditions, i.e., those that involve the interaction of two or more genes and the possible added contribution of some environmental condition, and (2) the less complex single-gene Mendelian conditions, which lend themselves to specific efforts at control.

Genetics as a General Factor

For the great array of disease conditions wherein genetics is a contributing but not a defining factor, such as heart disease, cancer, diabetes, obesity, and schizophrenia, good health practices require that individuals check into their family history and seek professional advice concerning the need to take specific action to offset any apparent liabilities. In the case of heart disease, for example, a familial susceptibility may be transmitted by a specific tendency for hypertension or high cholesterol severe enough to require treatment; where the connection is more diffuse, a more general effort to reduce the controllable risk factors in order to offset the possible genetic factor may be in order. In most cases where genetics is a significant contributor to disease potential it generally accounts for less than 50 percent of the risk; moreover, it is frequently difficult to sort out aspects of family culture, such as eating habits or recreational patterns, from true genetic propensities. Consequently, people with threatening family histories need encouragement to offset liabilities with life-style changes and perhaps more frequent check-ups. There is plenty of work here for the health educator.

Protecting the Gene Pool

Presumably the world's biosphere—that is, the total complement of living organisms—evolved into its current form through a process based on genetic variation and natural selection. Genetic variation resulted from the natural assortment of genes during normal reproduction and the occasional mutations caused by such things as cosmic radiation and chemicals present in the natural environment. This process yielded a mixed bag of handicapped and gifted organisms that were sorted out by the process of natural selection as they struggled to survive in primitive environments. Only the more able survived to maturity and reproduced. However well the process of natural selection may have served humankind in the past, it is an inhumane process at best which measures any progress in millennia; it obviously has limited usefulness in terms of our present-day problems. Our hope of exerting some control over this situation, within the foreseeable future at any rate, does not seem to lie with genetic engineering. Schull and Hanis in their comprehensive review of "Genetics and Public Health in the 1990s" tell us that:

> Gene therapy, which has received so much attention and will be useful in some diseases, will not be a panacea. It is difficult to see what role it could play in diseases that stem from an interaction of genetic and environmental factors and in which some risk is associated with every genotype. (1990:118)

Two strategies offer more immediate results. The first is to increase our efforts to keep known or suspected mutagenic factors out of our environment. This effort can be part of a general goal of environmental protection; the same toxic substances that cause mutations in body cells and increase one's cancer risk also cause inheritable defects when sperm or ova are involved. The second strategy is to encourage individuals at risk, because of their individual history or membership in a high-risk group, to undergo genetic screening and counseling.

Targeted Programs

Many of the Mendelian, and to a lesser extent, the multifactorial and chromosomal, disorders can be controlled with varying degrees of success through specialized programs such as the following.

Genetic Counseling

Blood tests have been developed for several Mendelian disorders that can determine if prospective parents are carriers. If one member of the couple is found to be a carrier in the case of recessive disorders, such as sickle-cell anemia and Tay Sachs disease, the odds are that 50 percent of the prospective children will be carriers and 50 percent will be totally free of the condition. If both parents are carriers then the odds are that only 25 percent will be free of the trait whereas 50 percent will be carriers and 25 percent will inherit the disorder. If one prospective parent is a carrier (and thus also an eventual victim) of a dominant disorder such as Huntington's disease, 50 percent of any offspring are likely to be similarly afflicted whereas the other children will be completely free of the condition. All of these percentages are probabilities, not certainties; they will prove quite accurate for groups; however, the odds may go for or against specific couples. This fact further complicates an already delicate counseling task as each couple weighs such factors as the strength of their desire for children, their willingness to accept the task of raising a handicapped child, their feelings about adoption or artificial insemination, and their acceptance of abortion as a viable alternative in the possible event of a prenatal diagnosis of a severe condition. The counseling goal is to help those involved to understand all the important ramifications and alternatives and thus enable them to make a decision suitable to their particular situation.

Prenatal Diagnosis

Expectant parents who have reason to be concerned about the prospective child's potential affliction with a congenital abnormality can often seek a diagnosis in utero. Depending on the particular case, this may be done by amniocentesis, wherein a hypodermic needle is used to withdraw a sample of amniotic fluid for chemical analysis or microscopic examination, or by chorionic villus sampling, which accomplishes essentially the same thing; it involves the insertion of a tube (catheter) through the vagina. Either technique may be used to identify a variety of Mendelian or chromosomal disorders. More recently ultrasound imaging has proven to be safe and effective in identifying gross structural defects. The prospective parents who have appropriate need of such procedures need proper counseling to decide whether or not to seek diagnosis and how to act on any results subsequently obtained. In the case of a gross defect, the decision may be to abort; if the condition is more manageable, then preparations may be made for prompt treatment upon delivery of the child or, in some cases, for supportive treatment during pregnancy.

Screening of Newborns

A number of genetic conditions result in problems in the metabolism of food components and/or their subsequent derivatives. Such conditions, most notable of which is phenylketonuria (PKU), require prompt treatment if irreversible damage to the child is to be avoided. Consequently, most states require mandatory screening for a number of conditions such as PKU and galactosemia. Porter (1982) estimated, for example, that it cost approximately $80,000 to identify and treat a PKU patient as compared with approximately $900,000 for lifetime care for a severely retarded child if the condition is not diagnosed or not properly treated. Research continues on the development of effective screening tests to identify both carriers (prior to their decision to conceive) and affected infants promptly upon their delivery. Both the initial use of screening tests and suitable responses to their results often require knowledgeable and sensitive action by the procreating couple. There is a clear need for health education and health counseling at all stages of the situation. The *Healthy People 2000* document calls for increasing to at least 90 percent the proportion of women enrolled in prenatal care who are offered screening and counseling on prenatal detection of fetal abnormalities.

The Physical Environment

Probably from the time humankind was first able to conceptualize "health" as a desirable quality, people also were able to perceive it as related to certain features in the surrounding environment. Hippocrates reported the association between low swampy areas and malaria in his treatise *Air, Water, and Places* along with other similar observations. History is replete with accounts of the wealthy moving to warmer and/or drier locations in their attempts to improve their health. Currently, efforts to protect the environment (and thus ourselves) are the object of considerable attention both in the mass media and various legislative bodies.

Food and Water

Although public attention in recent years has been focused on the more exotic threats posed by synthetic chemicals and nuclear radiation, historically the greatest environmental problem has been waterborne infections and infestations. Throughout the early years of the United States and extending well into the current century such diseases as cholera, typhoid fever, and various types of diarrhea and enteritis were significant causes of death. Tuberculosis was frequently spread by milk from the grocer while the butcher's meat came with the risk of salmonella; periodic outbreaks of botulism from improperly canned food were not uncommon. The reduction of these historical scourges to their current low levels was a complex process with improved nutrition and medical treatment generally sharing the credit. But arguably more important were the legislative mandates and regulations that were necessary to provide the nation with water and food essentially free of infectious agents and parasites. Now, we must ask ourselves why these ancient foes still ravage the Third World; the most prevalent health problems in developing countries are infectious and parasitic diseases that are direct products of unsanitary water and waste disposal (Cunningham and Saigo, 1992). On a worldwide basis, the lack of clean water and adequate waste disposal are the greatest public health problems.

Today our efforts to protect our food and water supplies seem to be in an awkward stage of transition as we seek solutions to the more subtle threats posed by thousands of chemical additives and contaminants. Numerous surveys dating to the 1970s have identified a variety of carcinogens in public water supplies. Among these agents are organic chemical compounds such as chloroform, benzene, bis ether, and bromine, plus dangerous metals such as lead, mercury, cadmium, and arsenic, all of which are carcinogenic to some degree (Boyle, 1979). The major sources of waterborne carcinogens are (1) dumping by industry; (2) run-off from agricultural, forest service, and public applications of herbicides, pesticides, and fertilizer; and (3) waste from domestic sources. A great deal of the problem results from the seepage of toxic chemicals into the water supply from disposal sites. There does not seem to be any easy way to dispose of toxic chemicals or waste metals so that they do not find their way into the water supply.

Lead, for example, remains a serious problem despite the strong efforts directed at its control. Current restrictions on its use in gasoline or as the solder to seal the seams of canned goods, have kept our air and food relatively free of this metal. However, because of its widespread use in such products as automobile batteries, TV tubes, and power cables, it still finds its way into landfills, where it poses a threat to groundwater supplies. Lead paint provides another route to human tissue. Although such paint has been banned for almost 20 years, the renovation or simple deterioration of older homes and apartment complexes can expose layers of lead tainted paint which can spread in the form of airborne flakes and dust. In such situations household members, particularly children, can ingest enough of this toxic metal to incur some degree of neurological damage (Nadakavukaren, 1995).

While we still struggle with many of our traditional threats to the environment, the continual development of new synthetic chemicals presents new challenges. Lave and Ennever in a recent review pointed to the enormous size of the problem and expressed their uneasiness with the situation:

> We live in a sea of known (or suspicious) substances, both natural and synthetic. Of the 60,000 synthetic chemicals in use, only a few have received extensive toxicity testing. Thus the potential health effects of these exposures are largely unknown. (1990:70)

One bright spot in this whole picture is that, in regard to cancer, the disaster has not yet fallen upon us; thus far, the apparent toll in terms of death and disability has not yet approached the dimensions of that currently presented by deficits in living conditions or personal behavior. In 1981 the National Cancer Institute commissioned two British epidemiologists to conduct a thorough analysis of research in cancer etiology in the population of the United States. Foreign investigators were selected for this task in an attempt to improve objectivity. Quite surprisingly they found that the type of environmental toxins that typically created the most public concern, the synthetic chemicals, were contributing relatively little to cancer risk. They estimated that less than 1 percent of cancer incidence was attributable to food additives and little more than 2 percent to environmental pollution (Doll and Peto, 1981). Moreover, these unexpected findings were supported by a more recent study using a different approach (Gough, 1988).

Two quick points can serve to reconcile the apparent conflict between this evidence and the widespread and very genuine concern for environmental pollutants among other experts. First, Doll and Peto found diet responsible for 35 percent of cancer risk and tobacco for 30 percent. As noted, some broad definitions of environment include food and tobacco exposure and thus bring these findings in line with other estimates. They also are supported, in part, by the fact that mortality from all cancer, exclusive of lung cancer, whose causes are well established, shows a slight decline since 1950 with no great change in the body sites affected; colorectal and breast cancer are still the main runners-up following respiratory cancer. This pattern suggests that, for the moment at least, we are not in the midst of an environmentally induced cancer epidemic. What this probably means is that we have time—provided we don't waste it. As a society, we need less hysteria and more deliberate, systematic action to gain control of the problem. There is a typical time lag between broad exposure to a carcinogen and the onset of the disease. Cigarette smoking was quite common in the United States during the 1920s and 1930s yet the incidence of lung cancer was low. Later in the 1950s and 1960s we paid the price for these earlier indiscretions. Many of the sometimes seemingly irrational efforts we now make to protect the environment from suspicious substances, which may have required massive doses in rodents to prove their carcinogenic nature, may be preventing the cancer epidemic of the next century.

Air

Air pollution is a widely studied environmental problem and the focus of great public health concern and effort. Its control poses even more difficulties and complexities, perhaps, than does water pollution. During the 1960s lead and carbon monoxide posed the greatest threat. Public concern reached a level of intensity that eventually resulted in the Clean Air Act of 1970. It took considerable time to get its many provisions implemented; however, since 1977, for example, lead and carbon monoxide in urban air have been reduced 87 percent and 32 percent respectively (Bingham and Meader, 1990). This was accomplished despite increases in the number of automobiles on the road and average number of miles driven.

These early efforts were relatively successful and there has been periodic tightening of the regulations, but these victories have been largely offset by population growth and industrial expansion both in the United States and around the world. The most serious air pollution problems are now global in nature. Among the more challenging ones are (1) acid rain, (2) depletion of the ozone layer, and (3) global warming.

Acid rain results from excess emission of sulfur dioxide into the atmosphere from coal-fired power plants and, to a lesser extent, from automobiles. The most visible of the deleterious effects is damage to trees and to the plants and wildlife of freshwater lakes. The problem could be largely controlled by installing the proper equipment in power plants, but the costs are high and public aversion to higher prices for electric power has delayed serious efforts to correct the problem. Another difficult obstacle is that the acid deposition often occurs in locations, and thus political jurisdictions, remote from the source of emission.

Ozone depletion appears to have more serious consequences. Paradoxically, in the lower levels of our atmosphere this active form of oxygen (O_3) acts as a dangerous irritant to the respiratory system; whereas in the stratosphere, it serves as a beneficial shield filtering out some of the most harmful wavelengths of ultraviolet radiation (Doll, 1992). The main ozone depleters appear to be a class of chemicals termed **chlorofluorocarbons** (CFCs), commonly used in air conditioners, refrigeration equipment, and in the manufacture of certain plastics, and various oxides of nitrogen, resulting mainly from auto and aircraft emissions. Once they escape into the atmosphere, these substances migrate to the stratosphere and destroy molecules of ozone. This effect appears to be a significant contributor to the rising incidence of the common basal and squamous cell skin cancers and may increase the risk of the more deadly melanomas as well.

The validity of the global warming threat is less well established; however, the preliminary evidence is persuasive and the potential long-term consequences serious and extremely difficult to control. The evidence suggests that the release of large amounts of carbon dioxide, methane, and CFCs into the atmosphere creates a "greenhouse" effect. The heat that would normally dissipate into space during the night is trapped by the gaseous cover and over time the average temperature rises to produce disruptive climate change and erosion of shoreline areas due to increased melting of the polar ice cap. A review of weather records over the past 300 years reveals a small but significant warming trend; the world on average is approximately 0.5 degree Celsius warmer (Jones and Wigley, 1990). Currently it is difficult to determine how closely this rise is linked to the greenhouse effect, whether or not it will accelerate, and how serious the consequences will be. Carbon dioxide, the main suspect, is emitted in large amounts from virtually all forms of combustion; because it results from complete combustion or the full oxidation of the fuel, it is normally regarded as one of the more desirable by-products. Unfortunately, there is no apparent way to avoid its release as long as we continue to rely on fossil fuels. Basic energy conservation and the continued development of "soft" sources, such as solar power, may be the ultimate solution.

Global problems require global solutions. Fortunately, there is at least a start in this direction. The most notable example occurred in 1988 when the Montreal Protocol was signed by representatives of the United States, Canada, and most of the European community; this agreement calls for a 50 percent rollback in the release of CFCs by 1999. This agreement, of course, does not include all the industrial nations and enforcement is always a problem in such arrangements; however, it is a promising start and could set a pattern for the future. More recently, in June 1992, the United Nations Conference on Environment and Development, often termed the "Earth Summit," was held in Rio de Janeiro. Progress at this conference was marred by the refusal of the United States to sign the agreement on biodiversity because of certain concerns over patent rights. However, several more countries agreed to phase out ozone depleting chemicals and more than 150 countries signed a treaty designed to reduce the danger of climate change.

Currently, the world's ecology is showing serious signs of strain mainly as a result of pollutants generated by the one billion or so people of the industrial nations; meanwhile, the approximately 4.5 billion population of the developing countries is growing rapidly and its members are doing everything possible to emulate our style of living. Moreover, it does not appear to be either possible or desirable to hamper their efforts if we are to ever achieve a more peaceable world. A well-established and commonly observed phenomenon termed the **demographic transition** presents the world with a serious dilemma. It refers to the tendency for population growth to decline with higher levels of economic development, the very activities that strain the world's ecosystem. Yet, population growth also places a tremendous burden on our natural resources. Thus, countries that are in the midst of struggles to free themselves from the urgent, "here and now" problems of poverty are understandably slow to put a priority on environmental efforts—the benefits of which won't be realized until the next century. Consequently, it behooves the United States and the other "middle-class" nations to develop both the technology and policies that offer the chance to achieve a high standard of living that does not embody the seeds of its own destruction.

Unintentional Injuries

Another category of health problems that has proved hard to classify is that of unintentional injuries, commonly termed accidents. We have long been conditioned to treat injuries as a problem of personal safety behavior, or as a product of "risk-taking" behavior. As always, personal behavior is an important part of the problem whose role should not be minimized. But arguably it accounts for less of the problem than do environmental conditions. Moreover, even when some ambiguity exists as to the primary cause, public health workers have found environmental conditions far easier to change than human behavior.

Statistics confirm the need for concern about safety; clearly, we live in a very hazardous society. Except for the first year of life, injuries are the leading cause of death for the first four decades of one's existence in the United States. In 1990 approximately 93,600 people were killed and probably three times that number were permanently disabled by accidents in the United States (U.S.

Bureau of the Census, 1993). Close to one-half of the deaths and disabilities were associated with motor vehicles. In addition to the loss of life and human suffering, the accident toll also places a heavy economic burden on society. During this same year, approximately $174 billion in costs were attributable to unintentional injuries (U.S. Bureau of the Census, 1993). This total is more than was spent for all the nation's colleges and universities during the same year. The young, poor, and elderly suffer disproportionately more from injuries than do others. Miners, industrial workers, and farm laborers suffer a disproportionate number of disabling injuries. All of this represents a tremendous cost to society in lost work, increased medical costs, and unnecessary suffering.

Most of these accidents are preventable and many of the resulting injuries can be eliminated or minimized. Smith and Falk (1987) advocate the use of a framework devised earlier by Haddon (1980) which identifies three phases of accident control:

1. Pre-event phase—preventing the occurrence of injury-producing events.
2. Event phase—reducing the extent of injury.
3. Postevent phase—reducing the consequences of injury.

Within each phase efforts are made to improve (1) human behavior, (2) vehicles and equipment, and (3) the environment. In regard to auto safety, for example, these factors can be illustrated by seatbelt use, crashworthy vehicles, and improved highway construction. These authors emphasize the use of measures that protect the individual without any action on his or her part. These "passive" interventions are considered more effective than "active" approaches that depend on individual responsibility.

The Social Environment

The study of social factors and their relationships to health problems is commonly termed **social epidemiology**. Such social factors as race, income, education, gender, family composition, and occupation are examined by social epidemiologists to determine their influence on and their associations with health. Through a variety of methods, researchers attempt to determine the individual, interactive, and collective impact of these and other social factors on health outcomes. Research in this area has shown that social variables are predictors of general health status or of specific health problems. It is instructive to take a broader look at those variables as a category before discussing specific aspects.

Social factors reflect the way a society is organized, for example, who marries whom and how many children they have; who works for whom and how much autonomy, power, and income workers are allowed; who makes policy decisions on local and national levels on major issues such as health, war, poverty, discrimination; and how well these policy decisions are carried out. The authors firmly believe that society has the power to create healthy or unhealthy environmental conditions and it is these conditions that are reflected in the social factors we are about to examine.

Ironically, these powerful and all-pervasive factors are so much a part of our lives that they tend to be undervalued as health determinants in favor of physical and biological threats. However, in actual fact, the health of a nation depends to a large extent on the social structure of society. John Ratcliffe comments:

> Over time . . . socially designed systems have become more important than the physical environment to individual survival *because* they control the distribution of and access to those very factors that now determine mortality levels . . . . To be sure, the physical environment still exacts a certain toll through such incidents as earthquakes, tidal waves, floods, and long-term climatic changes. Nevertheless, the socioeconomic systems created by and for people constitute, to all intents and purposes, the human individual's "natural" environment. (1980:45)

Among the most important social factors in terms of impact on health are the critical influence of income and the recurrent human phenomenon of war. Because of its closer relationship to community health programs, our discussion will concentrate on income levels and their health effects. Among other well-studied variables are occupation, gender, religion, and race. Some social factors account for conditions unique to the time period of one's life; war and the economy are two such factors. Others (e.g. personal income and occupation) divide society into certain strata or classes that tend to persist over time. Factors such as gender and race are immutable, genetic conditions; their influence, however, relates to the structure of society including opportunities afforded to minority groups and the behavior patterns assigned to specific social roles. The common thread among all of these factors—the state of the economy, the advent of war, discrimination by occupation or race or sex—is their social nature.

For purposes of analysis it is useful to distinguish between socioeconomic factors as a health determinant and the equally important category of personal behavior; however, the intimate relationship between these two aspects should be recognized. When for example, a single mother is attempting to provide for two children with the income from a low-paying job and neglects routine dental care and other more serious aspects of her health, it is difficult to distinguish between poor personal choice behavior and the restraints of economic deprivation. Generally, some combination of the two are probably involved. The concept of "life-style" is emerging as an increasingly well-defined term that combines these two considerations. According to Green and Simons-Morton, "As a behavioral concept, life-style generally implies more complex, repetitive (if not habitual) patterns of behavior conditioned by living standards but still under the control of the individual or family within their economic means" (1991:189).

Socioeconomic Status

The distribution of wealth within a society is at the heart of any discussion of social influences on health. Socioeconomic status has demonstrated an extremely strong and persistent relationship to health status regardless of historical period or cultural setting. This fact was revealed quite clearly by Antonovsky, who in 1967 completed a landmark review of research on this topic involving both Europe and the United States and extending, in some cases, back to the 1600s. A few years later Kitagawa and Hauser (1973), based on an extensive nationwide survey in the United States, found that, whether socioeconomic status was measured by income, educational level, or occupation, the higher the level the lower the rate of mortality. More recently Marmot and others (1987) drew a similar conclusion on the basis of an extensive review of studies focused mainly on England and Wales but including several cross-cultural comparisons. Although they approached the topic from the broader perspective of social class, they found differences in income levels to show the most consistent relationship to health status. Syme (1991) drew similar conclusions but noted that despite this strong relationship we still know very little about the mechanisms by which this array of factors may affect individual levels of health. He speculates that, somewhat paradoxically, its very strength causes researchers to control it statistically, least it overwhelm any other factors under study, thus it seldom receives direct scrutiny.

The relationship between socioeconomic status (most easily measured by relative income) and health can be demonstrated in four ways. First, the striking disparity in mortality rates and other health measures between the wealthier and poorer countries shows the association of better health with higher economic status. For example, life expectancy at birth is a good measure of overall health status of a country; based on 1990 data, it is only 45.5 years in Angola, one of the poorest countries; in Ecuador, a more developed country, life expectancy is 66 years; and in the United States, a highly developed country, life expectancy is 75.9 years (United Nations Development Programme, 1993).

Second, as a country becomes more developed, it increases its Gross Domestic Product (GDP) and gradually the wealth is distributed broadly. Statistics measuring health status show improvements in health associated with this increase in GDP. Typically, society purchases health by improving access to medical care, adopting needed public health measures, and increasing the standard of living of its population. The increase in the living standard of the poorest people contributes most greatly to the improvement in health status of the country, for these are the people who are most susceptible to disease and therefore can most benefit from improvements in environmental conditions. Improvements in health status in the past century, as measured by infant mortality rates and other statistics, are largely a result of improvements in the living standard of the poorest citizens within a country (Powles, 1974). These trends are shown quite clearly in table 2.1.

Table 2.1 World Trends in Human Development

	Life expectancy at birth in years		Under-five mortality rate per 1,000 births		Daily calorie supply as % of req.		GDP per capita in purchasing power ($)	
	1960	1990	1960	1990	1960	1990	1960	1990
Developing	46.2	62.8	233	116	90	107	790	2,170
Industrialized	69.0	74.5	46	18	124	132	4,690	14,350
World	53.4	65.5	218	108	100	113	1,770	4,340

Source: United Nations Development Programme. *Human Development Report, 1993.*
         New York: Oxford University Press, 1993.

Third, the distribution of income within a country is associated with differences in health statistics within that country. For example, studies in the United States, England, and Wales have shown that average life expectancy is greater for those people in the higher socioeconomic classes and less for those in the lowest classes. Concomitantly, the mortality rates for the higher classes are less than for the lower classes. These relationships have held across many studies over many years (Antonovsky, 1967). The same type of relationship holds in the poor nations. The lowest socioeconomic classes in the poorest countries have the worst health problems as is demonstrated by the fact that they have the highest infant mortality rates and the shortest life expectancies in the world (United Nations Development Programme, 1993).

Fourth, there is evidence that within a country health status worsens during times of economic slump or upheaval. For example, in the United States mortality rates increased and life expectancies decreased during the Great Depression of the 1930s. Less dramatically, there are documented increases in suicides, depression, and other problems during times of national economic setbacks and high unemployment such as recessions (Brenner, 1977).

In a major review of the literature on socioeconomic status and health in the United States, Graham and Reeder (1979:76) concluded that "there appears to be two to three times as much serious illness among the poor as among the population as a whole." Specific studies have observed social class (income) gradients favoring the rich for the following health indicators: serious illness, number of patient visits, mortality, disability, and infant mortality. Among the factors that explain the greater magnitude of health problems among the poor are crowded living arrangements, poor nutrition, less access to health care, and lack of education.

Some attempts have been made to attribute the poorer health status of lower income groups to their generally reduced access to health care. This may have some effect, particularly in regard to preventive services such as immunizations and the early detection of cancer. However, as will be discussed in the later section on health care, it appears to account for a relatively small portion of the difference. Evidence for this view is supported by the fact that wide disparities in health status still exist among various socioeconomic groups within a number of industrialized nations that have managed to provide a generally adequate level of health care to their total population, regardless of income level.

One's educational level is also highly related to health status. Winkleby and others (1992) studied the effects of income and education on cardiovascular risk factors and found that education showed the strongest and most consistent relationship. In an earlier study, Pincus and associates (1987) found a straight-line relationship between lower levels of education and number of chronic disease conditions among adults between 18 and 64 years of age with 65 percent of those with eight years or less of schooling reporting at least one major condition as compared with only 33 percent of those with twelve or more years. Researchers do find that education is so closely related to income level that it is difficult to separate out the individual effects. This may be a moot point because probably the most effective and politically viable strategy to get people out of poverty is to provide them with better education and occupational training.

In the United States, income is also highly correlated with race—income for nonwhites is lower than income for whites. Figure 2.1 presents the difference in mortality rates by race. Nonwhites had considerably shorter life expectancy than whites in 1900, and slightly shorter life expectancy in 1989. However, nonwhites with moderate to high incomes tend to take on the vital health characteristics of their income peers, demonstrating the impact of social factors over genetic or racial factors. Of course, cultural characteristics should be taken into account for a more precise assessment, but the broad picture is this—race (nonwhite versus white) is related to income (low versus high) which, in turn, is related to mortality (early versus late). A similar picture emerges when morbidity is compared by race. The formulators of the *Healthy People 2000* report found the disparities in health indices among different racial and ethnic groups to be so striking and consistent as to merit a major set of goals for their reduction (USDHHS, 1990).

Religion

The members of many religious denominations, such as Seventh Day Adventists, Mormons, and Jews, often share several common cultural characteristics. Predictably, these cultural subgroups have unique health habits coupled with variations in health statistics. For example, Seventh Day Adventists, most of whom are lacto-ovo-vegetarians (nonmeat eaters who consume dairy products and eggs), and who neither smoke cigarettes nor drink alcohol, have about half the rate of cancer and heart disease when compared to the national average (Phillips, 1975). Rural Mormons, who subscribe to similarly prudent health habits,

Figure 2.1 Life Expectancy at Birth by Race, U.S., 1950–1990

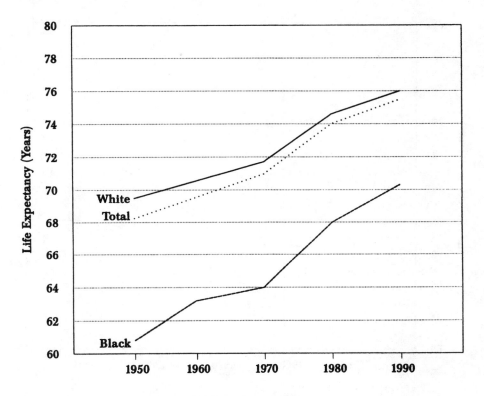

Source: National Center for Health Statistics. *Health, United States, 1991.*
Hyattsville, MD: Public Health Service, 1992.

have modest rates of cancer and cardiovascular disease (Enstrom, 1975). More recently, Goodloe and Arreola (1992), as part of an effort to clarify the concept of spiritual health, reviewed several studies of the effects of religion on health and found, along with a few negative effects, a preponderance of beneficial relationships such as lower risk of cardiovascular disease, less hypertension, and higher thresholds for pain.

Gender

Health statistics also show important differences related to gender that present an interesting pattern of biological and sociological implications. Syme (1991) found that females had lower mortality rates and consequently longer life expectancies than their male counterparts throughout all the developed countries of the world. Figure 2.2 shows the life expectancy at birth for males and females

Figure 2.2 Life Expectancy at Birth for Males and Females, U.S., 1950–1990

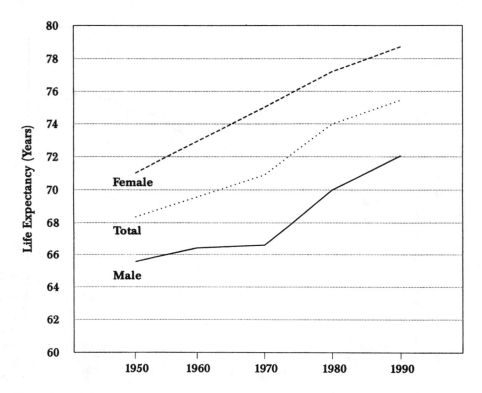

Source: National Center for Health Statistics. *Health, United States, 1991.*
Hyattsville, MD: Public Health Service, 1992.

in the United States from 1950 to 1990. Note that life expectancy was greater for females than for males during the entire time period, presumably because of the male's greater susceptibility to work related accidents, homicide, and heart disease. However, prior to about 1945 the female advantage was partially offset by the hazards surrounding pregnancy and childbirth. After World War II the steadily escalating mortality from lung cancer among males together with improvements in the quality and availability of obstetrical care resulted in a greater rate of improvement for females within the context of general gains for all population groups. Since 1980, however, the gender gap in life expectancy has narrowed slightly because of increases in the number of female deaths from respiratory cancer and a slower rate of improvement in mortality from heart disease. Consistent with the lower life expectancy for their gender, males have higher mortality rates than females at all ages. But females have more physician visits, longer hospital stays, greater disability, more surgery, and more absences from work and school. This pattern prompted one observer to remark that "women get sick and men die." However, it is still unclear whether or not females experience more illness or if the differences result from a tendency to consult physicians more promptly and to incur more absences because of their traditionally heavier burden of child care responsibilities.

Both the medical care establishment and the massive biomedical research enterprise in the United States tend to be male dominated despite recent efforts to correct this situation. Ruzek (1993) noted a recent increase in funding for research into women's health problems by the National Institutes of Health but also viewed the goal of placing women's health on the national agenda as only partly realized. There appears to be a need for vigilance to insure that the health issues of particular importance to women receive their fair share of attention.

Health Care

It seems clear that the general public credits medical care for most of the historic gains in the nation's health and continues to view it as the main vehicle for continued improvements. It is not unusual for TV commentators and print journalists to use phrases such as "Due to modern medical technology the average life expectancy has increased . . ." or ". . . the proportion of elderly citizens has increased . . ." This prevalent belief is also apparent when we consider the lower health status of certain groups, such as migrant laborers, particular minority groups, or the unemployed. We tend to see the culprit as their limite l access to medical care. We feel that if we can somehow provide these low-incom groups access to regular medical attention their health problems will dissipate.

Historical Record

As will be discussed in this section, this popular view is highly questionable. As a society we have, indeed, experienced large gains in health during the twentieth century. Life expectancy, for example, rose from 47 years in 1900 to approximately 75 years in 1990. When this situation is closely examined we find, quite predictably, that the immediate cause of this dramatic progress is the greatly reduced mortality from infectious diseases. This factor explains the bulk of the difference between the very low levels of health that prevailed throughout the world at the turn of the century (and that still exist today among most of the poorest Third World countries), and the relatively healthy state of society within the modern industrialized nations. Tuberculosis, diarrhea and enteritis, and pneumonia were and continue to be major killers of young people where primitive conditions prevail. But the key point is that the record clearly shows that the death toll from such causes dropped sharply *before* the development and widespread application of effective medical technology.

Powles (1974) presented dramatic data showing that in Great Britain, mortality among children from such common airborne infections as whooping cough, measles, and diphtheria had declined more than 95 percent from the extremely high levels of 1860 before the widespread introduction of effective treatment or immunizations, which occurred in 1945. A similar pattern is found in historical data for the United States. Tuberculosis, for example, was the second leading cause of death in 1900, killing approximately 185 of every 100,000 people. Although efforts were made to isolate those infected, no truly effective treatment became available until the introduction of streptomycin and izoniazid in the early 1950s. However, by this time, the mortality rate had dropped more than 86 percent to 30 per 100,000, presumably because of better nutrition, a shorter work week, and safer working conditions. Moreover, the rate was still declining when effective medical measures were introduced, thus modern medicine does not even have a clear claim to the further reduction of the mortality rate. Mckinlay and Mckinlay (1986) present evidence to make the same point in regard to other common infectious diseases, such as measles, scarlet fever, and influenza, which caused significant mortality in the early 1900s but declined to a fraction of their former rate prior to the development of effective drugs or vaccines for their control. These revelations raise the obvious question as to what actually caused these large declines.

The evidence suggests that the most important factor is the improved levels of nutrition that naturally occur as modern societies become more affluent; well-nourished babies, for example, typically survive the occasional bout of diarrhea with or without antibiotics, particularly if the simple practice of keeping them well hydrated is observed. Today's generally robust adolescents, with little more than fluids and bed rest, typically survive attacks of influenza that frequently progressed into deadly pneumonia among young people in years past. Improved working conditions also have played a major role. Early in the century 50- and 60-hour work weeks were common and had a debilitating effect on poorly nourished adults and particularly on children, who were often pressed into service at young ages. In addition to shorter hours, dust and noxious chemicals in the workplace are now better controlled; within the community, drinking water and food are generally free of infectious agents and most women do not have to bear the burden of frequent childbearing that was common in the early part of the century.

Thomas McKeown, a notable English physician, summarized the historical aspects of these issues quite well in a widely quoted article (1978):

> Health improved, not because of steps taken when we are ill, but because we become ill less often. We remain well, less because of specific measures such as vaccination and immunization than because we enjoy a higher standard of nutrition, we live in a healthier environment, and we have fewer children.

Current Performance

Clearly, the historical contribution of medical care has been overrated. But admittedly, modern medicine provides distinct benefits, even as presently structured. It frequently plays a crucial role in the lives of individual patients; here and there it works a miracle or two that makes the difference between life and death. It does a particularly good job in the care of trauma victims and, even when its technology falls short, it still provides a measure of comfort and hope. However, it is not realizing more than a fraction of its potential contribution to health progress; even at best, it cannot offset shortcomings in the other health determinants; and, as currently managed, its huge appetite for money and personnel is consuming resources that are needed to provide the many other things needed for a healthy society.

Free Access and Poor Health

There are a number of modern countries that have succeeded in providing a reasonably high level of health care to their total population. If access to health care were the key determinant of health status, then one would expect few major differences in health status among the various socioeconomic groups of such countries; however, this is not the case. For example, a national health service was established in Great Britain in 1948 that made tax supported medical care available to the total population. Although there have been some complaints about long waits for elective surgery and other less essential procedures, it is generally agreed that the important medical needs have been met. If medical care were a strong factor in determining health status one would expect that the more than 40 years of free access would have given Great Britain's poorer people the chance to move closer to the level of the more well-to-do. However, Marmot and others (1987), after an extensive review, found that the gap was still substantial. Higher rates of infant mortality and deaths from coronary heart disease were prime contributors to a large difference in the standardized mortality ratio. With an index of 100 representing the average, among adult men 137 deaths were observed among the lowest socioeconomic group for every 74 deaths in the highest group. Other comparisons for women and children showed the same pattern as did measures of long-standing illness and restricted activity days.

In a society even more similar to that of the United States, Canada instituted a system of national health insurance in the early 1970s that provided tax supported medical care to all its citizens. Although the system has been popular and has undoubtedly corrected a social injustice, here too the gap between the health of rich and poor has remained essentially unchanged (Terris, 1990).

High Cost

The average citizen seems generally aware that medical care costs are very high. There is much complaining and, since the mid-1970s, several efforts have been made to control the rate of increase. Thus far, however, these cost containment efforts have taken the form of patchwork solutions put into place by individual segments of the system acting to protect their own interests. At various times the federal government, the state governments, employers, or insurance companies have adopted strategies designed mainly to shift costs to some other sector. At this writing, it appears that we may experience more of the same piece-meal strategies. The major reform effort undertaken by the Clinton Administration during 1993–94 failed mainly because of its inability to gain the support of the general public, a task that was hampered by the very effective opposition of the health insurance industry. One major benefit of this struggle was that health care providers and pharmaceutical companies voluntarily held price inflation for their products and services to its lowest level in several years. It remains to be seen, however, whether this effort can be maintained over time, particularly in the absence of any serious governmental threat to intervene.

Given the dismal history of past reform efforts, this recent failure was not surprising. The task of rallying public opinion to this cause is a daunting one mainly because the bulk of the costs are hidden. They come in the form of reduced salaries from employers, who bear the direct burden of ever rising costs for employee health insurance, and subsequent higher prices for the goods these companies produce as they seek to recoup these costs. In addition to the explicit payroll deduction to support Medicare experienced by working Americans, their paychecks are reduced further by higher state and federal taxes to support Medicaid. This complex financial apparatus, which developed over the years in a hit-and-miss fashion, seems almost ideal for collecting massive sums of money without causing undue public ire. During 1991, for example, $752 billion was spent for health care, a sum equal to 14.1 percent of the nation's gross national product (National Center for Health Statistics, 1991). This amount equals $2,868 per capita and is the highest in the world; it is more than twice that spent in Denmark ($1,151) or Japan ($1,267), countries that have achieved better overall health status than the United States. If our health care system were giving us decent value for our money, then we could well afford its high cost but, unfortunately, that is not the case.

It would be unfair to blame medical care costs for the fact that more than 35 million people in our society have incomes below the official poverty line and that at least an equal number of the "working poor" live in substandard conditions. However, it is clearly a significant contributor to this problem. It absorbs much of the profits of business and industry and subsequently inhibits the expansion and modernization needed to create good paying jobs. The reduction of profits also directly reduces tax revenue that otherwise would be available for better education and job training to help the underclass work their way out of poverty; the whole array of social services such as food programs, low income housing, and public assistance also suffer. Meanwhile, the burden of this "invisible tax" puts middle-class America in no mood to increase its taxation to improve the situation.

Poor Administrative Efficiency

Both hospitals and physician's offices, as they try to collect their fees, are currently faced with a bewildering array of third-party providers; one patient

Figure 2.3 Trends in Health Costs as a Percent of GNP and Life Expectancy in the U.S., 1950-1990

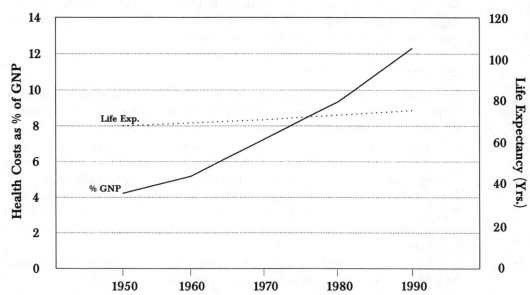

Source: National Center for Health Statistics. *Health, United States, 1991.*
Hyattsville, MD: Public Health Service, 1992.

may present a Medicare card, the next a Medicaid card, while another may be covered by any one of a multitude of private insurance plans. In addition, people may arrive in serious need of attention with no coverage or means to pay at all. Each year literally billions of dollars in costs result from the excessive paperwork required by this patchwork system. Liberal medical economists advocate a move toward a Canadian-style national health insurance with one set of forms for all; conservative experts maintain that many of these problems could be solved if true competition were introduced into the system. It would appear that any change would be worth the gamble.

Unnecessary Medical Procedures

Under the best of conditions it is often difficult to decide whether surgery is needed or whether an equally good result could be obtained by less expensive treatment; surgeons whose income depends on the volume of operations they perform often have difficulty making unbiased judgments in the many borderline cases. Leape, following an extensive review, found it "reasonable to conclude that 10 percent or more of surgical procedures are unnecessary. For controversial operations, the fraction may be substantially higher" (1992:374). Patients also are frequently subjected to unnecessary inconvenience, expense, and occasional danger by diagnostic tests ordered, not to guide treatment, but to preclude possible legal action against the physician in the event of an unhappy outcome. Many suggestions have been made to make economic and legal changes that would remove the incentives for these wasteful actions.

Treatment Orientation

Several factors in the current health care system are biased toward treatment rather than prevention. For example, many of the nation's poor lack health insurance and thus tend to let medical needs go untended until they become expensive emergencies. A serious chronic condition, such as hypertension, may go undetected until it produces a severe stroke. In another common occurrence, a young woman working at minimum wage may find herself disqualified for Medicaid yet unable to afford the $400 or $500 that prenatal care may cost. This lack places her at risk for the delivery of a low birth weight baby that may require several thousand dollars worth of added medical care, usually at public expense.

Even the more well-to-do find their physicians more interested in treating their illnesses than in preventing them. Much could be done both in medical education and in restructuring the economic aspects of our health care system in a manner that would give physicians a vested interest in our health rather than our illnesses. Such measures, in combination with improved education of the public in regard to preventive services, would enable medical care to make its full contribution to the nation's health status.

A Modern Role for Medical Care

As noted, modern medical care has not made the substantial impact on mass health statistics for which it is commonly credited. However, in the ideal system it could provide considerable help "at the margin" after the more important factors had been improved and had thus reduced the serious health problems to a small percentage of the population. Few would deny that good medical care can make a crucial difference in certain individual cases. And while these cases may be limited in number, this fact does not matter to those persons directly involved. Moreover, with considerable restructuring the medical care system in the United States could help a much larger portion of the population reach and maintain higher levels of health status without diminishing its traditional role of providing intensive treatment to seriously ill and injured patients.

This larger and more effective contribution to the nation's health would require that (1) inflation in health care costs be brought under control, (2) access be expanded to the total population, (3) both the financial incentives to providers and their mode of training increase the attention given to preventive services, and (4) both health care providers and health educators help the individual become emotionally less dependent on health care and develop a sense of personal responsibility for his or her own health.

In a review of the potential value of health care for the general task of health promotion, Roemer decried the dichotomy that had been created between prevention and treatment as a view that "not only overlooks the many benefits derived from medical care, but also ignores the great value of the medical process as a major channel for the delivery of preventive health services" (1984:245). He notes that a rationally planned health care system would enhance progress in both prevention and treatment. More recently this concept was strongly endorsed by the *Healthy People 2000* initiative that seeks to "achieve access to preventive services for all Americans" as one of its three major goals (USDHHS, 1990). The specific national objectives for these services were based on the recommendations of the U.S. Preventive Services Task Force. This 20-member, multidisciplinary panel reviewed more than 2500 studies over a five-year period in order to determine the most effective procedures (U.S. Preventive Services Task Force, 1989). Health care has much to offer; however, the effective realization of its great promise is going to require many changes.

Personal Behavior

The great health progress made during the first half of the century in overall nutritional status, improved working conditions, and better community sanitation was brought about mainly by the collective action of labor unions, legislatures, and city health departments, as well as by general economic progress. Throughout this struggle the individual was generally too busy trying to make a living and pay the bills to give much thought to health matters, particularly in regard to prevention. The average citizen was generally a passive recipient of the steadily improving health conditions. Fortunately, this passive role is changing in favor of a more active one both in response to improved public awareness of health practices and the changing nature of the health threats we commonly face.

The second half of the century presented a different pattern of major health threats which, among other things, highlighted the role of personal behavior in achieving and maintaining health. The Surgeon General's 1979 report stated unequivocally that "you the individual can do more for your own health and well-being than any doctor, any hospital, any drug, any exotic medical device" (USDHHS, 1979:120). Its successor, *Healthy People 2000*, has perhaps stressed individual behavior to the neglect of other determinants in its call for a "'Culture of character,' which is to say a culture or way of thinking and being, that actively promotes responsible behavior and the adoption of life-styles that are maximally conducive to good health" (USDHHS, 1990:v).

The role of individual patterns of behavior in regard to such modern problems as chronic disease, substance abuse, and the many problems surrounding sexual behavior, procreation, and child rearing is clear; however, what is not so clear is to what extent the individual has effective control over behavior under various degrees of economic and social duress. Also, it is often useful to distinguish between occasional, episodic behavior and behavior that is habitual and repetitive. As noted, the term "life-style" has evolved as a more narrowly defined aspect of personal behavior that is complex and repetitive; in our discussions of either life-style or personal behavior the reference is to practices over which the individual has reasonable control. As will be shown, many such actions have major effects on health.

Cigarette Smoking

During the early part of the century Americans began forsaking their less harmful pipes and cigars for the more deadly cigarette. This trend greatly accelerated among men because of the circumstances surrounding World War I; a similar acceleration occurred among women some 20 years later during World War II. As early as the 1930s, surgeons began to notice that the large majority of their lung cancer patients were heavy smokers; however, definitive evidence of the health risks associated with this habit was not available until the late 1950s. Finally in 1964 the U.S. Public Health Service, under the direction of Surgeon General Luther Terry, published a thorough review of all the significant studies in a report entitled *Smoking and Health* (USDHEW, 1964), which had a strong impact on both the general public and subsequent legislation. The role of cigarette smoking as a definitive cause of lung cancer and emphysema was reemphasized and new evidence linking smoking to mortality from coronary heart disease was later confirmed in an update of the Surgeon General's report (USDHEW, 1972) and in the findings of the Framingham Study (Dawber, 1980). Current estimates attribute 115,000 or 23 percent of the deaths from cardiovascular heart disease and 107,000 or 79 percent of all lung cancer deaths to cigarette smoking along with another 57,000 smoking related deaths from emphysema, chronic bronchitis, and other chronic obstructive pulmonary conditions (Fielding, 1991). Cigarette smoking is also related to a host of other problems ranging from increased risk of colds and influenza to cancer of the esophagus. *Healthy People 2000* noted that cigarette smoking is associated with an estimated 390,000 premature deaths each year and emphasized that "tobacco use is the most important single preventable cause of death in the United States accounting for one of every six deaths . . ." (USDHHS, 1990:57).

Dietary Practices

In terms of health effects, American eating habits appear to have come full circle from the ravages of dietary deficiencies in the early part of the century to the ravages of excess in recent decades. The role of excess dietary fat and cholesterol as significant contributors to heart disease is well established. Saturated fats, such as those provided by beef, pork, and many dairy products, tend to raise serum cholesterol levels and thus have been branded as a coronary risk factor. However, the unsaturated fats common to most fish and vegetable sources tend to lower cholesterol and thus may have a positive effect. Also, serum cholesterol levels, while highly related to heart disease, do not seem to be raised as much by dietary intake as by the body's own metabolic process which in turn is affected by other food components (Dawber, 1980). Hypertension (high blood pressure) also shows a clear relationship to heart disease. This condition is often exacerbated by excessive sodium intake and obesity; therefore, efforts to restrict both salt and overall consumption of calories are appropriate. The National Research Council published dietary recommendations which they estimate, with considerable confidence, could reduce mortality from coronary heart disease by 20 percent (National Research Council, 1989). Moreover, because coronary heart disease, stroke, and a number of other serious problems share a common root cause, namely atherosclerosis, the dietary implications are very similar.

The possible contribution of dietary factors to the development of cancer has been largely ignored for many years as investigators concentrated their attention on chemical toxins, radiation, and other substances known to cause abnormal cell division. However, in a major review of research on cancer risk, Doll and Peto (1981) identified dietary factors as a major and perhaps the leading cause of cancer in the United States. They concluded that 35 percent of all cancer in the United States was attributable to dietary factors—an estimate based mainly on comparisons of specific rates with those in other cultures. Diet maintained its status as the main factor even when other major suspects were controlled for; however, the search for the exact mechanisms linking diet to cancer has proved to be very difficult. Nonetheless, the National Research Council (1989), in a major report on diet and health, also views eating habits as a major factor in the etiology of cancer and cites estimates that anywhere from 10 percent to 70 percent of the deaths could be prevented by dietary modifications, especially for cancers of the stomach, the large bowel, and to a lesser extent, the breast, the endometrium, and the lung.

Although our dietary problems are more often those of excess, hunger and malnutrition still exist. Within many low-income groups American children display high incidences of stunted growth, increased susceptibility to infectious diseases, and such preventable conditions as pellagra and rickets. Brown and Allen (1988) cite evidence that 20 million American citizens suffer from hunger, a situation made more disturbing by the fact that this problem had been virtually eliminated during the 1970s. In this case, the problem is not one of ignorance but of lack of means, another legacy of our persistent problem of poverty.

Alcohol and Drug Use

Depressant drugs such as alcohol, morphine, heroin, and barbiturates (e.g., sleeping pills) are capable of producing addictions among susceptible users. Although the circumstances surrounding addiction to a "street drug" such as heroin tend to produce greater risks of death (such as with heroin overdose), alcoholism represents the greater public health problem because of the larger number of persons affected. As of 1990, 61 percent of the adult population of the United States reported at least occasional use of beverage alcohol and of these 9 percent reported heavy use (National Center for Health Statistics, 1994). Although it is difficult to define and survey the number of alcoholics within this group, a common rule of thumb holds that one of every 10 users encounters some sort of serious drinking problem; by this formula we can place approximately 10 million adults in this category which includes alcoholics and heavy "escape" drinkers. Alcoholics invariably blight their own lives and severely affect the members of their families, thus creating a public health problem of truly monumental proportions. In a typical case of alcoholism, serious disruptions of work efficiency, social life, and family life drastically reduce the victim's quality of life long before any physiological damage occurs. However, if the disease continues for several years, cirrhosis of the liver may develop. This condition ranked ninth among causes of mortality, accounting for 25,815 deaths in 1990 (National Center for Health Statistics, 1993).

Figure 2.4 Alcohol Consumption of Persons 18 Years of Age and Over, U.S., 1988

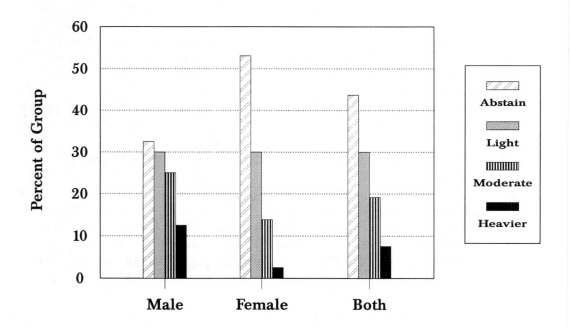

Source: National Center for Health Statistics. *Health, United States, 1991.*
Hyattsville, MD: Public Health Service, 1992.

Despite some recent progress, the role of alcohol as a cause of auto accidents remains a serious concern. Accidents (unintentional injuries) as a general category are responsible for approximately 100,000 deaths per year in the United States. They rank as the fourth leading cause of death overall, and as the first among people in the 14–44 age group. Because a disproportionate number of accident victims come from younger age groups, accident losses in terms of total years of life lost and total years of disability warrant the high priority placed on this problem. Laboratory evidence shows that only moderate blood alcohol concentrations are needed to produce a measurable reduction in judgment, coordination, and visual acuity; epidemiological studies have shown that 25 percent of drivers injured in serious crashes were legally intoxicated as were 50 percent of all drivers killed in auto accidents (Smith and Falk, 1987). Because motor vehicle accidents account for almost one-half of the total accident toll, reducing the practice of driving while under the influence of alcohol merits strong efforts both in law enforcement and education.

Although alcohol abuse has not been identified as a major cause of cancer, its effects apparently interact with those of cigarette smoking to increase the risks of cancers of the mouth, throat, esophagus, and liver. An estimated 7 percent of cancer deaths among men and 2 percent among women are clearly related to alcoholism when the interaction with cigarettes is included (Greenwald, 1980:261). People who use alcohol have also been shown to smoke more than abstainers; thus it is quite possible that drinking encourages more smoking as well as exacerbating its harmful effects.

Interestingly, Colsher and Wallace (1989) in their extensive review found some limited evidence of health benefits from alcohol use. Studies of longevity have shown that moderate users of alcohol live slightly longer than those who abstain. These additional years appear to result primarily from a reduced susceptibility to coronary heart disease but it is not known whether or not this effect is a direct result of alcohol use or the effect of some related factor such as personality differences between moderate users and abstainers. Moreover, Colsher and Wallace also noted that the general absence of "dose-response relationships" offers little support for an overall health-promoting effect of low to moderate alcohol intake.

The use and abuse of various street drugs is a particularly troublesome health problem in terms of blighted lives and economic cost. Schuster and Kilbey (1991) cited evidence based on a large national sample of people 12 years of age or older that 37 percent of this population reported using illegal drugs at least once in their lifetime, including 11 percent who reported using such substances during the past month. Moreover, an estimated 3.3 million people reported the use of crack cocaine 12 or more times during the past year. These same reviewers cited estimates of $75 billion in direct care and other costs associated with substance abuse in the United States in 1988. The fact that these distressing numbers persist after years of vigorous law enforcement suggests that we, as a society, should make a stronger effort to reduce demand for street drugs though a more intense educational approach.

Unintentional Injuries

As noted in a previous section, the prevention or control of accidents, or more precisely, unintentional injuries, requires careful attention to road construction, vehicle design, working conditions, home construction, and a host of other environmental factors. Personal behavior is, of course, the other main factor in the etiology of this problem. Efforts within both these realms have enjoyed reasonable success for, despite the increasing exposure of our population to industrial technology and modern means of transportation, mortality rates for unintentional injuries have declined throughout most of the twentieth century. For example, 72 people per 100,000 died from all forms of unintentional injuries in 1900 as compared with 33 in 1990. Even our modern nemesis, the automobile, appears less threatening when the increase in miles traveled is taken into account. In 1924, for instance, 20 motor vehicle deaths occurred per 100 million passenger miles but by 1989 this rate had dropped to slightly more than one per 100 million passenger miles. Comparable progress also has been made in the rates for the other common accident sites, namely homes, farms, and industrial settings. Although the trend towards improvement on a passenger mile basis seems clear, exposure to accidents has increased greatly because more and more people own cars and drive more miles and thus offset much of the improvement in rates.

Any reasonable analysis of the overall accident situation will reveal opportunities for significant savings in terms of premature deaths, crippling disabilities, human suffering, and economic cost with relatively small improvements in personal habits. Smith and Falk, following an extensive review of the available evidence, express the belief "that the gap between what is and what could be is larger for unintentional injuries than for any single disease" (1987:159). The ability of the average citizen to do much more for his or her safety represents a largely untapped source in the battle against accidents and thus a major challenge to the health educator.

Acquired Immunodeficiency Syndrome (AIDS)

Despite the considerable progress that has been achieved in gaining a scientific understanding of the HIV virus and the nature and progression of AIDS, the search for a truly effective treatment has proven to be elusive. Preliminary figures for 1991 show approximately 43,000 new cases and 33,000 deaths (National Center for Health Statistics, 1994). However, the number of cases and deaths are escalating so rapidly that any total will be hopelessly dated by the time it reaches the reader. David Rogers (1992) of the National Commission on AIDS notes that the cumulative death toll from this disease already exceeds the lives lost in the Korean and Vietnam wars combined. He also suggests that upwards of one million people in the United States are HIV positive and thus prime candidates for the eventual development of the disease itself. Because the victims are generally young, AIDS is one of the leading causes of years of life lost before age 65. Thus far prevention remains the best weapon. Such measures, however, require condom use; sexual abstinence; restriction to a safe, monogamous relationship; use of clean needles by drug addicts; and similar practices, some of which many people find difficult to follow. This situation presents a major challenge to health education.

Stress

The human organism seems to be constructed such that threatening stimuli trigger a complex set of neurological and endocrine responses to produce a high level of arousal. Hans Selye's pioneering research revealed much of the basic mechanics of the stress response, and prompted epidemiological and clinical research into the relationship of stress to various diseases (Selye, 1974). Although controversies abound as to the importance or size of its contribution, few researchers dispute the widespread involvement of stress in the etiology of a wide variety of illnesses. The list begins with reduced resistance to colds, influenza, and other upper respiratory infections, then proceeds to headaches, peptic ulcers, asthma attacks, and heart disease. There is even some tentative evidence that it may have a role in producing growth deficiencies and cancer. Finally, the fatigue and mental distraction it produces is believed to be a major contributor to accidents.

Prolonged stress, in addition to disrupting the healthy functioning of the body, is also subjectively unpleasant for most people; consequently, they generally take some type of deliberate or intuitive action to reduce their stress. This coping behavior may be beneficial, such as recreational exercise, hobbies, or religious activity or meditation; but often it is detrimental, such as excessive drinking or eating, excessive reliance on tranquilizers or similar medications, or the abuse of street drugs. In such cases the coping behavior often becomes more threatening to one's health than the original stress. Although our understanding of human behavior is incomplete, it seems clear that stress plays a role in child abuse, spouse abuse, and other various forms of antisocial behavior.

There is an obvious need to take action to reduce the incidence of stress-induced disease and other untoward responses. The type of intervention programs needed tend to be almost global in scope and amount to a broad based effort to improve the overall quality of life in our society. Starting with the psychosocial environment we can collectively support social security programs, job training, unemployment insurance, and similar measures to reduce economic stress. Threats of physical violence can be reduced by our support of efforts to combat street crime in our own neighborhoods as well as to defuse international tensions throughout the world. As individuals, we can seek to meet our personal responsibilities to friends and family members and so foster stress-reduction techniques such as time management, differential relaxation, and meditation. In the event stress symptoms become unmanageable we can seek professional attention and follow through with the prescribed regimens. Clearly, there is much the well-informed individual can do both to prevent harmful stress reactions from occurring and to deal effectively with those that do occur in spite of preventive measures.

Exercise

The case for the health benefits of exercise is based on a combination of epidemiological and experimental research as well as clinical observations. For many years it has been observed that men working at active occupations tended to have less heart disease than those in sedentary jobs. Laboratory investigations have revealed that long-term exercise tends to strengthen and enlarge the heart muscle and increase the volume of blood pumped during each contraction. This internal change is commonly manifested in a lower resting pulse rate. Preliminary evidence suggests that the arteries supplying the heart are enlarged and new capillaries, the small blood vessels that directly nourish body cells, are generated. Blair and others (1991), on the basis of an extensive review of completed research, cited evidence that regular exercise reduces blood concentrations of cholesterol and increases the proportion of beneficial high density lipoproteins; insulin sensitivity and utilization is enhanced; and the tendency for blood to clot is reduced. These and other changes in structure and blood chemistry yield a variety of health benefits including increased physical fitness, some reduction of emotional stress and depression, reduced risk of coronary heart disease, less obesity, and less risk of osteoporosis. Although less well established, the functioning of the immune system may be enhanced as evidenced by a slight reduction in cancer risk. A major conference on the health effects of exercise held in Toronto during 1988 attracted several prominent researchers. In a consensus statement the value of exercise was quite clearly expressed:

> In addition to an improvement in overall lifestyle, potential societal benefits of greater personal physical fitness may include a reduction in demands for acute and chronic medical services, lower indirect costs of illness, and less costly physical dependence during the retirement years. (Bouchard et al., 1990:27)

Although the benefits of regular intensive exercise over a grossly sedentary life-style are easy to demonstrate, it is less clear as to what level of activity is required for a beneficial effect. It was once popular to believe that one must reach a certain threshold to achieve any noticeable benefit; there is little evidence to support this view (Blair et al., 1991). The average person may be well advised to think of activity level as existing on a continuum extending from bed rest, through normal daily activities, to the intense aerobic program.

The educational needs of the average individual in regard to personal exercise patterns are many and varied: people need to know what sort of exercise is beneficial and how much is most valuable; they need help in handling the motivational aspects, such as by finding a partner or group to provide support; they need to be advised of the importance of medical clearance when there is any threat of a pre-existing heart condition; and they need to know how to reduce the risk of both minor nuisances, such as blistered feet and pulled muscles, and accident hazards such as those associated with bicycling and swimming. These needs are currently being addressed somewhat haphazardly in the mass media and by the health club industry. However, much more could be done in a systematic way through health and physical education to capitalize on the nation's rather stable trend toward more active life-styles.

Use of Preventive Health Services

As discussed in a previous section, the vast health care delivery system in the United States contributes only a fraction of its potential for improving health status. Although the industry itself must take the larger share of responsibility for this poor performance, the individual consumer's inability or reluctance to use available preventive services is also a major factor.

Although a number of effective methods of pregnancy control exist, they are grossly underutilized. The best current estimates reveal that 56 percent of all pregnancies are either unwanted or occur earlier than desired (USDHHS, 1991a). Under such circumstances prenatal care is often neglected and any subsequent infants face both undue biological risks before birth and psychosocial risks afterward. Many parents also neglect routine pediatric care and thus deny their child such benefits as proper monitoring of nutrition and growth, as well as immunization against common childhood diseases such as measles and pertussis. Among older children and adolescents, many remedial conditions, ranging from simple vision problems to severe orthopedic defects, go untreated despite the screening and parental notification efforts of school nurses.

Hypertension, more commonly known as high blood pressure, is an important risk factor contributing to both cerebral hemorrhage (stroke) and coronary heart disease. A major problem in the detection and subsequent treatment of this condition is its failure to produce any discomfort or noticeable symptoms in the large majority of cases, a quality that earns it the title of the "silent killer." Despite considerable recent progress at detection and control, many Americans still are believed to have blood pressure above the 160/90 level that usually indicates the need for intervention; this threatening condition is almost 100 percent controllable when detected and treated.

Cancer mortality is another problem that could be greatly reduced with better consumer behavior. The American Cancer Society estimates that more than 100,000 of those who die from cancer each year in the United States could have been saved with earlier detection. Although the benefits of early detection vary considerably according to the type of cancer and the organ affected, the chances for survival are nearly always improved. A clear example is the 70 percent reduction in deaths from uterine cancer that accompanied widespread use of the Pap smear. During 1990 approximately 81 percent of women over the age of 18 years reported having a Pap test within the past year; however, only 47 percent of the women over 50 years of age had received a clinical breast examination and mammogram within the past year (USDHHS, 1991a). Routine screening tests for rectal and colon cancer as part of an annual medical examination for older adults, and age-appropriate mammograms and breast self-examinations by women appear to merit particular attention. The success of these aspects of cancer control clearly depend both on service accessibility and individual willingness to seek out preventive medical services and to perform self-examination.

Only the priority areas with proven effectiveness within the total array of preventive services have been addressed in this section. There are many other underutilized opportunities such as the monitoring of blood cholesterol levels, immunization of at-risk adults for influenza and pneumonia, and health counseling for diet and weight control. The utilization of these and other services fostering health promotion and disease prevention could result from the wider availability and more intelligent use of good primary health care.

Summary

The factors that exert strong effects on individual and community levels of health status may be logically categorized as (1) genetic aspects, (2) the physical environment, (3) the social environment, (4) health care, and (5) personal behavior. Although opinions differ considerably among various health authorities as to the relative importance of each of these factors, evidence was presented in this chapter to show that the role of health care was secondary in importance to such factors as socioeconomic level and personal behavior. At the beginning of the twentieth century, various infectious diseases were leading causes of mortality; as the years passed the rates for tuberculosis, pneumonia, influenza, and many others declined to a small fraction of their former size, and this occurred prior to the introduction of effective antibiotics or vaccines. Such astute observers of these trends as McKeown and Dubos feel that improved nutritional status occurring as a normal result of the historic trend to higher income levels was the primary factor. Child labor laws, shorter work weeks, and improved working conditions also contributed to the decline.

Currently the many millions of Americans who live in poverty, or near poverty, experience higher rates of mortality and morbidity in several categories including infant mortality, drug addiction, and homicide. This relationship is equally apparent in Canada and the United Kingdom, where the poor presumably have free access to government supported health care.

As heart disease, cancer, and unintentional injuries become relatively more prominent health threats, the role of health behavior in the form of better eating and exercise habits, avoidance of cigarette smoking, safe driving practices, and the early detection of disease becomes crucial. Protecting the physical environment from synthetic chemical pollutants is necessary to preclude any long-term increases in the incidence of cancer or birth defects; however, the detrimental effects of environmental pollutants thus far appear to be moderate in comparison to the ravages of economic deprivation and unhealthy life-styles.

Genetic factors are very important to one's health status; however, the means of control are limited. Currently, genetic counseling, screening of newborns for genetic disease, and protecting the environment from mutagenic or teratogenic substances have been employed to reduce the impacts of genetic defects.

Health Professions and Organizations

*Once upon a time, and perhaps even now, there
lived a handsome Greek god named Asclepius.
According to legend he was the first physician—a
noble healer skilled in the use of both medications
and surgical procedures. Although his immortal
patients no doubt complained about the size of his
fees, he was nonetheless hailed and revered for his
miraculous cures. His beautiful associate, Hygeia,
who was alternately depicted as his daughter and
as his wife, depending on the vagaries of Greek
mythology, was also a health practitioner with a
large clientele. But unlike Asclepius, whose style
was to treat illness after it occurred, Hygeia
encouraged her followers to live balanced and
reasonable lives—to avoid toxic substances and to
provide their bodies with proper nourishment, rest,
and exercise. Furthermore, during their occasional
bouts of illness, her followers were to rely on their
own natural recuperative powers rather than on
medical or surgical intervention.*

Introduction

As would many modern Americans, the ancient Greeks found Hygeia's rules
and recommendations too confining. They preferred to work and play to excess
and then run to Asclepius for help when their abused bodies or personalities
broke down, as they frequently did. They recognized Hygeia's wisdom but held
Asclepius in greater esteem because he helped them when they were in need—
when they were in pain and fear he brought them relief. Hygeia's popularity
was threatened not only by the curative abilities of Asclepius but also by her
sister Panacea, a celebrated herbologist who barnstormed around Mount Olympus
advertising a potion for every ill. Panacea's extravagant claims were very
troublesome to Hygeia, and her own sensible advice proved to be very difficult
for others to follow.

Medicine and Public Health: Contrasting Approaches

Although the myths in the preceding story may be somewhat distorted, the
basic ideas illustrated are accurate in terms of the current health care situation

in America. Virtually all of our personal and collective activities have some effect on health; however, the people who approach the task of health improvement directly—that is, health professionals—tend to fall into two basic groups: there are (1) those who dispense personal health care, a vast group of physicians, dentists, counseling psychologists, and similar health professionals and their support personnel and (2) the public health professionals, a considerably smaller group who do their most visible work in city and county health departments and such federal agencies as the Centers for Disease Control and Prevention. The first group, like Asclepius, tend to wait until after the illness occurs before taking action; their approach is **curative**. The second group, like Hygeia, attempts to **prevent** illness and increase health among those free from illness. Although many public health officers hold medical degrees, they usually acquire additional training in schools of public health whose technology base is similar to that of medicine but whose traditions, orientation, and modes of application differ greatly. In this chapter we will examine some of the fundamental differences between these two groups, discuss the contribution of each group, and show how they relate to health education and health promotion.

Fundamental Differences

Three important differences serve to distinguish the medical from the public health establishment. First, in regard to the relationship with the people served, physicians generally deal with people one at a time; the doctor-patient relationship is revered and it is seldom if ever appropriate to place the interests of other persons or groups above that of the individual patient. Public health workers, however, tend to think in terms of population groups rather than individuals. They see themselves in a global war against massive disease threats and, because they must fight with limited resources, they work to accomplish the greatest good for the greatest number with what means they have.

A second major difference is found in the attitudes toward the health problems themselves. Despite the considerable rhetoric concerning preventive medicine, the basic style of physicians is to wait in their offices for the problems to come to them, or more precisely, to wait until the patients schedule appointments and present their complaints. This may be very appropriately termed a **reactive** strategy. Granted, some physicians, such as many of those based in health maintenance organizations, take a more **proactive** approach and encourage their patients to develop good health habits and return for routine medical examinations. Health maintenance organizations (HMOs) contract with their clients to provide any care they might need for a prepaid fee and thus acquire, in theory at least, a vested interest in each member's health. Although more committed to prevention, HMOs currently serve only 20 to 30 percent of the nation's population. In contrast to the traditional medical care system, public health agencies use the mass media to inform the public on health matters, encourage good health behavior, provide immunizations when not otherwise available, and generally take a proactive approach to preventing health problems.

A third quite important and sharply defined difference pertains to the respective political and economic ideologies of the two categories of health workers. Physicians and the political action committees of their various professional organizations tend to be stronger advocates of the concept of free enterprise. They tend to react negatively towards government involvement in health care, whether it be regulation, financial support, or the direct dispensing of services. The opposition of the American Medical Association (AMA) to the enactment of the Medicare and Medicaid legislation of the 1960s is a case in point as is their current opposition to any serious proposal for health care reform. The enactment of Medicare and Medicaid was a historic turning point in the funding of health care—it channeled billions of dollars of public funds into the health care system and provided effective care for millions of elderly and poor citizens who were previously underserved. Despite the obvious need, these programs were vigorously opposed by the medical establishment. In fairness we must note some recent softening among individual physicians towards various liberal proposals, such as national health insurance; but, as a group, they remain opposed. The public health establishment, on the other hand, is a virtual creation of local, state, and federal governments. Tax dollars constitute its main source of support; it exists in an environment of regulation, with its activities defined by legislative mandates and the bulk of its members working as salaried government employees. Furthermore, public health workers generally support government-funded health services for populations, especially for those people who may not have access to these services in our free enterprise system.

Similar Goals

Although these two groups of health professionals often find themselves in serious disagreement on specific issues, any logical analysis of their functions and responsibilities suggests that they should be complementary components of a single system. This observation raises a series of questions crucial to any practical understanding of society's overall efforts at health protection and promotion. How much does each of these entities contribute to this effort? How close are they to making their optimal contribution? And what changes, if any, either in public policies or within the conduct of the respective professions, would move them closer to these ideal goals? The search for answers properly begins with a review of the historical development of these two groups which use quite different methods to pursue very similar goals.

Historical Development

As one reviews the history of the practice of medicine or the various collective efforts that might be classified as public health activities, the most obvious phenomenon is the impact of modern science on the effectiveness of these two fields. This is not to say that significant events did not occur earlier than the nineteenth century; however, this turning point does serve to divide the historical account into two periods with some distinctive features: the prescientific and the scientific.

Prescientific Period

As one reviews the historical accounts of the great civilizations of the past it soon becomes apparent that the efforts to preserve and maintain health have been a priority as far back into the past as historical records extend. The ancient cultures of Babylonia, Egypt, Greece, and Rome, as well as Europe during the Dark Ages and the Renaissance, all show evidence of having made strong, persistent efforts to cope with disease and to promote health as they understood it. Written evidence in the form of laws, administrative decrees, religious customs, and professional codes of conduct are the most common legacy of these endeavors; however, more concrete manifestations also abound in the form of surgical instruments, hospital buildings, and, at least in one instance, aqueducts and sewers that have been functioning for more than two thousand years. Physicians, medicine men, or their equivalents appear in virtually every culture for which we have any reasonably well documented historical account.

Such a long and complex history lends itself to a variety of interpretations depending upon the thoroughness of the observer's scholarship and the nature of his or her biases. Lewis Thomas, for example, suggests that "the history of medicine has never been a particularly attractive subject in medical education, and one reason for this is that it is so unrelievedly deplorable a story" (Thomas, 1980:132). By modern standards of effectiveness this harsh assessment is admittedly accurate, but the striking thing about humankind's efforts in both medicine and public health throughout the many centuries before modern science was not the many failures but the fact that these efforts were, on balance, a positive force for health. The ancient practitioners lacked any accurate knowledge of why various treatments or preventive measures succeeded or failed, yet their efforts brought much comfort and often some tangible help to those in need.

Ancient Healers

Despite its shortcomings, the practice of medicine has always enjoyed respect and prestige seemingly out of all proportion to its real value. Consider the ancient Asclepiads for example. Somewhere around the year 500 B.C. this group of healers who ascribed their origin to Asclepius, the legendary Greek god noted earlier, established a medical cult that spread throughout the Greco-Roman world and flourished for perhaps a thousand years. These practitioners were more priests than physicians as they plied their craft in impressively designed temples whose walls were typically filled with the inscribed testimonies of grateful patients who had presumably been restored to health. As the apparent result of a process of suggestion that may have been outright hypnosis, many of those seeking help reported that Asclepius himself came to them in a dream and ministered to their ills. Understandably, many who experienced this phenomenon and recovered their health joined the ranks of the true believers.

Modern research investigations tend to show that approximately 50 percent of the illnesses that are presented to the average physician are based either entirely or in significant part upon psychogenic causes. Although physicians who practiced before the advent of modern psychiatry lacked any sophisticated understanding of psychosomatic etiologies, they observed that "believing often made it happen" or that the more faith the patient placed in the treatment, the more effective was the result. Even in cases of traumatic injury or infectious disease the assurance of the physician tended to reduce shock and anxiety, promote rest, and materially assist the patient's own recuperative powers. Hippocrates, who was a contemporary of the Asclepiads, adopted some of their methods, but not their religious theories. As Magner (1992:68) noted, "The Hippocratic physician rejected superstition, divination, and magic." However, Hippocrates's writings also reveal a recognition of the pragmatic value of the patient's faith in the cure. In his description of the demeanor physicians should adopt he states: "He [the physician] must always remain calm, and must make his behavior inspire the patient with confidence" (Durant, 1936:347). Thus, during this early period, physicians learned that a good "bedside manner" not only aided their popularity but their therapeutic effectiveness as well. This was an example of the healing power of the mind, now known as the **placebo effect**, a technique that remains extremely useful today.

A second and closely related device that physicians have used throughout history is described by Thomas: "The great secret, known to internists . . . but still hidden from the general public, is that most things get better by themselves. Most things in fact are better by morning" (Thomas, 1975:100). And even when the illness is more extended, the wiser physicians have always known that the natural recuperative power of the body was usually the safest and most reliable treatment. Admittedly, there are examples of the successful use of medication, with digitalis for heart disease being perhaps the prime example next to opium for palliative relief. Also, some ancient surgeons had fair success in opening inflamed sinuses and removing tumors (Bender, 1961:5). But throughout all of history prior to the current century, the patient was best served by the conservative physician who counseled rest and appropriate nourishment, administered inert drugs which were, in effect, placebos, and brought hope and confidence. This was not a very dramatic way of healing but it was genuinely useful. It often included an element of *care* frequently lacking in modern high-technology medicine.

Ancient Sanitarians

The genesis of the modern public health movement probably began when the first tribal chieftain hiked several paces downwind from camp and established a common latrine. This example is crude but nonetheless valid; while the prescientific physicians were tuning in on the emotional state of their patients, the ancient sanitarians were relying on their noses, their taste buds, and their other basic senses as they responded to aversive stimuli within their communities. They knew nothing of viruses or bacteria, but they knew that garbage and sewage gave off disagreeable odors which they suspected were causes of disease; therefore, they made provisions for the removal and disposal of these noxious items. They found that the local surface water was often foul tasting, and consequently, they dug deep wells or rigged flumes and aqueducts to bring in water from the mountains. They were offended by weevils in their flour and maggots in their meat, and so they enforced laws to ensure proper storage and transport of food items.

These measures did not require scientific knowledge; however, considerable political will and organizational ability were required to allocate resources and carry out these measures, which were, in general, technologically simple but logistically difficult. The ancient Romans, for example, were not as renowned for their technological innovations as for their administrative skills; however, their sewers and aqueducts represented both an engineering and an organizational triumph in view of the considerable labor and material resources needed for their construction. In addition, many of their other health-related activities, which brought significant benefits to the citizenry, were more directly attributed to this essential talent for administration. As Hanlon relates:

> At its zenith it [the Roman Empire] had laws for the registration of citizens and slaves, for a periodic census for the prevention of nuisances, for inspection and removal of dilapidated buildings, for the elimination of dangerous animals and foul smells, for the destruction of unsound goods, for the supervision of weights and measures, for the supervision of public bars, taverns, and houses of prostitution, and for the regulation of building construction. An uninterrupted supply of good and cheap grain to the population was assured. (1974:14)

Although one suspects that even in this golden age the Roman community was far from utopian, it is interesting to note that its success was based on efficiencies in areas that represent the most troublesome obstacles to modern health progress. Within the general area of public health and human services we have useful technology that is underutilized because of a lack of public support and continuing vacillation among our political leaders; once past these barriers, even well-conceived programs may often founder on the rocks of administrative inefficiency.

Scientific Period

Many of the respective ideologies and value systems of modern medicine and public health establishments have roots in the ancient past; however, the whole array of technology that defines their modern character began to take shape in the nineteenth century and came to fruition in the twentieth century. Within the short span of perhaps 150 years a technology was developed that worked with reasonable, and at times amazing, effectiveness. Health-related fields were, of course, not unique in undergoing such a miraculous development. The way people farmed, produced goods, traveled, and conducted their everyday affairs as recently as the early 1800s was more similar to the ways of the Romans and Greeks two thousand years ago than to the ways of their twentieth-century descendants. The developments within this short span—this historical pressure cooker—provide insights useful in the understanding and interpretation of many modern enterprises, including those of medicine and public health.

Medicine Goes to School

Wisdom often begins with a confession of ignorance. "Like a good many revolutions this one [modern medicine] began with the destruction of dogma. It was discovered, sometime in the 1830s, that the greater part of medicine was nonsense" (Thomas, 1980:132). In other words, the more astute physicians of the time finally realized that most of their great stock of medications and surgical procedures were of little value and that some were harmful.

Although this new insight perhaps marked the beginning of something better, it still took a while for new developments to occur. Throughout the entire nineteenth century medicine improved by discarding many of its dubious treatments and moving toward a more supportive, naturalistic approach. This appeared as a strange response to the advent of modern science, which was just coming into its own. During the nineteenth century, Claude Bernard of France ushered in the study of modern physiology with his study of the homeostatic balances that regulate bodily processes. Rudolf Virchow of Germany laid the groundwork for the science of pathology with his careful study of diseased tissue at the cellular level. Louis Pasteur moved a step beyond Edward Jenner, who earlier had developed a naturally occurring cowpox inoculation, by creating the first laboratory-produced vaccine, which protected against anthrax. A prerequisite for modern surgery was put into practice when William Morton, a dentist from Massachusetts, discovered the use of ether as an anesthetic. A bit later Joseph Lister, an English surgeon, killed germs in the operating room with carbolic acid and thus began the concept of **antiseptic** surgery. This practice was soon improved upon by an American, William Halsted, who devised the modern technique of **aseptic** surgery in which the surgical field is kept germ free in the first place.

These were indeed major advances but attempts to apply them proved difficult. Although considerable technology had been developed, much of it existed only in the laboratory or the hospital where it had originated. The dissemination of these new advances was painfully slow for a number of reasons, not the least of which was the low training level of the average physician. This problem was particularly acute in the United States, where the large majority of physicians were trained in private, profit-making, proprietary medical schools. Ebert assesses the quality of these schools as follows:

The proprietary schools were shockingly bad by modern standards. The only requirements for admission were the tuition and the ability to read and write. Education from the viewpoint of the students was entirely passive: the teacher lectured and the students listened. The schools had no laboratories, and frequently "chairs" of medicine and surgery were sold to the highest bidder. (1973:139)

Two closely related events did much to improve this disturbing situation. In 1893 Johns Hopkins, a Baltimore whiskey merchant, provided seven million dollars in his will for the development of a university and a medical school as part of the same institution. Although common in Europe, this combination was unique in the United States. In 1908, Abraham Flexner, who graduated from Johns Hopkins University as an educator, was commissioned by the Carnegie foundation to study American and Canadian medical schools. Flexner carried out this assignment very thoroughly and effectively; in 1910 he published a scathing and well-documented report that, in essence, recommended that the proprietary schools be closed and that medical education in North America follow the European and Johns Hopkins model of basing medical schools in universities so that the curriculum could benefit from the typical university resources in the basic sciences. In addition, he advocated more stringent admission requirements, the hiring of full-time rather than part-time professors to head clinical departments, and a curriculum more closely attuned to histology, pathology, bacteriology, and other medically related sciences.

The Flexner Report was a prime example of the right document being published at the right time. Many carefully prepared cases for professional reform are greeted by apathy or by fatal opposition from vested interests but, in this case, a nucleus of powerful individuals within the medical profession saw the value of the recommendations and, because of their own training in Europe or at Johns Hopkins University, had a vested interest in promoting this pattern as the norm within the profession. The outstanding reputation of Johns Hopkins also contributed to the strength of the new movement for reform. Very soon after its establishment this unique school recruited two famous clinicians, William Osler and William Welch. Osler, who came to Hopkins from Montreal after a short tenure at the University of Pennsylvania, was known for his great skill at diagnosis and for his innovative clinical applications of scientific discoveries. Welch, who quickly became renowned as an educator, was credited with developing a curriculum for medical training that was used almost exclusively by American schools for most of this century and that has only recently undergone significant modification.

According to Welch's curriculum, medical students study normal physiology, anatomy, and biochemistry during their first year and emphasize pathology, diagnosis, and pharmacology in their second year. These first two years are primarily didactical in nature (i.e., lecture sessions) and are based squarely on the life sciences. The latter two years, although still including some classroom work, are much more clinical and applied. Despite the widespread adoption of this pattern, Flexner's ideal of a medical school closely integrated with the science department of a university's main campus proved to be an elusive goal. Medical schools have typically established their own science departments and have remained some distance from the main university both geographically and administratively. However, even this somewhat tenuous relationship still managed to nourish this new scientific emphasis and enabled medical education to utilize much of the rapidly developing technology of the twentieth century.

Public Health Begins a Revolution

Just as a "crisis of ignorance" initiated the revolutionary changes leading to the modernization of medicine, a "crisis of social consciousness" is credited in large part with sparking the development of the modern public health establishment. During the latter part of 1831 and most of 1832, England suffered a major epidemic of cholera that had particularly devastating effects on the urban poor. This prompted Parliament to appoint a commission to investigate the administration of the "poor laws" that had been enacted to help this population group. Edwin Chadwick, an ardent social reformer, served on this commission and became acquainted firsthand with the deplorable living conditions of the working class and their consequent vulnerability to disease. He found neighborhood wells located near gutters and streams that functioned as open sewers, and food markets full of flies and vermin. In addition to these living conditions, work days extended for fourteen or more hours and salary levels were insufficient to provide adequate diets. The work of this commission led to a more ambitious study, climaxed in 1842 by Chadwick's extremely influential *Report on the Sanitary Condition of the Labouring Population and on the Means of Its Improvement* (Hanlon, 1947:19).

Chadwick's report included both impressive statistical analyses (see table 3.1) and vivid examples of the appalling living and working conditions that prevailed. It was widely publicized and quoted to the extent that significant support for a solution developed among the English landed gentry who held the bulk of the political power. Consequently, Parliament enacted legislation that mandated major improvements in community sanitation and, in addition, addressed such areas as factory working conditions, child welfare, and care of the aged.

There had probably been many such "reports" released to the public that presented their case and were written as well as Chadwick's, but which never produced any results. The difference in this case appeared to be a matter of timing. Liberal political philosophies had been on the rise throughout the Western world during the 1700s and, among other things, provided the rationale for the American and French revolutions. The climate for reform was aided by the writings of such men as Locke, Rousseau, and Voltaire, who were advocates of the inherent dignity and integrity of the common man; perhaps even more effective support was provided by Jeremy Bentham, a Utilitarian philosopher who championed a "social engineering" approach to public problems which argued that the health and well-being of the work force was essential

Table 3.1 Death by Social Class, London, 1840

Class	Proportion of Deaths from Epidemics to Total Deaths of Each Class (%)	Proportion of Deaths of Children under 1 Year to Births in That Year	Proportion of Deaths of Children under 10 Years to Total Deaths of Each Class (%)	Mean Age of Death of All Who Died— Men, Women and Children	Mean Age of All Who Died Above Age 21 Years
Gentry, professional persons, and their families	6.5	1 to 10	24.7	44	61
Tradesmen, shopkeepers, and their families	20.5	1 to 6	52.4	23	50
Wage classes, artisans, laborers, and their families	22.2	1 to 4	54.5	22	49

Source: John S. Hanlon, *Public Health Administration and Practice* (6th ed.). St. Louis, C. V. Mosby Co., 1974. Modified from Chadwick as quoted in B. W. Richardson, *The Health of Nations: A Review of the Works of Edwin Chadwick* (vol. II), London: Longmans, Green & Co., 1887.

to the economic well-being of the merchants and country gentry. This dissemination of liberal concepts among the literate members of English society had greatly influenced Chadwick as well as other political leaders and intellectuals. Although radical for its time, the resulting liberal reform movement was quite modest by modern standards. Great Britain was perhaps the most democratic of the great powers, yet voting rights had been extended to no more than 5 percent of the population. In view of this narrow distribution of political power it is even more remarkable that Chadwick's ideas gained support.

Although the political struggle was difficult, the combination of righteous indignation and enlightened self-interest that developed within this small but influential segment of the population resulted in a steady stream of legislation and administrative action on behalf of the working class. These political efforts achieved an important goal in 1848 with the establishment of a General Board of Health for England. By this time public passions had cooled considerably and progress might have correspondingly slowed had it not been for the entry of John Simon upon the scene (Rosen, 1958). He was appointed as the first medical officer for the city of London and soon after was chosen as a member of the General Board. Later in 1858 he became the medical officer for the Privy Council, which is roughly analogous to our president's cabinet. These appointments kept Simon in the forefront of the reform movement and throughout his long career he raised issues and made proposals based on meticulous review of the relevant facts. When his ideas were supported, as they often were, he saw to it that they were carried out. Unlike Chadwick in his report on sanitary conditions, Simon forsook flamboyant rhetoric in favor of concrete and persistent action. Hanlon provides Richardson's (1887) description of progress in London—progress that reflects Simon's influence as the medical officer in charge of the city's health department:

> The foot-pavements, the lamps, the water supply, the fire plugs, the new sewers, defective enough by later standards, were admired by all. . . . Beneath the pavement were vast subterraneous sewers arched over to convey away the waste water which in other cities is so noisome above ground, and at a less depth are buried wooden pipes that supply every house plentifully with water, conducted by leaden pipes into kitchens or cellars, three times a week for the trifling expense of three shillings per quarter . . . (Hanlon, 1974:20)

As one notes these accomplishments of more than one hundred years ago, it seems strange to review studies of the health needs of today's Third World cities. Here we find that the simple provision of a safe water supply remains one of their most pressing health concerns (Mahler, 1988).

The advances in Great Britain were watched closely by those in the United States who were concerned with the health of the general public. A somewhat similar scenario was played out in Massachusetts, where Lemuel Shattuck chaired a committee of the state legislature for the study of health and sanitary problems within the state. He was a very talented person with a very diverse background, qualities which, in 1850, were reflected in an extraordinary *Report of the Sanitary Commission of Massachusetts*. As Hanlon writes:

> With remarkable insight and foresight the report included a detailed consideration not only of the present and future public health needs of Massachusetts but also of its component parts and of the nation as a whole. This most remarkable of all American public health documents, if published today, in many respects would still be ahead of its time. (1974:22)

Among its many progressive recommendations was a proposal for an ambitious program of health education within the public schools. Altogether, the report constituted a precise blueprint for a state department of health. But unlike the Chadwick report, it did not find a receptive audience. It was generally ignored until 1869, when its still valid provisions guided the establishment of the Massachusetts State Board of Health.

During this period of time, Congress established a National Board of Health, but the agency soon became caught up in political crosscurrents that led to its demise. However, the need for such an organization was fulfilled by a different route. A national Marine Hospital Service was created by Congress in 1798 to provide medical care for sick and disabled seamen. The scope of this organization's activities was gradually expanded by successive legislative efforts throughout the 1800s until, finally, in 1902, Congress retitled it the Public Health and Marine Hospital Service (Mullan, 1989:40). It subsequently evolved into the present-day U.S. Public Health Service, the principal public health agency of the federal government. Although it got off to a slower start than in Great Britain and many of the European countries, by the turn of the century the modern public health movement was well established in the United States.

Public Health and Health Education

During the period from 1900 to 1950 a political trend toward an expanded and more proactive government combined with rapid progress in the development of disease-fighting technology to generate dynamic growth in the size and scope of public health agencies. Because of the excesses of the entrepreneurs of the late 1800s; the swearing in of Theodore Roosevelt, a president with liberal views; and a variety of other reasons, it became politically popular during the early 1900s for government to assume a broader role in society's overall pursuit of human well-being. During 1906 this new public mood was exemplified by both the publication of Upton Sinclair's novel, *The Jungle*, which dramatized the deplorable conditions existing throughout the meat packing industry, and the enactment of the Pure Food and Drug Act. The federal government's Children's Bureau was established in 1912, followed by the first federal child labor laws in 1915. In this nurturing environment State Boards of Health were strengthened and city and county health departments became more numerous and grew in size and stature.

Growth of Governmental Health Agencies

This political popularity of public health departments was accompanied by improvement in their technological effectiveness. The work of Pasteur and Koch during the latter 1800s had firmly established the germ theory of disease; subsequent discoveries led to effective means of control for many of the common water- and foodborne infections such as cholera and typhoid fever, as well as such mosquito transmitted diseases as malaria and yellow fever—significant causes of illness and death during the previous century. Somewhat later in the 1930s and 1940s vaccines for diphtheria, pertussis, and tetanus were developed and refined to a point where they could be used with confidence by public health personnel, school health workers, and private physicians to protect children against these conditions.

By 1950 the threat of communicable diseases had been drastically reduced with consequent reductions in mortality and gains in longevity. With benefit of hindsight we now know that much of this progress should have been attributed to improvements in working conditions and in the general standard of living resulting from the efforts of labor unionists and other social reformers, as well as the normal growth the economy. However, the various local, state, and federal public health agencies made a substantial contribution to this achievement and, as the most visible agencies in the struggle, they became firmly established as protectors and promoters of health.

Rise of Nongovernmental Health Organizations

As noted earlier, health care workers and public health workers comprise the bulk of our nation's health professionals. Both groups formed strong and enduring professional associations during the nineteenth century, namely, the American Medical Association and the American Public Health Association. These were soon followed by similar organizations formed by other health-related professionals, all of which served a variety of functions designed to strengthen and improve the performance of their respective professions. Typically, conventions would be arranged, journals would be published, standards would be established, and legislation favorable to the group's work and/or economic well-being would be advocated. During the first half of the twentieth century many organizations for health professionals grew and matured to exert strong influences on modern health issues.

During this period **voluntary** health organizations also grew in importance in the United States. The first of these, the Pennsylvania Society for the Prevention of Tuberculosis, was organized in 1892 by Lawrence Flick, a Philadelphia physician. Similar organizations were soon established in other states, which led to the eventual formation of the National Tuberculosis Association (Rosen, 1958). This organization, now the American Lung Association, was followed by a number of other such private, voluntary health organizations: the American Cancer Society, the American Heart Association, the March of Dimes, and many more, all of which were dedicated to the fight against specific diseases.

Although the first voluntary health organizations originated in Europe, their growth has been most prominent in the United States. In the recent national planning effort, *Healthy People 2000* (USDHHS, 1990), for example, 275 private professional and voluntary organizations took part. Each organization has its own unique history and pattern of activities; however, they typically include (1) education of the public, (2) service to those stricken with the specific disease, and (3) research into methods of treatment and control. Because of their private status, such organizations can often act more quickly and innovatively than our sometimes cumbersome governmental agencies. They can provide research funding for new, perhaps even radical, approaches to the search for causes, treatment, or prevention of disease; governmental agencies, on the other hand, must answer to the public and therefore might be reluctant to support a new program or may be forced to move more slowly.

Role for Health Education

Throughout this period in the development of the public health establishment, health education had played an important role. With the traditional focus on communities, public health officers were always faced with the task of stretching limited resources to protect and improve the health of large numbers of people. Early in this struggle they found that disseminating information so that people could help themselves was a highly cost effective way to carry out a portion of this vast mission. Public health nurses taught young mothers how to protect their infants from intestinal infections; media releases advised people to get sufficient rest and avoid crowds during periodic flu epidemics; in rural areas people were instructed as to the proper construction of pit privies to keep flies from carrying fecal matter to kitchens and dinner tables. This important educational role had been presaged by Lemuel Shattuck in his 1850 report in which he delineated the functions of a public health department; later Winslow's widely endorsed updating of these functions reinforced this commitment to health education (Hanlon, 1974). Health education found a home both in the rhetoric and the actions of the public health establishment.

But while accorded a place of importance in the early years of the twentieth century, the role of health education was clearly secondary to the more direct "hands on" efforts in community sanitation and the dispensing of community health services. Directly or indirectly, virtually all public health efforts were focused on the control of communicable diseases. Although there was much that well-informed individuals could do to protect themselves, the nature of this task lent itself to actions directed at the environment rather than at people. Rather than teach people how to purify contaminated water and prepare tainted food, it was obviously more effective to treat public water supplies and enforce regulations governing the commercial preparation and sale of food. Another serious limitation for health education during this period was the lack of any strong theoretical base for behavior change strategies. Most health education was presented on the somewhat naive assumption that if you told people what they should do they would probably do it. Information was often delivered, but not in a manner that would encourage anyone to act on it.

From Bacteria to Behavior

Although it is difficult to identify the beginning of a trend, it appears that sometime during the 1950s interest among public health personnel started to shift from communicable to chronic diseases. Interest in reducing infant mortality also accelerated and broadened from a narrow focus on intestinal infections to concern for the many factors that contribute to low birth weight babies, which is the immediate cause of most preventable infant deaths today. As mortality from communicable disease subsided, the death toll from accidents, particularly auto accidents, became relatively more important. The heightened interest in these problems were part of a general shift in attention from infectious agents and vaccines to personal behavior and life-style factors. Research findings began to accumulate that implicated saturated fats, cholesterol, cigarette smoking, and lack of exercise as risk factors for heart disease; consuming more dietary fiber and avoiding cigarettes were behaviors found to be important in the battle against cancer; avoiding unplanned pregnancies or pregnancies at too early an age, and avoiding toxic substances during pregnancy became important factors in reducing infant mortality; seat belt use and, more recently, stiff penalties for driving under the influence of alcohol became key strategies for reducing traffic deaths.

Research on Behavior Change

With so many modern risk factors tied to personal behavior, the need for increased emphasis on health education became obvious. Fortunately, health educators were becoming increasingly better prepared to meet these new challenges. During the 1950s the research of Hochbaum and Rosenstock, funded by the U.S. Public Health Service, resulted in the development of the **health belief model**, which was the first comprehensive explanation of the dynamics of health behavior (Becker, 1974). From this modest beginning, work on the scientific bases of health education continued at a steady pace. By the early 1980s McGuire (1984) recognized the expanded scope of both theory and practice in health behavior with his **contextual perspective**; here he identified 16 theories that could be applied depending on the specific situation involved. Also in this period, the earlier work of B. F. Skinner and the other behaviorists was revisited to develop more effective ways of dealing with addictive type problems such as obesity, cigarette smoking, and drug abuse. Somewhat later the development and application of social learning theory (now social cognitive theory), with its emphasis on modeling and contracting, provided additional strategies for promoting behavior change. Although these new theories did not invariably improve program effectiveness, they provided a structure to program planning that enabled health educators to go about their work with more confidence and creditability. Research activities were also helped considerably. Aspects and factors could be systematically studied and modified; this represented a major improvement over the trial and error approach that had prevailed.

Extensions of Health Education

As the research and theoretical bases improved, a number of informal extensions of the concept of health education became more clearly defined. The early researchers soon realized that such **internal** characteristics as knowledge and attitudes were not the only factors that influenced health behavior. People were influenced in a powerful way by **external** factors in their immediate environment. A young mother's decision to seek immunizations for her child, although influenced by her knowledge and feelings about such procedures, depended as much on the location of the clinic, the hours it was open, and how much, if anything, it charged for its services. Thus, during the late 1970s and early 1980s these **situational factors** that had been viewed as obstacles to help people overcome were redefined as elements to be modified in order to enhance behavior change. Accordingly, a business firm's new health education program might combine conventional education with an on-site jogging/walking path, new offerings in the cafeteria, restrictions on cigarette smoking, and/or changes in work rules to reduce job related stress. This new strategy of combining educational efforts with environmental modifications created a new, more powerful approach termed **health promotion**.

Defining Health Promotion

Currently health promotion seems to be evolving as a more comprehensive form of health education. Certainly, the move toward this broader approach is the predominant trend among health educators with a public health orientation, whereas many school health educators are more comfortable with the more traditional concept of health education.

The term "health promotion" is a venerable one. Winslow, in his 1920 definition of public health, identifies one of its basic purposes as "promoting health and efficiency through organized community effort" (Hanlon, 1974). However, at this writing there is not yet a consensus as to its exact meaning. Some health professionals, for example, use the term to indicate the goal they are seeking, i.e., positive health; they prevent disease but promote health. More commonly, the term is used to connote differences in methodology, i.e., combining environmental modifications with educational efforts. Green and Kreuter, in a definition that appears to reflect mainstream thinking among health educators, state: "Health promotion is the combination of educational and environmental supports for actions and conditions of living conducive to health" (1991:4). But though the process of health promotion is still evolving, it is clearly a powerful tool that has become available at a time when the nation, as witnessed by the *Healthy People 2000* initiative, seems poised to make a concerted effort to improve health through behavior change. This important concept will be discussed more fully in the following chapter.

Organizational Change

In addition to the development of greatly improved behavior change technology, health education/promotion has also expanded along other dimensions. As noted, one of the basic tenets of health promotion is that environmental factors should often be modified to encourage more favorable health behavior on the part of individuals. However, in many situations such changes may be needed simply to create a more healthy environment for the people involved. For example, a health educator specializing in stress management may be hired as a consultant by a factory manager who feels that job-related stress may be reducing worker performance. The traditional remedy would call for teaching relaxation exercises; providing audiotapes of soothing sounds from mountain brooks, the seashore and the like; and other measures designed to help employees deal with the stress that results from their work. But a careful review of the situation may reveal that the most efficient approach is to allow the workers more flexibility in the sequence of their tasks, improve communication between workers and managers, and make similar changes in the work environment that will prevent much of the stress from developing in the first place.

In other situations the unhealthy aspects of the environment may be physical rather than psychological, such as exposure to noxious fumes or dangerous machinery. Such cases require the primary intervention of a safety engineer rather than a health educator; here, the health educator's role would revert to the more secondary task of encouraging compliance with the safety recommendations. But when the problems involve social interaction or role relationships as with manager to employee, employee to employee, or employee to customer or client, then a health educator often provides the expertise needed to improve the situation. The methods and procedures that have been developed to make needed changes within organizations represent an additional extension of the modern concept of health education/promotion (see chapter 12).

Community Organization

In another modern extension to the scope of its applications, health education/promotion is now used to encourage more favorable community, as well as individual, behavior. Traditionally, health education efforts had been generally restricted to improving individual responses related to personal hygiene, food selection, use of tobacco or alcohol, and other such personal choices. This pattern typically prevailed despite the fact that it has always been known that many health problems, such as those related to pollution or the lack of available health services in a particular area, lent themselves to collective, rather than personal, action. If there is too much sulfur dioxide in the air, too many drug pushers on the streets, or too few physicians in the neighborhood, individual citizens, no matter how well-informed or motivated, may have difficulty correcting the problem by themselves. Such situations are best attacked through organized community action (see chapter 13). Public health departments often find themselves in a delicate situation when tempted to lead such efforts, as they are often part of the government that is being attacked; however, voluntary health organizations and ad hoc community groups can raise funds and hire health educators well versed in community organization to lead such efforts.

Training Other Health Professionals

In yet another extension of its scope, health educators often are called on to help professionals from other fields become skilled in health education or health counseling. Nurses, physicians, elementary school teachers, and other related professionals often must adopt the role of health educator in addition to their primary tasks. Nurses and dental hygienists, in particular, have always taken their education responsibilities seriously: school health education, as noted, arose from a separate but parallel movement. However, within the past 20 years or so, representatives from these diverse fields have joined with public health educators to form a more clearly defined field of health education. As will be discussed in chapter 14, health education—with its professional organizations, specialized degree programs, research base, and credentialing process—is rapidly developing into an independent profession that is not only training its own practitioners but training related professionals who provide health education incidental to their main tasks.

Public Schools and Health Education

The historical development of health education within the public schools roughly paralleled its rise within public health organizations. In many instances the public schools served merely as another setting or opportunity for public health officials, who came to the school and initiated programs for students. In other cases, school personnel interested in health started their own programs, thus giving the school health movement a chance to find its own direction.

Early Developments

During the Colonial Period and throughout the early history of the United States, the concept of tax-supported education gained public acceptance at a slow pace. The various public school systems did not begin to assume anything resembling their modern form until late in the nineteenth century. Some of the earlier developments, however, had important effects on the eventual shape and structure of the modern system.

Horace Mann

Health education was fortunate to have a supporter in Horace Mann, who is generally considered to be the father of public education. He established the first public "normal school" for the training of teachers and later, in 1837, he became the first secretary of the state board of education of Massachusetts, the nation's first such organization. Throughout all his public actions and pronouncements he was a strong advocate for health and the need for "common men to understand the laws and functions of the healthy body" (Means, 1962:32).

Temperance and Sanitation

As previously noted, the Shattuck report made specific recommendations for school health education which, while ignored at the time of publication, had important effects in later years. During the late 1800s as scientific evidence accumulated on the effectiveness of sanitation, early detection and isolation, and other aspects of disease-fighting technology, the schools were seen as natural sites for their application. In 1872 a "Sanitary Superintendent," whose duties included inspecting schoolchildren, was appointed for the city of Elmira, New York; soon afterwards, school physicians and school nurses became common additions to many of the larger systems. In an event more pertinent to instructional programs, the politically powerful Women's Christian Temperance Union succeeded in persuading many states to require school instruction on the health threats related to tobacco and alcohol; these legislative mandates were frequently broadened to include other health content (Means, 1975).

Starting a New Century

The shift in political sentiment toward a broader role for most public and governmental organizations that occurred in the early 1900s provided support for expanding health-related activities within public schools. Consequently, school-based programs made substantial contributions to the dramatic progress in communicable disease control, which was the main challenge of this period.

Health Education and Physical Education

Early recognition of the need for the medical inspection of schoolchildren and for school sanitation gave rise to a system of school health services that traditionally had strong ties to local public health departments. Health education, however, soon became linked to programs of physical education that developed internally within the various school curricula. Thomas Dennison Wood, who previously had developed programs of "Physical Education and Hygiene" at Stanford and later at Columbia University, was one of the originators and the first chairman of the Joint Committee of the National Education Association (NEA) and the American Medical Association (AMA) on the Health Problems of School Children. This prestigious committee became extremely influential and essentially defined the role schools were to play in society's effort to promote health. During his tenure as chairman (1911 to 1938), the committee developed and propagated the modern concept of the school health program as one giving attention to health instruction, health services, and a healthy school environment. In the course of these advances, however, a virtually permanent bond was formed between health education and physical education within the schools—a pattern that often makes it difficult for current school health educators to establish their own identity.

Communicable Disease Control

During the early 1900s school health workers, like their public health counterparts, were occupied mainly with efforts to control communicable disease. Most school districts throughout the nation developed effective health services, including the full- or part-time services of a school physician and a staff nurse. The quality and comprehensiveness of these programs varied, as they do now, depending on the size and financial strength of the particular school system and the pressure of state mandates; however, most provided for the identification and referral of children with disease symptoms, the conduct of periodic immunization campaigns, and the maintenance of health records. In addition, school health personnel usually monitored growth by use of weight and height measurement, screened children for vision and hearing defects, provided emergency care for injuries, and other similar services.

While programs of school health services were being established by physicians and nurses, instructional programs were being developed somewhat independently within the framework of the school curriculum. Although school nurses provided considerable incidental health instruction in conjunction with their primary concern for health services, the day-to-day program of health instruction developed in most school systems as part of a combined health and physical education program staffed by teachers trained in both disciplines. The various voluntary health agencies often developed programs targeted at school aged children and thus provided considerable support and assistance to school programs. One of the most prominent of these was the "Modern Health Crusade" sponsored by the American Tuberculosis Association. This complex movement, which generally took the form of a nationwide health club for school children with pamphlets and "chore cards" for monitoring health habits, was very influential during the early part of the century (Means, 1975).

Model School Health Curricula

As the threat of communicable disease receded in the 1950s and 1960s, school health curricula adopted a broader focus with increased attention to such topics as human sexuality, drug abuse, and consumer health. The School Health Education Study (1964) contributed significantly to this transition (Sliepcevich, 1964). This study involved a nationwide survey of school health education programs, including assessments of student knowledge, attitudes, and behavior, and the subsequent development and testing of a model curriculum. This model further inspired the development of many local health curricula and several other national projects.

Accountability

Although the need for health education in schools has always been relatively easy to demonstrate, evidence as to its effectiveness has been more elusive. Actual improvements in health behavior have proved difficult to accomplish, difficult to measure when successfully achieved, and difficult to link to specific programs when accurately measured. Consequently, the success of the School Health Education Evaluation project, as reported in 1985, was particularly encouraging. Here, specific instruments for the measurement of knowledge, attitudes, and practices were developed and used to evaluate four different model curricula. In every case significant improvements were found in all three variables among the four curricula (Connel, Turner, and Mason, 1985).

Despite such evidence of its effectiveness, the development of health education within the public schools has lagged in recent years because many school districts are facing financial problems, while at the same time they are being pressured to emphasize academic subjects. Also, the lack of coordination among the three components of traditional school health programs has served as an obstacle to their optimal development. In some school systems there has been a high level of cooperation and communication among school nurses (responsible for health services), teachers (providing health instruction), and administrators (who oversee the total school environment) whereas, in other systems, these three groups might be barely aware of one another's activities.

The Comprehensive School Health Program

In an effort to increase the effectiveness of the overall effort to promote health within the public schools, many health educators are advocating a broader, more comprehensive role for school health programs. This expanded role would include more components of the current school structure, additional functions, and better coordination of its activities. For example, in addition to its traditional functions of education, services, and environment, this broader program would incorporate physical education, food service, and counseling programs. Moreover, community health activities would be integrated with those within the school. Another addition would be school-based health promotion programs for faculty and staff (Allensworth and Kolbe, 1987). Such programs would combine environmental changes within the schools with classroom instruction to improve the prospects of behavioral change. This innovation represents an extension of the modern concept of health promotion into the public schools. Environmental changes, in this case, refer to such things as modifying the offerings in the school cafeteria to reduce fat-ridden and other "junk food" items and increase the choice among more nutritious selections; in a similar fashion, school policies on smoking would become more restrictive, opportunities for healthful exercise would be increased, and so on.

When systematically applied, the combination of instructional efforts and environmental modifications has proved effective in producing favorable changes in behavior. Simons-Morton and others (1991) combined classroom health instruction and vigorous physical education with changes in the school lunch program in a well-coordinated program that resulted in significant reductions in pupil intake of fat and sodium and increases in the time spent in moderate to vigorous physical activity. Particularly encouraging was the fact that these results persisted over a two-year period. Although the coordination of the various components of the school health program has been uneven since Wood's formulation of the concept early in the century, this modern reformulation clearly has exciting possibilities. Two challenges to its implementation, however, are the need for central direction, such as might be provided by a school health coordinator, and firm administrative support. Given these two conditions, the schools could make a substantial contribution to the achievement of the nation's ambitious health goals for the year 2000.

School Health Education as Related to Other Settings

During the early part of the century when infectious diseases provided the main challenge, the schools provided a means by which health professionals could

Figure 3.1 School Health Promotion Components and Outcomes

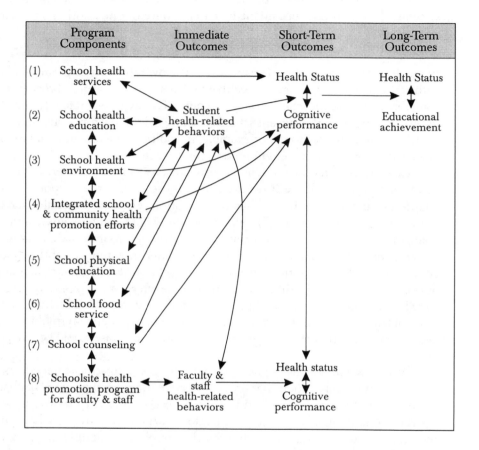

Source: Lloyd J. Kolbe, "Increasing the Impact of School Health Promotion Programs." *Health Education* 17:5 (Oct/Nov), 1986.

gain access to a broad and particularly vulnerable segment of the population. Although health instruction was important, health services in the form of screening and immunization campaigns had a somewhat higher priority. Today, the reality of drug abuse, alcohol abuse, suicides, homicides, unplanned pregnancy, and other behaviorally related health problems among young people has tended to tilt the emphasis toward programs of health education and health promotion. Well-conceived school programs can bring about short-term behavior change and, because of their long duration from kindergarten to grade 12, are unique in their potential for instilling lifelong health values and developing a reservoir of health knowledge. This knowledge, in turn, can make children receptive to, and capable of responding to, the appeals of programs presented years later in worksite, clinical, or community settings.

Summary

As with many other important and complex tasks, the preservation and enhancement of health is best accomplished by a combination of individual and organizational activity. Numerous organizations in modern society have important health-related functions; however, those devoted exclusively to health are generally divided into organizations related either to health care or to public health. In general, health care professionals focus on individuals rather than groups, and treatment rather than prevention. They also tend to favor free market approaches to the delivery of health care and remain skeptical of governmental programs or encroachments. These priorities differ from those of public health professionals, who typically think in terms of communities and population groups rather than individuals and emphasize prevention rather than treatment. They usually work in public, tax-supported organizations and thus have confidence in the effectiveness of public sector approaches, particularly as applied to disease prevention and health promotion. Although a certain degree of rivalry and tension exist between these two major groups, ideally they both should form part of a comprehensive system.

The concept of the informed individual acting in behalf of his or her own health, although always important, has become even more vital in the struggle against the current array of health problems. Such conditions as cancer, cardiovascular disease, AIDS, unintentional injuries, and drug and alcohol abuse, all require informed individual choices for their prevention and control. As the main societal tool for improving personal health behavior, health education has gained increased status and recognition, particularly during the past ten or twenty years. Moreover, with the recent expansion of health education to incorporate health promotion, its value in effecting changes within organizations, communities, and society in general through political action has been enhanced. This new capability has enabled health educators to go beyond their traditional role of changing individual behavior, which frequently carries the risk of "victim blaming." Now they can often facilitate improvement in working conditions, the physical environment, the availability of preventive services, levels of material support, and other such factors that help empower individuals so they can better meet their own health needs.

Historically, school health education has evolved as a separate entity somewhat distinct from health education as practiced in other settings; the development of the modern concept of health education along with the advocacy of comprehensive school health programs, with their focus on health promotion, has tended to bring school health educators back into the general arena. Health education is, however, a young and dynamic professional field; we can expect frequent changes in the relationships of its various components.

Health Education

Health education is concerned with the health-related
behaviors of people. Therefore, it must take into account the
forces that affect those behaviors, and the role of human
behavior in the promotion of health and the prevention of
disease. As a profession, it uses educational processes to
effect change or to reinforce health practices of individuals,
families, groups, organizations, communities, and larger
social systems. Its intent is the generation of health
knowledge, the exploration of options for behavior and
change and their consequences, and the choices of the action
courses open and acceptable to those affected (SOPHE,
1976).

Introduction

The profession of health education is concerned with promoting healthful behavior and with altering the conditions that affect health behavior and health directly. The term **health promotion** refers to a set of processes that can be employed to change the conditions that affect health. **Health education** is the profession principally devoted to employing health promotion processes to foster healthful behavior and health itself. While many other professions also are involved in health promotion, health education is the only profession devoted to health promotion and whose practitioners are specifically trained in the range of health promotion change processes. This chapter describes health promotion concepts and processes and considers the role and practices, responsibilities, and foundations of the profession of health education.

Health Promotion

Health promotion and public health share the primary goal of improving health. Public health, of course, is a broader concept and field than health promotion because it includes a wide range of health assessment and surveillance procedures; technology, policy, and environmental controls and protections; and health care services, as well as health promotion. Health promotion is concerned specifically with the sociobehavioral processes for improving personal health behavior and for implementing public health measures.

Health problems have multiple, interrelated causes that are the targets of public health and health promotion programs. These causes may be personal health behavior, environmental conditions, the lack of appropriate policies, or deficiencies in programs and services. For example, the causes of early death due to lung cancer include smoking, a personal health behavior; air pollution, an environmental factor; the lack of smoking control programs, a deficiency in the availability of public health programs; unfettered tobacco marketing, a public policy deficiency; and inadequate screening and referral to early treatment, a health services deficiency. Resolution of these problems frequently requires attention to at least several of these causes. Intervention aimed at only one cause is not likely to be successful because the causes are interrelated. For example, with respect to lung cancer and most other health problems it is impossible to separate personal health behavior from marketing, or health services from public policy because they are hopelessly interrelated. Hence, in public health multiple intervention approaches are commonly employed to address the multiple causes of a health problem.

Health policies, technologies, and services are examples of public health measures for improving health. These same measures, however, are also health promotion objectives because getting them in place requires changes in human behavior. For example, public health measures for preventing lung cancer include controls on access to cigarettes and restrictions on smoking in public places, air pollution technology, screening, and smoking prevention and cessation programs. While health promotion is most closely identified with actual smoking prevention and control programs, it is also concerned with implementing policies and technologies that support nonsmoking. Hence, many public health measures become the objectives of health promotion efforts because their accomplishment requires behavior change on the part of patients, citizens, technocrats, and policymakers. Consequently, the targets of health promotion efforts are not always the people whose health is in question. Instead, the targets of interventions frequently are policymakers or health and education professionals because the objectives of health promotion are to foster the adoption of healthful policies, encourage healthful changes in the environment, improve health services, and foster healthful personal behavior change.

Health promotion objectives can focus on several societal levels, as shown in table 4.1. Indeed, many health promotion programs target intervention objectives at multiple levels. For example, health promotion programs to prevent lung cancer may target individuals for smoking prevention and cessation, organizational decision makers and practitioners to implement smoking control programs, community activists and policymakers to enact smoking restrictions, and government officials to support research and enact public policy favoring nonsmoking.

Health promotion change processes can be directed at various intervention objectives. A range of powerful change processes are available for use by the health educator or health promotion specialist. These processes, which are the major focus of chapter 7, include education and training in personal behavior change; using media, persuasive communication, media advocacy; organizational change and program implementation; community development and social change; policy advocacy; and the empowering of people to exercise control

Table 4.1 Multilevel Health Promotion Objectives

Level	Objective
Individual	Knowledge
	Attitudes
	Behaviors
	Physiology
Organization	Policies
	Practices
	Programs
	Facilities
	Resources
Community	Policies
	Practices
	Programs
	Facilities
	Resources
Government	Policies
	Programs
	Facilities
	Resources
	Legislation/ordinances
	Regulation
	Enforcement

over their environments. Hence, health promotion is about behavioral intervention directed toward changing personal health behavior and the social and physical conditions that affect people's health.

Evolution of the Concept

We have just described health promotion as a set of change processes, but the term "health promotion" means different things to different people. For some it is synonymous with health education; for others it is the same as public health. Some define it in terms of wellness, while others define it in terms of market-oriented programming or wellness. While considering the evolution of the concept of health promotion, keep in mind its definition as a set of change processes that can be directed toward the causes of health problems.

The term "health promotion" came into common usage with the publication of *Healthy People: The Surgeon General's Report on Health Promotion and Disease Prevention* and continued in the current document, *Healthy People*

Table 4.2 Health Promotion Change Processes

Teaching	Media and advocacy
Training	Policy development and advocacy
Counseling	Organizational change
Consulting	Community development and social change
Communications/media	Diffusion

2000: National Health Promotion and Disease Prevention Objectives (USDHHS, 1979, 1990). In *Healthy People* health promotion is defined in terms of life-style improvements of essentially healthy people. This is consistent with a conceptualization of health promotion as focusing on getting healthier, as in a progression from tertiary prevention to secondary prevention, to primary prevention, to health promotion.

> Health promotion begins with people who are basically healthy and seeks the development of community and individual measures which can help them to develop lifestyles that can maintain and enhance the state of well-being. (*Healthy People*, 1979)

While this definition has the advantages of including both community and individual measures, its focus on people who are basically healthy has tended to generate among some enthusiasts a "wellness" type of attitude toward health promotion (Dunn, 1977; O'Donnell, 1994). Of course, there is nothing wrong with the wellness concern for improving individual health. But the essential concern in health promotion is improving the health of the public, which is not necessarily inconsistent with wellness, but may not always be the same as a concern for the higher-level wellness of individuals. That is, public health tends to honor a long tradition of focusing on measures that can improve the general health of the population, for example, water fluoridation and water purification, and measures directed at the neediest or most at-risk populations, for example, health services for indigent populations or pregnant teenagers. A wellness program, on the other hand, might focus on improving individual health through improved nutrition and physical activity, or along other mental and spiritual dimensions. This is an absolutely important concept and enterprise. Indeed, because the preponderance of exposure to health-damaging or health-enhancing experiences contributes greatly to longevity and quality of life, it is a logical public health goal to alter the nature of these exposures. In an age in which a major impediment to improved longevity and quality of life is the failure of most Americans to engage in health-enhancing lifetime behaviors such as exercising; eating a low-fat, low-calorie, vegetable-intense diet; and moderating stress—an age in which many people retire in their early sixties and live well into their eighties—wellness is clearly an idea whose time has come. Nevertheless, wellness is just one of many health promotion emphasis areas, and should not be considered the same thing as health promotion.

In *Healthy People 2000* (1990), public health is divided into preventive health services, health protection, and health promotion. Preventive health services are concerned with such conditions as maternal and infant health, heart disease and stroke, cancer, diabetes and chronic disabling conditions, HIV infection, STDs, immunizations and infectious diseases, and clinical preventive services. Health protection covers unintentional injuries, occupational safety, environmental health, food and drug safety, and oral health. Health promotion encourages physical activity; good nutrition; avoiding tobacco, alcohol and other drugs; family planning; mental health; controlling violent and abusive behavior; and educational and community-based programs.

The separation of service, protection (or environmental controls), and behavior components, although less severe than in the 1979 report, has, nevertheless, been unfortunate. Most health problems do not fit nicely into one of these categories, but instead require services, protection, and promotion. For example, the primary means of controlling HIV infections is through education and behavior change, not through health services. Similarly, accidental injury control does not belong exclusively under health protection, although environmental controls are a very important part of it, because health services and health behavior considerations are also important in injury control. Tobacco use and violent behavior will be controlled only when health services, environmental protection, and personal behavior change interventions are coordinated. Health promotion, defined in terms of change, plays a role in each of the priority areas listed in *Healthy People 2000*. Hence, the artificial categorizations adopted for this report are not completely satisfactory.

The emphasis in *Healthy People 2000* on health behavior, however, has increased recognition of its importance to health and has advanced the cause of health behavior change. The linking of health promotion with selected personal health behaviors rather than behavior change processes, however, has been an unfortunate impediment to progress in health promotion. Primarily, its focus on personal health behavior seems partly to blame people for behavior that is largely the result of exposure to environmental influences. Secondarily, it fails to emphasize change processes for altering related health services and environmental controls. An unintended side effect of equating health promotion with health behavior has been the neglect of the concept of health promotion as a set of change processes concerned with the broad range of causes and solutions to health problems.

Sadly, the *Healthy People* (1979) definition of health promotion as behaviors or topics has encouraged professionals narrowly trained in areas like nutrition, exercise physiology, and nursing, as well as people completely untrained in health, to claim expertise in health promotion. The problem is not that these professionals should not be involved with health promotion; they should be and health educators want them to be. But interest in and knowledge about a particular health behavior or health topic is not adequate preparation in health promotion. Sadly, in too many cases, people without an adequate background in health promotion are responsible for such programs in schools, hospitals, and corporations.

Moreover, to embrace a definition of health promotion as a list of target health behaviors is inconsistent with its focus on populations, limits the scope of practice, promotes victim blaming, undermines the broader objectives of health promotion, and encourages the assignment of untrained professionals to manage and deliver health promotion programs. Indeed, equating health promotion with health behavior is, perhaps, the single most damaging misconception to the advance of the field.

Green and Johnson (1983) defined health promotion in terms of supports for healthful behavior:

> Health promotion is any combination of educational, organizational, economic, and environmental supports for behavior conducive to health.

This is perhaps the most widely employed definition of health promotion, and it does have decided advantages over the definition given in *Healthy People*. In particular, the emphasis on a *range* of supports is good, because each of these is needed for improvements in public health. But the definition can be faulted in two ways. First, the emphasis on supports for ". . . behavior conducive to health," rather than on health itself, is limiting because health is our goal, with health behavior as only one of several intermediate outcomes. Second, the definition confuses objectives with measures or approaches. In our view, the educational, organizational, economic, and environmental supports in the definition are public health measures and health promotion objectives, but clearly, they are not health promotion processes. For example, there are a number of organizational supports that are conducive to healthful behavior or to health itself, such as smoke-free and ventilated workplaces, safety equipment and regulations, and so on. In our view these are health promotion objectives, and organizational change is the process by which health promotion accomplishes them. If we think of health promotion as a set of change processes, then educational, organizational, economic, and environmental supports are best thought of as objectives. Health promotion, then, is a set of processes to change knowledge, attitudes, skills (educational outcomes); practices, programs, policies (organizational outcomes); and conditions (environmental outcomes). We propose the following modification of the Green and Johnson definition:

> Health promotion is any combination of change processes directed at educational, organizational, economic, and environmental supports conducive to health.

Minkler (1989) takes particular issue with conceptualizations of health promotion that emphasize personal health behavior. Recognizing that programs based on personal health behavior may well be creative and effective, she regrets that they too often focus on containing health care costs or increasing profits. She believes health is a social good, not a commodity, and programs should not be reimbursed on the basis of how much health behavior change they produce. She argues against the concept of health promotion as profit-oriented wellness programming, whether it is located in corporations, hospitals, or health departments.

Instead, Minkler encourages us to think about health promotion in terms of Dorothy Nyswander's admonition to focus on empowering individuals and changing systems (1982). For Nyswander, the success of health education programs would not be measured in the conventional way by assessing the amount of health behavior or health status change, but by the extent to which they increase meaning, control, and quality of life.

Minkler calls our attention to an early WHO definition of health promotion as "a process of enabling people to increase control over and to improve their health . . . as a mediating strategy between people and their environments, synthesizing personal choice and social responsibility in health" (WHO, 1984). The WHO document focused on the determinants or causes of health, including personal health behavior, but emphasized socioeconomic, environmental, and health service causes, and recognized the importance of a range of health promotion approaches, including education, public participation, organizational change, and community development.

Minkler's comments reflect the view that health promotion is not just health behavior, it is not only wellness, and it is more than a set of change processes: it is a concept about health. Minkler (1989) and others (Freudenberg, 1981) are attempting to keep alive Nyswander's idea of focusing on health within the context of democracy and social empowerment. She would have us concern ourselves not only with health and health behavior outcomes, but also with social and political outcomes. The success of health promotion, according to Nyswander, would be measured not only by improvements in health behavior, mortality, and morbidity, but also by changes in the social structure and the actual and perceived control that people have over their lives. It is critical that the profession not lose sight of the basic principle that people should have maximum control over their behavior and their social and physical environments. Changing health behavior at the risk of reducing personal control and participation may be shortsighted and unethical, even if it is efficient.

Nevertheless, in our view, the tension between those who favor an emphasis on personal health behavior and those who favor an emphasis on community or environmental aspects of health problems is largely unnecessary. Ecological approaches to health promotion (Simons-Morton BG et al., 1989; McLeroy et al., 1988) encourage a concept of health promotion in which all causes and solutions are recognized and those that are most important, changeable, or otherwise of highest priority are selected for programmatic attention. Hence, any particular health promotion program might emphasize changing knowledge, attitudes, and skills; implementing programs; facilitating the adoption of practices, policies, and technologies; advocating socioeconomic improvements conducive to the population's health; improving access to health care; or fostering a healthful environment by strengthening social networks and social supports.

Indeed, health promotion, thus conceptualized, could focus on empowerment, control, and participation as primary outcomes, not just intermediate outcomes. Clearly, it is in the interest of the public's health that individuals, families, and communities maintain maximum autonomy, control, and influence consonant with public health.

Dwore and Kreuter (1980) defined health promotion as follows:

> The process of advocating health in order to enhance the probability that personal (individual, family and community), private (professional and business), and public (federal, state and local government) support of positive health practices will become a societal norm.

This is an excellent definition that captures the sense that health promotion is about change. The strengths of this definition include its emphases on advocacy, multiple societal levels, and social norms. The emphasis on social norms is particularly noteworthy, considering that social norms exist among population groups, organizations, neighborhoods and communities, and decision makers. Public health is often distinguished from medicine—with its emphasis on high technology cures of individual health problems—by its emphasis on achieving small amounts of change among large numbers of people. Such changes are largely the product of what becomes normative in a society, for example, smoking or not smoking, tobacco marketing practices, restrictions on smoking in public places, and economic incentives for tobacco production. Hence, the focus on social norms is very relevant, and norms are shaped by education, as well as by private and public policies and practices.

The Joint Committee on Health Education Terminology lumped together the terms "health promotion" and "disease prevention" in the following definition:

> Health promotion and disease prevention is the aggregate of all purposeful activities designed to improve personal and public health through a combination of strategies, including the competent implementation of behavioral change strategies, health education, health protection measures, risk factor detection, health enhancement and health maintenance.

This is a useful definition. Appropriately, it emphasizes improvements in health. Also, its emphasis on purposeful activity and competent implementation reminds us that health promotion should be programmatic rather than haphazard or incidental.

A famous scholar remarked that there is nothing more practical than a good theory. Relatedly, there is nothing more practical than a good definition. Definitions reflect concepts and concepts drive programs. Good concepts are more likely to lead to good programs. In the following section we explore how defining health promotion as a process of change can lead to enlightened health promotion programming.

Tobacco Control: A Health Promotion Example

Smoking, a leading cause of cancer, cardiovascular disease, and respiratory infections, has been labeled the number one preventable chronic disease risk factor. Let's examine how smoking can be prevented.

To be a major cause of mortality, a risk factor must be highly prevalent. The prevalence of smoking among American adults is 29 percent, down from 40 percent in 1965 (USDHHS, 1991a). The prevalence of smoking has been in decline among all age groups, although initiation has increased recently in the United States among teenage girls.

The decline in smoking can be attributed largely to a general acceptance by Americans of the fact that smoking is hazardous to their health and to an increase in the availability of effective smoking cessation programs. But close examination of the smoking problem reveals that smoking control involves a wide range of initiatives, like waging a war across a number of important fronts. Table 4.3 shows the range of target outcomes or objectives that might be addressed in a smoking cessation campaign (Simons-Morton DG, Parcel, and Brink, 1987). These include individual objectives, for example knowledge about the hazards of smoking, attitudes about smoking, peer resistance skills, and self-management skills. Organization-level objectives include no-smoking policies and smoking cessation programs. At the local community/government level

Table 4.3 Smoking Control Intervention Matrix: Desired Outcomes for Three Targets in Four Settings

	School	Worksite	Health Care Institutions (HCI)	Community
Individuals	students' nonsmoking	employees' nonsmoking	patients' nonsmoking	residents' nonsmoking
Organizations	school policies, programs, practices, and facilities to foster nonsmoking by students	worksite policies, programs, practices, and facilities to foster nonsmoking by employees	HCI policies, programs, practices, and facilities to foster nonsmoking by patients	policies, programs and practices of community-serving organizations and institutions to foster nonsmoking by community residents
Governments	legislation, regulation, and enforcement affecting schools to foster nonsmoking by students	legislation, regulation and enforcement affecting worksites to foster nonsmoking by employees	legislation, regulation, and enforcement affecting HCIs to foster nonsmoking by patients	legislation, regulation, and enforcement affecting community sites to foster nonsmoking by community residents

Source: Simons-Morton DG, Parcel, and Brink. *Smoking Control Among Women: A CDC Intervention Handbook*, 1987.

objectives include restrictions on cigarette sales, limits on public smoking, and media messages. At the state and federal government level objectives include taxes on cigarettes, restrictions on advertising, and support for smoking control activities. Naturally, these objectives can be specified for school, health care, worksite, and community settings to improve specificity.

Health promotion efforts might focus on any number of these objectives in one or more settings. Some health promotion programs focus mainly on smoking prevention among students in school settings. Some health promotion programs are concerned mainly with community and government/policy approaches to smoking control. Other programs focus on smoking cessation. Indeed, much current smoking control effort focuses on interventions involving advice by health professionals and referral to a smoking cessation program. Another important area of smoking control involves community approaches that seek to alter the commmunity's normative acceptance of smoking. Some initiatives have attempted to empower communities to combat the advertising and lobbying influences of tobacco companies.

Each of these actions is important and each involves somewhat unique health promotion processes. They share a concern about the health consequences of smoking and an appreciation of the causes of smoking. Some programs are comprehensive, involving individual, organizational, and community actions, but most are specific to one level and/or setting. A variety of health promotion processes are involved, including media, education, skills training, program implementation, community organization and development, policy advocacy, and empowerment. An ecological approach to the problem allows a variety of programs to contribute to the overall control of smoking. Programmatically, health educators might focus on any one or several of these outcomes, but widespread change will only occur when many of these target outcomes are in place, affecting large numbers of people.

Smoking control nicely illustrates the complex nature of health promotion efforts. A strictly personal health behavior approach to smoking cessation, while important and appropriate in some contexts, would not adequately address the range of critical objectives. In the same manner, an approach geared solely to the community or government level, which ignored prevention and cessation activities, would also be inadequate.

Health Education

The profession of health education is devoted to promoting public health. Health education is the primary profession devoted to health promotion, defined earlier as a set of change processes. While health educators are concerned about a wide range of health topics, smoking control serves as a useful illustration of the range of change processes health educators employ. Health educators concerned about smoking cessation may find themselves involved in the following health promotion activities:

- A high school health education teacher develops her lesson for the day on cigarette smoking. She knows that many of the teens in her class soon will experiment with smoking if they have not already done so. She recognizes smoking as a behavioral problem, not just a knowledge problem. Today's lesson is on peer resistance; previous class sessions have focused on the health effects of smoking and on the tobacco industry's clever marketing techniques for recruiting new smokers.

- A hospital-based health educator meets with physicians and nurses to plan a major smoking cessation initiative. Under the program all patients who smoke will receive advice and referral from their primary care physician to nurses, PAs, or health educators with special training who will conduct a brief smoking cessation workshop and administer a self-help program that motivated patients can follow.

- A health educator at the corporate headquarters for a major oil company reviews the media materials that are about to be produced for the many small work units that are geographically dispersed around a four-state area. These materials are designed to encourage smokers to avail themselves of self-help materials that will be dispersed by a safety officer in each local unit who has received special training in their use. The media and self-help materials are part of a campaign designed specifically with the corporate culture in mind that will emphasize competition between local units based on the number of sustained quitters.

- A health educator at a local health department prepares to meet with the city council to provide testimony about a proposed policy to ban cigarette vending machines from all public establishments except those that do not admit minors. The proposed policy is the product of the tireless efforts of a coalition of groups who worked for years on its development, found support for it among council members, and got endorsements for it from city leaders and community representatives.

Each of these scenarios reveals something different about the practice of health education. As a health educator you might have responsibility for planning programs, teaching or training, developing community interest and resources, serving as a coalition representative, advocating policy, or evaluating outcomes. You might do this in a public school, an industry, a public health department, a hospital, or elsewhere. Your primary concern might be a special content area, a specific health problem, or a specific health behavior. Such diversity of activity makes the discipline of health education a fabulous career.

Because the term "health promotion" has come to envelope the processes that health educators employ, the term health education is best applied strictly to the profession of individuals trained to employ these processes, rather than to a specific process such as education. Of course, health educators do not hold a monopoly on these processes because many other health and education professionals, applied social scientists, and public health activists who are not formally trained in health education are involved in important ways in health promotion. Nevertheless, health education is the only profession devoted to health promotion and whose practitioners are specifically prepared to employ the entire range of health promotion processes, depending on the health problem.

The many definitions of health education proffered over the years provide an interesting historical perspective on the profession and the evolving role of health educators. Some of these definitions are included in Appendix A.

Role of Health Educators

The role of the health educator has been the subject of considerable discussion and debate. In response, several instructive documents have been developed. In a paper entitled "What is a Public Health Educator?" (SOPHE, 1976) distributed by the Society for Public Health Education, the following description was offered. In our view this description presents the role and function of the health educator in a clear and succinct fashion.

> Why do people suffer from illness that could be prevented? Why do they fail to behave in a way that will promote good health? Why, in short, doesn't everyone use the health knowledge available? These questions concern every health worker. The health educator, though, is a specialist on the health team who diagnoses these problems from an educational point of view, and helps to solve them through the selection and use of sound educational methods tailored to particular educational needs.

> Sometimes it is simply a lack of information which keeps the public from taking needed action. When this is the case it is the job of the health educator to translate scientific achievements into everyday usable form. Health education of this type is as old as health knowledge, and every health worker shares responsibility in spreading that knowledge and getting it used. The health educator helps each health professional do this part of his job better, however, by teaching his colleagues to recognize education needs and potentials in various situations and the effective use of educational methods. In addition, because the health educator is a specialist in the techniques of getting health facts accepted and used, he works closely with all kinds of community groups who are interested in health projects and programs.

> Still, facts alone are not always the answer. The social sciences have shown clearly that human behavior is affected by a multitude of forces in addition to knowledge. Applying insights from psychology, sociology, and anthropology, the health educator analyzes the reasons people might not be following good health practices and organizes intensive, well-planned health education programs to remedy the problem. Skills in many fact-finding techniques, such as interviewing, surveys, and community study, help him in this process. The people he wants to educate, however, are his most valuable resource, for they, more than anyone else, know what is important to them and why. Then, too, being involved in fact finding is educational in itself. The health educator knows that people learn by thinking through their own problems.

> A basic tenet of the public health educator is that final decisions about health practices must be made by the individuals involved. Nevertheless, he accepts a responsibility to provide access to sources of information and experience needed by the individual in relating desirable health practices to his motives, goals, aspirations, and values.

The health educator thus serves as a psychological stage-setter stimulating people in the community to recognize health problems of which they may be unaware and to work for their solution. Such problems might have to do with pollution of the environment, chronic disease, over-population, drug abuse, or any of hundreds of ills which plague our society today.

Depending upon the situation, the health educator is prepared to use very different methods of communication. He is expert in a variety of individual, group, and community educational approaches, as well as knowing which educational media and materials can be used most effectively. Sometimes he helps a group create its own educational materials—an experience which often leads to greater learning than could ever result from exposure to the most polished professional teaching aids.

Sometimes the problems in taking health action lie not with the community, however, but with the people *providing* health services. The health educator also has an important role to play in helping other health personnel plan and deliver health care in ways which the community can and will use. His skills in education and communication are required just as much to teach professionals how the community *feels* about health, as to teach the community what professionals know about health.

Health educators, then, are modern pioneers—ever seeking new understanding into human behavior, new ways to apply this knowledge in solving individual and community health problems.

The Role Delineation Project (National Center for Health Education, 1980), which was an early step leading to credentialing (described in chapter 14), analyzed the role of the entry-level health educator in terms of responsibilities, functions, skills, and knowledge. A health educator was defined as follows:

> An individual prepared to assist individuals, acting separately or collectively, to make informed decisions regarding matters affecting their personal health and that of others.

Thus, the responsibilities and functions that the health educator may be called upon to discharge provide a useful description of the role of health education.

According to the Report of the Joint Committee on Health Education Terminology (1990):

> A health educator is a practitioner who is professionally prepared in the field of health education, who demonstrates competence in both theory and practice, and who accepts responsibility to advance the aims of the health education profession.

Hence, a health educator is a professional trained in health education.

Contemporary health education theorists have described the role of the health educator ecologically (Simons-Morton DG et al., 1988a; Simons-Morton BG and Simons-Morton DG, 1989; McLeroy et al., 1988). Accordingly, the health educator is problem oriented, selecting appropriate intervention approaches to fit the health problem, program objectives, setting, target population, and societal level. Hence, it is the role of the health educator to address important health determinants by educating the target population, training health and education practitioners, conducting community development activities, advocating for appropriate health practices and policies. Education is an essential component of each of these processes, but the change processes employed and role of the health educator vary according to the objective and the target population.

Health Education Practice

According to the Report of the Joint Committee on Health Education Terminology, the health education field:

> . . . is that multidisciplinary practice . . . concerned with designing, implementing, and evaluating educational programs that enable individuals, families, groups, organizations, and communities to play active roles in achieving, protecting, and sustaining health. (1990)

Health education is conducted in a planned, programmatic fashion. It is not merely informing people about health problems and instructing them to change their behavior. It is the product of careful program development. Indeed, the practice of health education is best understood in terms of its major responsibilities and functions, which include program (1) planning, (2) implementing, (3) conducting, and (4) evaluating. A health educator may be involved in all these functions for a particular program, or may primarily be responsible for only one or two functions. As these responsibilities are covered in more detail in a later chapter, they are described only briefly here.

Planning and Administering Programs

The success of any program depends upon thorough planning. Resources are too scarce and the problems too complicated for unplanned activities to be very productive.

> A health education program is a planned combination of activities developed with the involvement of specific populations and based on a needs assessment, sound principles of education, and periodic evaluation using a clear set of goals and objectives. (JCHET, 1990)

Planning includes the gathering of baseline data needed to give the program direction. Needs assessments determine the extent of the health problem, the causes or determinants (which become the program objectives or target outcomes), and the extent to which various target populations are at risk. The efficacy of various approaches to intervention and their potential for quality implementation are assessed and methods are selected for use. The evaluation is designed. Administrative aspects of the program are considered and program components and materials are developed. Staff are selected and training is organized. Administrative responsibilities may include (1) personnel and resource management; (2) scheduling; (3) preparing reports, budgeting and allocating funds, and developing policies; (4) developing program components, curriculum, and educational materials; and (5) coordinating the activities of the program, providing staff support, promoting cooperation and feedback among staff, and otherwise facilitating the conduct of the program activities.

Implementing Programs

Programs may exist in the form of bulky curricula and planning documents. However, any program exists in a real sense only to the degree that it is effectively "delivered" to the learner. This process of bringing programs into reality, termed **implementation**, is a challenging task. It may include selecting and training staff; procuring facilities, materials, and teaching aids; and recruiting learners (students, clients) into the program. Indeed, program implementation may be the main focus of the intervention, particularly in settings like schools, health care facilities, and worksites, where the health educator is largely responsible for developing interventions and facilitating their implementation rather than conducting them directly. One of the most important responsibilities of health educators is to develop, select or adapt interventions that other health and education professionals, or in some cases laypersons, can conduct. Implementation is a behind-the-scenes activity and is a vital component of a successful health education program.

Conducting Program Activities

Health educators are known for their ability to conduct interventions, serving in such roles as teachers, trainers, group process facilitators, communication and media specialists, and the like. In short, health educators are responsible for the change processes that are at the core of the health promotion program. The purpose of nearly every health promotion intervention is to provide new knowledge and skills, whether it is about personal health behavior or community control of HIV infection. Most health educators teach or counsel a specific target population of students, patients, workers, or other learners. Other health educators foster changes in organizational policy, organize community groups, or advocate for policies and practices. Many health educators are responsible for reaching large audiences by selecting, developing, and employing media. Either by direct contact or indirectly, health education interventions provide new information and skills in support of healthful living.

> The *health education process* is that continuum of learning which enables people, as individuals and as members of social structures, to voluntarily make decisions, modify behaviors, and change social conditions in ways which are health enhancing. (JCHET, 1990)

Evaluating Programs

Evaluation in health education is both an integral function of health education practice and an area of specialization. Some health educators who are specially skilled in research design and statistical analysis serve as outside evaluators of health education programs. Carefully designed health education programs provide measurable outcomes for program evaluation and feedback for program revision. There are three basic forms of program evaluation: process evaluation, impact evaluation, and outcome evaluation.

Process evaluation asks the question, "How well is the intervention addressing the objectives?" In order to answer this question, the appropriateness of the learning activities is examined as well as the delivery of those activities. Methods to perform this assessment include observing the conduct of the learning activities, obtaining feedback from the students, and obtaining feedback from the instructors. Areas of weakness and areas of strength are pinpointed in order to modify and improve the curriculum. In addition, process evaluation provides information useful in the assessment of ultimate program goals; that is, it enables the evaluator to determine to what extent program failure was due to inappropriate or poorly conducted learning activities.

Impact evaluation asks the question, "To what extent were the objectives achieved?" Thus, the focus is on the "impact" the program has on the learner in terms of knowledge, attitudes, and skills. The classic example of impact evaluation is the test given at the end of a course. Impact evaluation can identify areas of the curriculum which did not produce an adequate effect on the learners. In doing so, impact evaluation works hand in hand with process evaluation to pinpoint areas for improvement. In addition, impact evaluation enables the evaluator to determine the appropriateness of the educational objectives and, in turn, the extent to which program success or failure is due to achievement of the objectives.

Outcome evaluation asks the question, "Were the program goals achieved?" In health education programs the goals are concerned with health behaviors and with health status. In order to determine if the goals were met, the learners can be questioned as to health behaviors and health status at some time after the completion of the program. This type of information is necessary in order to measure the success of the program and to make decisions as to its continuation.

The three basic forms of evaluation—process, impact, and outcome—are interrelated and work in conjunction with each other to provide feedback enabling revision of the program. Chapter 8 presents a more detailed description of the evaluation process.

An Illustration

In practice, the relative importance of the responsibilities just described depends on the nature of the health educator's job. Not every health educator has equal responsibility in each area. To illustrate these responsibilities let's take the example of a health educator hired by the local cancer society to educate the public about cancer risk factors.

Sara graduated from the local university two years ago with a bachelor's degree in health education. As a senior she worked at the cancer society for her practicum. Soon after she graduated the health educator position became available and she got the job. The cancer society, like most voluntary health organizations, develops programs based on the national organization objectives. Local chapters have the option of selecting from among the available objectives and programs based on local needs and resources.

Recently Sara conducted a needs assessment, studying cancer prevalence and etiology by type and population characteristics to identify the most important cancers and the most important population groups in her geographic area. It became clear that lung cancer was a major concern and that smoking was the behavior most directly and importantly related to lung cancer. She determined that the factors associated with smoking initiation are somewhat different from those that perpetuate the habit. Concentrating on the initiation phase, she planned a smoking prevention program with public school teachers. She applied for and obtained support for the program from the national organization and from the local school district. With these resources, she hired a part-time staff—a former college classmate and a health education teacher who graduated a few years ago. Together they produced a curriculum, conducted a pilot test, and made appropriate revisions. They trained the school teachers in the use of the curriculum and in the conduct of the learning activities, and helped with the implementation. Each of them taught several classes to get firsthand experience with the curriculum.

Sharing administrative responsibilities—budgeting, coordinating, and promoting the program—with her counterpart at the school, Sara and her staff evaluated aspects of the curriculum and the quality of the teaching (process evaluation) by observation and by periodic teacher and student feedback. They prepared and administered to students pre- and post-tests to evaluate the program's impact (impact evaluation). They prepared a short questionnaire for a six-month follow-up of health behavior (outcome evaluation). A year later, they submitted a progress report to their funding sources. Due to the promising results of the evaluation, they were encouraged to seek funding to implement the curriculum on a broader scale.

Successful health educators require skill, industry, diligence, and creativity. As this example shows, the several areas of responsibility, each with its attendant functions and skills, provides the health educator with many professional opportunities and challenges.

Areas of Specialization

Health education is a diverse profession. Health educators may be involved with any number of practice settings, topics, target groups, and change processes. Table 4.4 includes four overlapping areas of specialization: (1) target group-specific; (2) setting-specific; (3) content-specific; and (4) process-specific.

Target group.   Many health educators, due to training, experience, or preference, are drawn to the profession by the desire to serve a particular target population. Some health educators work mainly with children and youth, while others work

Table 4.4 Areas of Health Education Specialization

Target population:

    Mothers, children, and adolescents
    Adults
    Older adults
    Minorities
    Special (e.g., low income, disabled, incarcerated)

Settings:

    School
    Worksite
    Health care
    Community

Content:

    Diet and nutrition
    Physical activity and physical fitness
    Family planning, sexuality, AIDS, STDs
    Injury and violence
    Tobacco, drugs, and alcohol
    Chronic disease (e.g., cancer, cardiopulmonary, diabetes)
    Mental health
    Oral health
    Immunization and infectious diseases
    Suicide, death, and dying

Process:

    Program planning/curriculum development
    Teaching/training
    Communications/media development
    Community organizing/development
    Media advocacy
    Policy development/advocacy
    Evaluation

mainly with a particular minority group, with women, the elderly, or other special populations. The advantage of target group specialization is that the health educator becomes highly sensitive to the needs of the population and the methods that are likely to be effective with its members.

Setting. Many health educators are interested primarily in one setting. School, community, health care, or worksite are the most popular setting-specific specializations. School health educators are linked by a common interest in children and adolescents and in the school as an intervention setting. They may work in schools as teachers or they may be employed outside schools yet interested in the school as a channel for reaching children and youth. Health educators who work in health care settings are primarily interested in patients and medical care providers. They are likely to be involved in teaching and group training; program planning, development, and evaluation; and materials development. Worksite health educators may work in corporate headquarters, wellness centers, the medical department, the employee assistance program, or a variety of other units. They are interested in workers and the potential influences of the worksite on health. Community health educators, probably the largest group, may work in health departments or other government agencies, volunteer agencies, or for-profit agencies. They are interested in citizen education and community development.

Content. Many health educators develop a content specialty or concentration. Still others develop several content specialties. Some health educators, due to professional requirements or personal preference, are content generalists. Content specialization may be fairly specific, e.g., smoking; somewhat broader, e.g., cancer control; or broader still, e.g., chronic disease.

Process. Certain methods or process specializations are also possible. For example, some health educators primarily are researchers; others are planners, evaluators, materials developers, teachers and trainers, group facilitators, community developers, or policy advocates.

Of course, these specializations are neither exhaustive nor exclusive. Indeed, many health educators eventually develop specializations within several or all four categories. For example, a health educator may specialize in children and youth, schools, tobacco control, and evaluation. Hence, these categories reflect the types of specialization possible. Most health educators are not specialists, but generalists with little opportunity or desire to specialize. Instead, these health educators must be able to address a variety of target populations and content areas in a variety of settings, employing a wide range of methods and processes.

Foundations of Health Education and Health Promotion

The success of any profession in serving its constituents, patients, clients, or students depends on its adoption of advances in scientific knowledge and efficient coordination with related professions and disciplines. No profession stands alone, least of all health education. In the tradition of other helping professions—teaching, nursing, medicine, social work—health education is practical and eclectic, drawing as needed on the ideas, theories, and methods of many other fields, but rooted in the basic sciences and in the study of humankind. As conceptualized in figure 4.1, the behavioral sciences, education, and public health

Figure 4.1 Foundations of Health Education

HEALTH EDUCATION		
Behavioral Sciences	**Education**	**Public Health**
Areas:	*Areas:*	*Areas:*
Psychology	Educational Psychology	Environmental Health
Sociology	Pedagogy	Population Dynamics
Social Psychology	Curriculum Development	Epidemiology
Anthropology		Biometry
		Health Services
Approach:	*Approach:*	*Approach:*
Operant Conditioning	Teaching, training	Health Planning
Information Processing	Counseling	Mass Media
Social Learning	Consulting	Community Development
Organizational Change	Group Process	Policy Development and Advocacy
Diffusion	Evaluation	
Social Change		

History	Political Science		Economics	
	Humanities	Philosophy		Biomedical Sciences

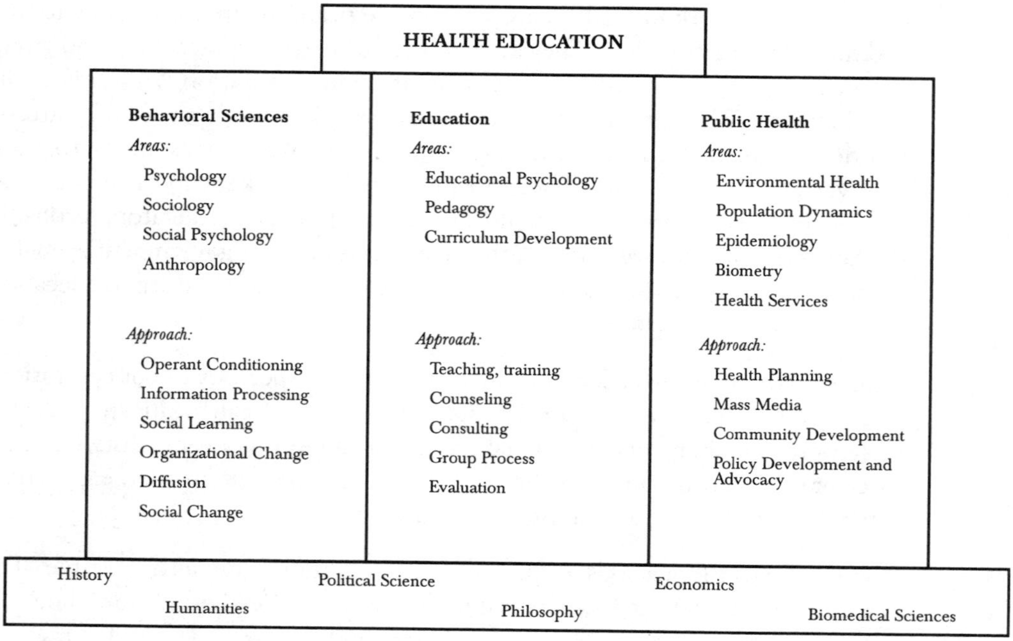

are the main foundations of health education. They in turn are supported by the humanities (especially ethics), political science, economics, philosophy, history, and biomedical sciences.

Behavioral Science

The behavioral sciences are concerned with how and why people behave as they do. Contributions from psychology, sociology, anthropology, and social-psychology in particular provide a substantial body of theoretical, conceptual, and practical literature on health behavior and change. The determinants of behavior can be categorized as psychosocial, sociocultural, or environmental. **Psychosocial** factors include characteristics that reside within or are owned by the individual—knowledge, beliefs, attitudes, concepts, values, skills, experiences, ability, and personality. **Sociocultural** context includes the influence of prevailing societal conditions and norms, especially with respect to accepted beliefs, attitudes, and practices, but also including economic and cultural conditions at local, regional, and national levels. **Environmental** factors may be supportive and reinforcing, or unsupportive and unreinforcing. The most important environmental factors are **proximal**, which are near and immediate—home, school, work, relatives, friends, coworkers, and teachers. Social and physical environmental reinforcement, whether intentional or unintentional, is a primary influence on behavior.

There are six broad theoretical/conceptual orientations that provide the bases for health promotion change processes and approaches. They are operant conditioning, information processing, social learning, organizational change, diffusion, and social change. Each offers unique interpretations of the relative contributions of psychological determinants, sociocultural context, and reinforcement. These approaches are discussed in part III.

Operant conditioning is primarily concerned with the role of reinforcement on behavior (Kazdin, 1989). The goal is to understand human behavior and foster self-control and self-management of behavior. Operant conditioning concentrates on the influences of stimuli and reinforcement on observable behavior. Reinforcement is perhaps the single most useful educational method and is part of virtually all approaches to behavior change. Change is measured in terms of individual or group behavior change.

Information processing (McGuire, 1984) is concerned primarily with the influence of information on internal cognitive and affective dispositions—knowledge, beliefs, attitudes, and values. Health educators draw heavily from the literature on information processing, memory and recall, and the relationships between knowledge, attitudes, values, and behavior. Information processing is concerned about what goes on inside a person's head and how various types of informational messages and images can influence behavior through mediation of cognitive variables. Outcomes are measured in terms of knowledge gains and changes in beliefs, attitudes, values, and self-concept.

Social learning approaches attempt to bridge operant and information processing theories. Social learning theory refers broadly to the theories of Lewin (1951), Rotter (1954, 1972), and Bandura (1977), but in modern practice, Bandura has come to dominate the thinking of most health educators interested in the interplay of individual psychological dispositions and the social environment.

Organizational change is a planned process by which organizations evolve. Organizational change can occur as a reaction to internal pressures, for example, worker demands for changes in work conditions. It also can occur as a reaction to external pressures, for example, market demands for changes in organizational products or services. Planned organizational change generally occurs in stages that include assessment, preinitiation, initiation, implementation, and institutionalization. A variety of strategies are effective in changing institutional policies and practices (Goodman and Steckler, 1990).

Diffusion theory is concerned with the rate of adoption of innovations (Rogers, 1983). Health educators are interested in increasing the rate of diffusion of healthful innovations, such as wearing condoms during intercourse as protection against AIDS and STDs, and inhibiting the rate of increase in the adoption of health-damaging innovations such as drug use and weapons carrying.

Social change is concerned with altering the conditions of people's lives rather than their personal health behavior (Rothman, 1970). Social change is interested in changes in institutions, systems, and policies that affect people. Success is measured not only in terms of improvements in health, but also in terms of improved access to health care, increased income and employment, levels of participation in the decision-making process, and other social, economic, and political indices. Sometimes the social change is directed toward organizing and developing population groups so that they may better obtain resources or control their environments. Just as often, however, the targets of social change are decision makers who control policy and resources.

Within each of these broad theoretical orientations there are several narrower theoretical applications. For example, there are a number of theories that focus on attitude formation and change and a variety of social change theories. However, each of these theories comes out of the same tradition of attempting to explain and interpret behavior based on what goes on inside the individual's head. It serves our practical purpose to discuss them in terms of this basic orientation. Also, as mentioned, our category of social learning theory combines somewhat distinct theories because they all share a common interest in the interplay of the individual and his or her social environment. Although by no means the only contributions of the behavioral sciences to health and education, these approaches are essential to health education practice.

Behavioral science provides information about how people actually behave at individual, organizational, and social levels. As such it provides important theoretical perspectives on health behavior. It forms an important foundation upon which health education practice stands.

Education

Education is the study and practice of teaching, learning, and change. Education is concerned with how learning can be achieved in various settings, for a variety of learners, through the most efficient means and useful methods. As such education is an important cornerstone to health education practice. Naturally, health education draws heavily on this foundation for its program development and intervention approaches.

Several educational foundations are important in health education. Learning theory is concerned with how people learn, the conditions that impede or facilitate learning, the order and style of presentation, the importance of practice, and learning styles. Human development and the unique cognitive and behavioral characteristics of children, adolescents, adults, and older adults is an important area of study for health educators. Measurement and testing is an area of educational psychology concerned with assessing aptitude, attitudes, knowledge, and behavior. Curriculum development is an important area of study for health educators.

A variety of educational approaches are important in health education. Teaching includes formal classroom instruction, as well as adult and informal approaches. Training is an important health education approach. Other educational approaches include group process, counseling, and evaluation.

Figure 4.1 presents education in fairly broad terms. This is not to ignore that health education is firmly rooted in public school education in terms of history and legislative mandate (Means, 1975). Among the early advocates of school health education were Benjamin Franklin, Horace Mann, John Dewey, and Henry Barnard, the first Commissioner of Education in the United States. Health is one of the seven cardinal principles of public education. Historically, health education as part of public school curricula has been advocated and supported by numerous groups including the National Education Association (1961), the American Council on Education (1944), the American Medical Association (Joint Committee, 1965), and the 1973 White House Conference on Health Education (President's Committee, 1973). At least some health instruction is required in nearly all states. In short, health education is an important and integral part of public school education, and school health education is a cornerstone of health education practices.

Health education practice in all settings has been profoundly influenced by school health education. Until very recently school health was the major focus of most college and university training programs for health educators (except at schools of public health). Health education in public schools offers the unique opportunity to teach health concepts and knowledge appropriate to the developmental stage of the student, providing the basic foundation upon which public health programs can build in later years or in other contexts. Schools provide natural environments for the evaluation of various programs and teaching methods; consequently, school health education is the focus of a great many of the published health education research papers. Finally, school teachers, by virtue of their tremendous potential for influencing health behavior, are important targets for health education training efforts.

However, in modern practice, health education is much broader than school health education. Because health educators operate in a variety of settings, with various target populations, in several different modes, concerned about a range of health problems and behaviors, the profession draws at least as heavily on adult and informal education, training, and consulting as from public education for theory, research, and methods. Furthermore, health educators are important contributors to this literature.

Public Health

Health education is influenced by the basic public health sciences. Environmental health is concerned with the physical environment as it affects health. Population dynamics is concerned with the growth, distribution, and concentration of humans. Epidemiology is the study of the distribution and causes of disease. Biometry is the study of statistics applied to the biomedical sciences. Health services administration is concerned with how services are organized and how they can best be organized. Biomedical sciences describe the mechanisms of the disease process.

Environmental health sciences, epidemiology, population dynamics, and the biomedical sciences are the major suppliers of information about the nature, type, and magnitude of problems that require public health education. Epidemiology and biostatistics provide important methodological bases for public health practice. Health education is often administered within a health services framework which influences the ways health education is organized and funded.

Epidemiology is concerned with the patterns of disease occurrence in human populations and of the factors that influence these patterns. Health education practice is particularly dependent on epidemiology and epidemiological methods for information needed to set priorities for programmatic attention. Epidemiological investigations yield results important to the development of priorities in health promotion and disease prevention; the most important health problems should have the highest priorities for programmatic efforts.

Epidemiology also seeks to determine the relative influence of various factors on the etiology and resolution of health problems. For practical purposes these factors or determinants are (1) environment, (2) public health and medical care, or (3) personal health behavior and life-style. These categories are also the channels through which health education and other behavior change approaches are initiated. Essentially, health education activities can be directed at the individual to influence his or her behavior and habitual life-style, or at public health and medical practitioners to improve care and promote patient and public health education, or at policymakers and institutions to bring about improvements in the social and physical environment affecting people's health. The relationship of health education to these categories of determinants is depicted in figure 4.2.

Figure 4.2

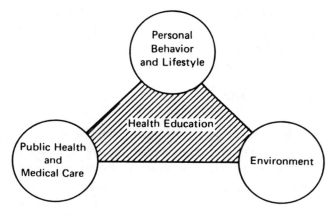

The relationship of health education to the three major categories of health and illness determinants.

Public health, often described as community health practice, includes a wide range of activities such as health planning, administration, and evaluation. Mass media, media advocacy, community development, and policy advocacy are other important public health approaches used by health educators.

Traditionally, public health has concerned itself primarily with prevention of disease and its sequelae. The term commonly applied to this is "health promotion and disease prevention." Disease prevention begins with an identified threat to health such as a disease or environmental hazard or a documented risk factor. Prevention is typically divided into three somewhat overlapping categories: primary prevention, secondary prevention, and tertiary prevention.

Primary prevention includes activities to prevent disease or ill health prior to its occurrence. One example of primary prevention is immunizations that are given to prevent communicable diseases. Another example is nutrition and fitness education programs designed to promote general health and to prevent ill health. The more directly a health behavior is linked to a health problem as a risk factor, the better candidate it is for primary prevention efforts. For example, individuals who are overweight or have excessive saturated fat or salt intakes are at risk of eventually having high blood pressure, heart attacks, strokes, and other cardiovascular diseases. These persons are prime candidates for primary prevention activities to decrease their risk of later disease. Of course, health promotion interventions to prevent smoking, unprotected intercourse, and violent behavior are primary prevention.

In **secondary prevention** action is taken to enable early detection of a health problem and to stop or modify the severity or extent of illness and disease. The dominant activities in secondary prevention are screening, diagnosis, and cure. People with chronic diseases, such as high blood pressure and diabetes, or who smoke are likely targets for secondary prevention. Patient and public education are vital parts of secondary prevention.

Tertiary prevention is disability limitation or rehabilitation. It includes both medical and educational approaches to help minimize complications and to facilitate optimum rehabilitation once a medical problem has progressed. Life-style counseling for postcardiac patients and patient education about appropriate exercises following stroke are examples of health education at the tertiary prevention stage.

Interrelated Domains

Behavioral science, education, and public health are more overlapping than independent. In particular, behavioral science is inextricably related to education and vice versa. Many of the ideas, theories, methods, and techniques developed by psychologists have found their greatest application in educational settings and situations. Educators and psychologists share a profound interest in individual learning. Other behavioral sciences, sociology and anthropology for example, are more interested in learning from a cultural or social perspective than from an individual one; educators, particularly those interested in how learning occurs or can be made to occur in natural settings, share this perspective. What unites the interests and contributions of the behavioral sciences and health education is the population-based perspective provided by public health, especially regarding priority setting and intervention approaches.

The health education profession, of course, is not limited to these three academic underpinnings. All professions must be grounded in the liberal arts. A profession that has no sense of history or does not understand politics or economics can not survive long. The humanities link the profession to the human condition. Equally important are the biomedical sciences which provide knowledge about the underlying mechanisms in health and disease that guide the direction of public health efforts.

Summary

Health promotion is a set of change processes that can be directed at individual, organizational, community, and government level target outcomes. Health education is a profession devoted to health promotion.

Health education must be considered in a social context. It exists as a profession because it is valued by society and supported by social institutions like schools, hospitals, and communities. School health education programs, for example, exist because society demands health education for its youth. The best such programs exist in communities with strong public support for health education. In every setting health education exists primarily as a product of its perceived importance to public health. Of course the better the profession represents and promotes itself, the more favorable its perception among the public and the public's representatives and institutions. Consequently, efforts to define and upgrade the profession are extremely important.

The problem of defining health education is really an academic one—who cares how it is specifically defined as long as the practitioners know what it is?—until you consider the political ramifications. If health education defines itself too narrowly it may exclude itself from the most interesting and important work. If it defines itself too broadly, it risks the criticism that, by trying to be all things to all people, it cannot deliver on its promises.

Our definition of health education as a profession is a departure from history in which health education was defined as a process. In our view, health education is better served if it defines itself as a profession dedicated to health promotion rather than as a narrow change process. Indeed, examination of the practice of health education clearly indicates that health educators practice a wide variety of health promotion change processes with a wide variety of target populations in a variety of settings.

Defining the profession is important not only conceptually, but also when it comes to writing legislation, mandates, requests for proposals, guidelines, and government and private documents. It is critical to the advancement of the profession that health education be defined broadly in national health legislation, in documents such as *Healthy People* (USDHHS, 1979), in curricula for public school education, and in guidelines for patient care and occupational health. When these documents call for something decidedly broader than health education—health promotion and disease prevention, for example—health education's role is clear because it has defined itself in relation to these broader concepts. The definition of health education advanced by the profession serves to define its areas of interest and to delimit the scope of its activities.

The four major responsibilities that constitute the practice of health education reflect the state of practice. Planning, implementing, conducting, and evaluating programs are the responsibilities practiced by health educators in the field. These areas, however, have only recently been accepted within the scope of the practice and only in recent years have professional preparation programs begun to revise their curricula to provide training in all these areas. However, no curriculum is adequate to the task of preparing students fully for the numerous functions they will perform and the myriad skills they will need to master in order to perform them. Much of this must be learned on the job.

In this chapter we emphasize the role of health education in health promotion and disease prevention. With the publication of *Healthy People* and related documents there has been a tremendous awakening of interest in health promotion and disease prevention. *Healthy People 2000* provides the health, health behavior, health services, and environmental objectives for the current decade. These high priority problems and target populations are the most likely ones to receive support and funding. *Healthy People 2000* is not only a statement of health needs and goals, it is a way of thinking about public health. The goals have been set, the rationale described, the data laid out, and the recommended actions stated, all of which present exciting challenges to health and education professionals. In accepting the challenge health educators will have to compete for scarce resources. They will have to review their planning documents and revise their curricula, further develop their practice skills, better document their success, and above all more effectively train their students. How health education will fare in the next decade, both in terms of contributing to people's health and advancing the profession, depends on the skill with which its practitioners produce evidence of improvements in behavior and health due to their efforts.

As always there are many difficult challenges ahead for health educators, but now is an especially exciting time to be a member of this profession. A great deal of excellent work has been done to establish priorities for action and to identify useful methods. Well-established professional organizations such as the Public Health Education and Health Promotion Section of the American Public Health Association, the Association for the Advancement of Health Education (AAHE), the Society for Public Health Education (SOPHE), and the American School Health Association (ASHA) have greatly advanced the cause of health education in recent years. Government agencies such as the Office of Disease Prevention and Health Promotion and the Bureau of Disease Prevention and Education, and private sector organizations such as the Center for Health Education perform important functions. Professional preparation programs in health education appear to be strong and growing. Health education journals reflect a growing sophistication in terms of both practice and research. All of this indicates that health education is healthy and vital and ready to meet the challenges of the present and future.

PART II

HEALTH EDUCATION AND HEALTH PROMOTION PROCESS AND PRACTICE

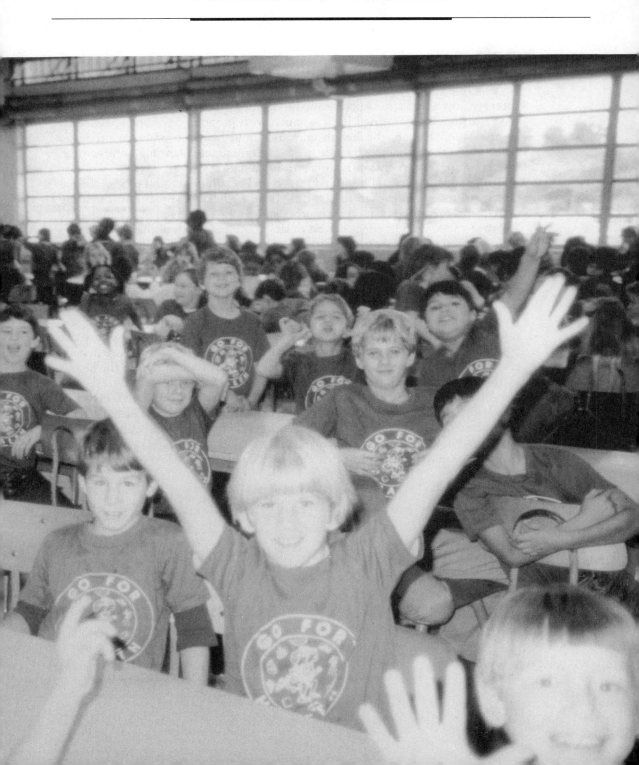

While we tend to think of health promotion in terms of certain intervention approaches such as media or policy advocacy, health education has traditionally concerned itself as much with program development as with intervention. Hence, the health education and health promotion processes described in these chapters include needs assessment and planning, intervention programming, intervention actions, and evaluation.

Planning is a central health education and health promotion process. Entire college courses are devoted to planning health education programs. Planning is frequently required by funding sources and a well-conceived plan can greatly improve the focus and effectiveness of the program. Much of planning can be thought of in terms of needs assessment, seeking to determine what population to target and what variables to address. This type of planning is integrally related to measurement and program evaluation. But there is another aspect of planning, which is addressed in chapter 6, that is concerned with developing health education programs once the target population and outcomes are defined. This aspect of planning, called intervention planning, is concerned with developing interventions for those who control the target outcomes, whether they are the population whose health and behavior the program is concerned with, or a teacher, administrator, or policymaker whose behavior is important to the health of the target population.

The broad range of available intervention approaches is what makes health education such an exciting and satisfying profession. At their most basic level all intervention approaches are educational; however, education can be manifested in a wide range of activities, including teaching, training, counseling, consulting, mass communications, and advocacy.

Needs Assessment and Planning

*A healthy program is like a healthy organism with the
planning process as a central nervous system responding to
the sensory feedback of evaluation and directing the muscles
of implementation.*

Introduction

At a glance, the task of health promotion appears to be simple and straight-forward. It consists of planning, implementing, and evaluating programs—then returning to the planning process to decide whether to modify, maintain, or terminate these programs. Planning is the process of making decisions as to what topic to address, or what problems to attack, and where to direct time and resources. Implementing is the process of actually presenting the program activities, providing the incentives, and otherwise making direct contact with students or clients. Evaluation is the process of monitoring client reaction, checking results, and otherwise assessing the quality and effectiveness of the program. Although these three subtasks have discrete roles, in good programs they are so interwoven and interdependent that the borders that separate them are indistinguishable; the interrelationships are similar to those among the processes of human biology. A healthy program is like a healthy organism with the planning process as a central nervous system responding to the sensory feedback of evaluation and directing the muscles of implementation. As one begins to plan a health education program, the initial impression of simplicity soon changes as the obstacles and complexities are encountered. Let's take a brief look at the principal factors.

- *Health* is the condition you seek to improve, but health has many dimensions and facets; different people tend to assign different priorities to these various components. Which is more important? Saving the lives of infants? Preventing premature deaths among middle-aged citizens? Preventing child and spouse abuse?

- *Risk factors and protective factors* are the variables you seek to reduce or increase if health is to be improved; but it is not always clear which of these factors are more important, how they interact with one another, or if they can be changed. If you wish to keep elderly citizens alert, active, and out of long-term nursing care facilities, do you focus on hypertension, cholesterol, diet status, or physical fitness?

- *Human behavior* is what you must change if you are to have any effect on the risk or protective factors, but few things are more complex. Which behaviors should be addressed? Smoking? Diet? Physical activity? Health care utilization? Which is the best approach to facilitating behavior change? Do you inform people? Make persuasive appeals? Provide models? Invoke sanctions? Or provide incentives?

When your target shifts from individuals to organizations or governmental agencies, as is often the case, then the complexities become even greater.

- *Health-related agencies* are the institutions that provide you with the authority and resources to mount your program, but they may also impose limits and constraints on the scope of your professional activities. If you are employed by an organization dedicated to reducing unwanted pregnancies among teenaged females, will they support your efforts to build competence, empowerment, and autonomous decision making? Will you be allowed to talk frankly about sex and contraception? Will you be allowed to distribute contraceptives? Or would the agency be more comfortable, and more likely to retain your services, if your program emphasized sexual abstinence and the negative consequences of single parenthood?

Overview of the Planning Process

Because of the complexity of these major aspects and their interaction with one another, planning becomes an imperfect, open-ended activity that could extend beyond the available resources. Obviously, at some point one reaches diminishing returns and it thus becomes more efficient to accept the current draft, along with its inevitable imperfections, put it into action, and rely on the ongoing evaluative process for mid-course or post-program refinements. This brings us to one of the important decisions to be made early in the planning effort: deciding how simple or how elaborate a process to undertake. As any working health educator knows, time, money, and other resources are generally limited. Too little attention to planning often results in efforts directed at relatively unimportant or intractable problems, or similar inefficiencies; excessive planning wastes time, money, and energy and thus debilitates the implementation of the program.

As will be described in this and the following chapter, there are a number of useful planning models; however, in actual field situations health educators frequently modify the various components to suit their own preferences and their assessment of the particular situation. But while many variations exist, certain elements are common to most of them.

Let's assume, for example, that the population of a resort community located in a ski area has become upset over the frequency of auto accidents involving drivers who had been drinking alcohol. During the ski season the community is visited by large numbers of predominately young adults; several taverns vie with one another for the lucrative after-ski business. By the time the crowds leave the slopes, the late afternoon sunlight is dissolving into dusk and the roads are frequently treacherous. Although most of the accidents that have occurred during this time period have been "fender benders," two recent collisions occurring later in the evening were lethal. The second of these claimed the life of a popular local resident and provoked a public outcry. An ad hoc citizens' committee was formed which promptly asked the Division of Health

Education and Community Involvement of the county health department to intervene. Using this hypothetical situation as a reference point, let's see how someone with planning responsibility might proceed. The purpose here is only to provide the reader with some general feeling for the process; more detailed descriptions will come later.

Reviewing the Externals

Every planning situation is surrounded by external factors that support or inhibit the process; these items are best considered earlier rather than later. The health educator in this case may need to determine if it is indeed appropriate to respond to this request. Does the division have a responsibility and a legal mandate to mount programs in this locality? If the community in question, for example, was an incorporated town with its own local health department, the intervention of county personnel might be inadvisable or subject to significant restraints. If we assume a clear mandate, then additional questions immediately arise. What resources can and should be devoted to this task? What other projects are ongoing? How much staff time is available? Are there sufficient funds to initiate the actual planning process? Given what is known about the community in question, what are the prospects for success? If, on the basis of these and similar considerations, our hypothetical planner decides to mount a program, this preliminary review will also guide its first tentative steps.

The Approach

The planner's selection of initial contact persons within the community, like so many of the early decisions, is particularly crucial. Perhaps the president of the local chamber of commerce is an influential community leader who can provide access to a network of active, concerned citizens. On the other hand, this person might be only a figurehead and thus unwilling or unable to offer help. Maybe the owner of the major ski facility is an entrenched and politically connected "player" in the community—any would-be leader who doesn't at least pay a courtesy call may find most other doors closed. Or, perhaps the facility is run by a newly hired manager struggling to lead his own staff much less the community. In some situations the selection is obvious; in others, intuition and luck must play a role in the decision.

Needs Assessment

The initial person or persons approached in the community may help guide the formation of a local planning group whose first task will be to assess the nature of the problem and the factors responsible. Also, any existing programs, policies, and so forth should be reviewed. This step will help determine if the fatal accident was the result of a lack of proper safety measures or merely an aberrant or freak occurrence. If safety measures or conditions are inadequate, what are the most important and most promising items to attack? The personal decisions of the skiers? The advertising and sales practices of the taverns? Law enforcement? The sanding and maintenance of the highways? Or, more likely, some combination of these? The answers to questions like these are the subject of much current research into health protection and the dynamics of health behavior, thus any answers will undoubtedly represent a best assessment of the situation rather than absolute certainty.

Formulation of Goals and Objectives

Once the available information is reviewed, the planning group should then decide what it seeks to accomplish and express these aspirations in clear statements. One or more goals should be formulated as a means of delineating the scope and general thrust of the program. For example, "Alcohol-related traffic accidents occurring within 10 miles of the community will be reduced 30 percent." The focus of the program could be sharpened further by health outcome objectives, for example, "Alcohol-related fatalities will be reduced by 50 percent." Because less frequent events such as fatalities can be influenced by chance factors, objectives for behavior should also be established, for example, "The use of designated drivers will increase by 50 percent." There may be objectives for organizational behavior also; in this case the planners might wish to encourage the taverns to require training in safety aspects for bartenders, waiters, and waitresses. At the governmental level, the planners might decide to seek better surveillance of the roads by the police and stricter enforcement of underage drinking laws.

Development of Program Components

The next step is to decide on the most efficient and practical way to accomplish the objectives. Here the planning group must consider what is known about individual, organizational, and governmental behavior, assuming all these elements are targeted by the objectives. This may involve a variety of components including distributing brochures to guests when they register at local lodges and motels; developing and marketing a training program for tavern personnel; devising a strategy for lobbying the county government for more police patrols; and planning an appeal to local radio stations for public service announcements.

Implementation

For a program of the type described, the principal challenge is often one of obtaining and making the best use of limited resources. During the implementation stage, funds may have to be raised for personnel, program activities, and materials such as pamphlets, fliers, signs, postage, and so on. It is essential to have one qualified professional to lead the program and be accountable for it; however, much of the work may require volunteers who must be recruited, trained, supervised, and encouraged. Most of the local citizens will have a vested interest in the area's reputation as a safe, yet friendly and well-managed place for recreation. The health educator should use this interest to get talented and energetic people involved in the program.

Evaluation

Early in the process of implementation program personnel may start to solicit feedback from lodge and motel managers and tavern owners as to how their customers are reacting to the program; a more arduous but very effective technique would be to conduct spot interviews with the visitors themselves. The findings could reveal that the campaign was unduly negative, poorly targeted, or inadequately implemented. In any case the early feedback could prompt program-saving corrections. As the season progresses, firmer evidence could be gathered by monitoring DUI citations and alcohol-related accidents. Depending on the volume of traffic, it might take more than one season to gauge the effect of the program on the number of deaths and serious injuries; however, over time, as the primary program goal, this outcome would be the ultimate criterion.

Revision, Maintenance, Termination

At the end of the ski season our hypothetical program leader will face yet another challenge. In a worst-case scenario, it may be found that the program had little impact, was very unpopular, or that the problem itself simply wasn't as bad as originally judged; here the decision might be to forget the whole project. However, assuming that the results were favorable, the program should be improved and institutionalized, i.e., adopted and maintained by the local community, thus allowing the health educator to move on to other problems. One solution would be to convince one of the involved community groups to take long-term responsibility for the program; a service club would be a likely choice. When circumstances are very favorable, a successful project may serve as a catalyst for the formation of a permanent organization with a board of directors and a commitment to conduct fund drives and maintain the program.

Planning Models

As health educators have struggled with the planning and implementing of programs over the years in a wide variety of situations, several efforts have been made to reduce the process to a formula, i.e., to develop planning models to guide development efforts so that each future planner does not have to "reinvent the wheel." The underlying principles that guide the development of the various models are very similar; however, there are important differences in sequence, emphasis, and the conceptualization of the major components that make certain models more appealing than others to individual practitioners.

Older Models

Because the ultimate quality of any program is undoubtedly influenced more by the skill and training of the personnel involved and the resources available to them than by the particular planning framework they use, many of the older, simpler models are still popular. One of the earliest examples in this group, as described recently by Breckon and others (1989), consisted simply of a graphically displayed timetable for the completion of the tasks necessary for the development and implementation of the program. The result was termed a PERT chart, an acronym for Program Evaluation and Review Technique. Although developed in the 1960s, various versions and modifications of PERT charts still find use in current applications.

A somewhat more complex model was described by Mico in 1966 and subsequently refined into six phases, namely, (1) initiation, (2) needs assessment, (3) goal setting, (4) planning/programming, (5) implementation, and (6) evaluation. Within each of these phases, attention is directed to the (a) content dimension, which indicates the information needed for the particular phase; (b) method dimension, which indicates the ways of gathering and analyzing the information; and (c) a process dimension, which indicates the purpose to be accomplished (Ross and Mico, 1980).

During the early 1970s Sullivan (1973) developed an even more elaborate model that still retains much of its popularity despite the advent of more current entries. This scheme organizes the process into six major phases, namely, (1) involve people, (2) set goals, (3) define problems, (4) design plans, (5) conduct activities, and (6) evaluate results. A suggested sequence of activities is provided for each phase. For example, within the design plans phase (4), the sequence carries planners from the listing of alternative approaches, through tentative selection and pretesting of the more promising ones, to final selection and securing of approval. Throughout the entire process, planners are reminded to view each aspect in terms of (1) the health problem(s) involved, (2) the individual behaviors involved and their dynamics, (3) the strengths and limitations of the health education process, and (4) the resources needed and available.

PRECEDE-PROCEED

The most popular and widely used of the current planning models was originally developed and titled PRECEDE by a group at Johns Hopkins university under the leadership of Lawrence Green (Green et al., 1980). The original title was, and remains, an acronym for Predisposing, Reinforcing, and Enabling Causes in Educational Diagnosis and Evaluation. Its recent modification is titled PRECEDE-PROCEED with the added term standing for Policy, Regulatory, and

Organizational Constructs in Educational and Environmental Development. This version parallels the development of the modern concept of health promotion which has broadened the scope of the health educator's responsibilities beyond the change of client behavior to include attention to environmental and organizational concerns. In response to this expanded role, the framework was revised to include attention to these aspects.

PRECEDE-PROCEED provides for a series of sequential steps designed to help the planner move from the recognition of problems or impediments to the overall quality of life through the analysis of these problems, and to the development of a program designed to address them. A major strength is its focus on a thorough assessment of the needs of each situation and the subsequent ranking or prioritizing of problems and possible responses at each step. Although it is sometimes a bit cumbersome in relatively small, circumscribed situations, its extremely broad scope is particularly appropriate for large projects with ample resources. A schematic diagram of this framework is presented in figure 5.1.

Figure 5.1 The PRECEDE-PROCEED Model

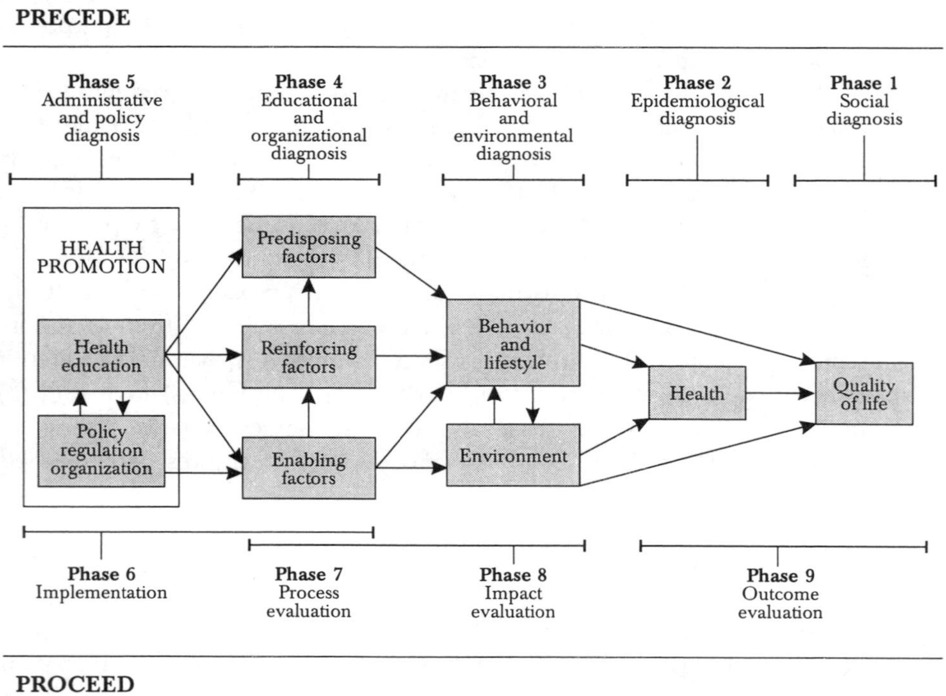

Source: Green, Lawrence, and Marshall W. Kreuter. *Health Promotion Planning: An Educational and Environmental Approach.* Mountainview, CA: Mayfield, 1991. Reprinted with permission.

Social and Epidemiological Diagnosis

During phase 1, social diagnosis, the planners generally research census data, mortality and morbidity data, and environmental assessments related to the particular community as a way to assess its quality of life and the general problems that diminish this quality. Ideally, this review would include current surveys of representative community members by use of mail-out questionnaires, house-to-house interviews, focus groups, town meetings, and so forth; however, this more direct approach is often difficult to implement. This whole process is, in effect, a review of the specific "symptoms" of community health or dysfunction.

In contrast to the data-gathering nature of social diagnosis, the epidemiological diagnosis (phase 2) is more of an analytical activity wherein the identified problems are sorted into health and environmental categories. This is, in effect, the first stage of the process of selecting specific problems to attack. Ideally, problems are considered purely in terms of their individual characteristics, although such factors as the mandate of the organization mounting the program and established national goals as provided in *Healthy People 2000* (USDHHS, 1990) may legitimately play a role in the eventual selection. Also, a specific problem's prospects for change given a reasonable effort merits consideration. The end result of this stage is a well-crafted set of objectives in the form of specific statements of the expected improvement in health status.

Behavioral and Environmental Diagnosis

With the key problems identified, phase 3 leads planners into a search for their root causes. If the preschool children within a particular community are found to be poorly nourished, for example, is it the result of poor meal planning by the parents (a behavior problem), or a lack of sufficient income to purchase proper food items (an environmental factor)? One assessment would prompt an educational approach whereas the other would suggest a lobbying effort to gain public funds or perhaps a drive to raise private support for some sort of food supplement program. The end product of this phase is a set of behavior objectives that states the desired changes in either individual or organizational behavior.

Educational and Organizational Diagnosis

With the needed changes in individual behavior and/or the policies and procedures of the employer, the clinic staff, or perhaps the town council thus identified, it is logical to question why such individuals or organizations are acting in an unfavorable manner in the first place. In other words, what are the behavioral determinants of the underlying individual or organizational behavior that is causing the health problem or problems?

The planners are encouraged to conduct this search for behavioral determinants within three categories. The first category, **predisposing factors**, includes such internal psychological variables as knowledge, beliefs, and attitudes that the subjects carry around "inside their heads"; psychologists refer to these items as **intervening variables** which, as part of the internal mental apparatus, lie between the external stimuli to which subjects are exposed and their subsequent responses (see chapter 9). The second category, **enabling factors**, generally includes those items in the external environment of the subjects that make it possible or convenient for them to actually carry out the desirable behavior. Here the planners examine such factors as the location of health care facilities and their hours of operation, the income level of the members of target group, and the availability of transportation.

The third category, **reinforcement**, refers to the influences of significant people on individuals or organizations. Here the planners must examine the social structure and power relationships in order to identify the most promising approach to change. The poor or inept policies that need to be changed may be supported by poor attitudes or misconceptions of managerial personnel, for example, or the they may result from external pressure from higher echelons. These and similar questions must be resolved before the specific content and activities of the implementation stage can be planned. The end product of this overall phase is a series of learning and resource objectives. Learning objectives are normally stated in terms of the things people will know or understand, or perhaps the attitudes they will display as a result of experiencing the program, whereas resource objectives are directed at material support, i.e., goods and services that program planners plan to obtain for the target group.

Administrative and Policy Diagnosis

During phase 5, decisions are made as to the exact nature of the program. Depending on the information generated by the preceding steps, the program may center on structured classes, mass media presentations, and/or distribution of pamphlets and brochures if the primary focus is on education; it may involve enforcement of rules or laws if a regulatory approach is deemed appropriate; or it may take the form of a multifaceted array of activities designed to mobilize local resources if community organization is the selected strategy. In many instances some combination of these basic approaches may be used. Within these various categories, specific decisions as to the nature and intensity of the program will be tempered by a careful analysis of available resources.

Implementation

Because it was designed as a planning framework, the PRECEDE-PROCEED model does not attempt to provide or describe any innovative methods for implementation (phase 6). It simply reminds planners of the importance of this step and challenges them to use state-of-the-art procedures. The planners and implementers are also asked to decide whether steps should be taken to "institutionalize" the program—making it part of the permanent structure of the organization mounting the program—or whether to terminate the program if it is no longer needed.

Evaluation

The authors of the PRECEDE-PROCEED model note that program evaluation is often an anxiety-provoking process, but suggest that this effect tends to be reduced when their model is used. They argue with considerable validity that such a strong emphasis is placed on data gathering throughout the entire process that much of the information will already be in hand by the time the implementation of the program has been completed. Phases 7, 8, and 9 are each devoted to a single aspect or dimension of evaluation.

Phase 7, process evaluation, calls for a specific review and assessment of the various program components both before and during their implementation in a effort to determine if they look and appear sound, logical, and appropriate. Although careful and systematic, this form of evaluation actually focuses on appearances rather than results. Phase 8, impact evaluation, asks the evaluators to examine the program participants rather than the program. Participants are examined to determine if they became more knowledgeable, their attitudes more favorable, and/or their personal behavior more conducive to their health. Depending on the nature of the program, this phase also may call for assessing any impact on organizational behavior. Did the employer add more rest breaks for the workers? Did the city council appropriate funds for a homeless shelter? Phase 9, outcome evaluation, involves a search for program-related changes in the actual health status of the target population. Did mortality decline? Were there fewer work days lost because of illness? Were there fewer accidents and injuries on the job?

PATCH

A unique planning framework, derived in part from the original PRECEDE model, was developed and refined by the U.S. Public Health Service (USPHS) during the early 1980s. Its title, PATCH, is an acronym for Planned Approach To Community Health. Throughout its history the USPHS has sought to promote health nationwide even though its financial resources have generally been minuscule compared to the size of the task. It soon found that it could make the best use of its limited funds by promoting and supporting grassroots efforts within state and communities willing to help themselves. Often the provision of a modest amount of technical assistance and expertise would serve as a catalyst that initiated an efficient and well-funded local effort.

In the past this general strategy had been used primarily to help with disease detection, pollution control, and other such problems within the physical environment. During the 1980s, however, as the role of individual behavior in health and disease became more apparent, the Centers for Disease Control of the USPHS developed the PATCH program "to create a practical mechanism through which effective community health education action could be targeted to address local-level health priorities" (Kreuter, 1992). One very helpful aspect of PATCH programs, which derives from their federal sponsorship, is the availability of a limited amount of start-up money for the participating local health organization. Also provided is information and literature and, in some cases, direct leadership for a planning process modeled along the lines of the original PRECEDE model (Green et al., 1980). Finally, PATCH programs have the unique advantage of bringing local planners into contact with state and federal agencies positioned to provide some degree of support to the health promotion effort. In many cases, this action enables the local organization to tap funds that had already been established for health promotion in appropriate situations.

MATCH

Whereas PRECEDE-PROCEED emphasizes formal needs assessment, MATCH, as formulated by Simons-Morton and associates (1988), is a framework that gives more attention to implementation. Increasingly, the health educator is required to look beyond individual behavior and seek changes in the organizations, communities, and governmental agencies that have significant and sometimes crucial effects on individual health status. A basic approach to this task is symbolized in the acronym, MATCH—Multilevel Approach To Community Health. This model does not ignore the importance of individual behavior change; however, its strength lies in the uniform attention it accords to the individual, organizational, community, and governmental levels. A detailed discussion of this model will be presented in chapter 6.

Needs Assessment

The first and most important step in a successful planning process is the gathering of accurate and comprehensive information concerning the target community. Health educators, by nature, tend to be action oriented and thus must resist the temptation to neglect the needs assessment process in their haste to get their programs up and running. Sufficient time and resources often may not be available for the kind of thorough and elaborate process described in this section; however, needs assessment should retain a high priority regardless of the level of support.

Even a superficial review of any town, neighborhood, work group, school population, or other community of interest will typically reveal a tangled web of social problems; a host of complaints and concerns varying from the trivial to the profound; a morass of unfavorable behavior patterns, deprivation, and poor environmental conditions all of which are intertwined with a group of salient health problems. As soon as the planning group has been assembled and its mandate clarified, the process of gathering information related to these various factors should begin. This search should be broad and comprehensive both in terms of the categories of problems and risk factors considered and the sources of data examined. The general purpose of this process is to identify the problems and their possible causes, and to analyze these items on the basis of their appropriateness to the planning organization's mission, their relative importance, and their changeability. When done properly, the needs assessment process will reduce this tangled web of information to a clear set of program goals and objectives.

Need Categories

As noted, there is a close, at times indistinguishable, relationship between problems and needs which makes fine distinctions counterproductive. The problems blend into needs and the needs blend into the strategies or devices required to meet the needs. It is useful, however, to distinguish between **health needs**, i.e., problems in health status such as disease, mortality, disability, and so on, and the things that need to be changed in order to alleviate these problems, commonly termed **educational needs** and **resource needs**. The assessment of educational needs answers the question, "What changes are needed in the knowledge, attitudes, or skills of the target population to facilitate more favorable behavior patterns or, perhaps, to shape policies on other ongoing programs to encourage better health behavior?" The answer should identify any specific lack of knowledge or information, any misconceptions, or perhaps a lack of appreciation for the seriousness of the health problems or the effectiveness of the health recommendations. The needs within this category may range from a rather superficial lack of information as to the availability of health services to a quite paralyzing sense of powerless and despair as a result of poverty, loneliness, or a host of other deprivations.

The assessment of resource needs also must cover a broad spectrum of alternatives, from low-cost batteries for smoke detectors to the funding and development of a professional fire department in a rapidly growing urban area. Also, within this phase of the assessment planners often must make difficult distinctions between genuine lack of personal funds or available public services, and the individual's failure to make efficient use of the resources available. Here, planners encounter a host of practical and philosophical considerations. Although they must be careful not to try to "educate" people to buy nutritious food which they cannot afford, it is equally undesirable to embark on a campaign for publicly funded food support if the current political conditions guarantee failure. Better to return to the "victims" and help them make the best of a poor situation.

Relationship of Needs Assessment to Program Objectives

Determining these three categories of needs should provide planners with the information needed to formulate an overall program goal and three parallel sets of objectives. The program goal typically is a broad, general statement; however, it should indicate clearly the problem that will be addressed. A series of health objectives subdivide this goal into more specific components, while behavior, learning, and resource objectives specify the changes that must be accomplished to achieve the desired improvements in health status. Examples of these components appear on pages 143–144.

Sources

The sources of data for a needs assessment vary according to the demands of the particular community; however, it generally includes information collected from such sources as (1) prior research studies and existing records, (2) individual members of the target population, (3) field professionals and staff, and (4) significant others such as friends and family members.

Prior Studies and Existing Records

The logical first step for acquiring information on any community or other target group is to search for data that already exists in the form of previous structured investigations or routinely gathered records or statistics. Although such information may have been based on a much broader population, such as census data or citywide morbidity rates, for example, it can nonetheless be quite useful when properly extrapolated to the target group (Kettner, Moroney, and Martin, 1990). A careful review of research investigations of similar groups in other locales can provide the basis for cautious assumptions. Such information can be far superior to mere guesswork in those frequent situations where the resources for new assessments of the target population are not available.

In many cases existing data may apply directly to the target population. When permission is obtained, patient or personnel records, for example, may provide considerable information relevant to needs assessment. From patient records, for example, one can determine the rates of control over long-term management problems such as high blood pressure and diabetes. Sometimes these records include information about patient knowledge of their medical regimen, their health behavior, even their rate of medication-taking, and other compliance with medical advice over time. Likewise, service or utilization data on the number of patient contacts in a public health clinic, for example, often shed light on local needs. Again, planners must consider the rights of patients and clients to confidentiality—they must be informed and willing participants even in the needs assessment phase.

In the hypothetical example presented earlier regarding a program to reduce the rate of accidents resulting from drunk driving, the types of records useful for an educational diagnosis include police reports, court records, surveys, records from courses for convicted drunk drivers, and school curricula. From these records and reports it may be possible to specify more narrowly the target population, the behavioral and environmental determinants, and the relevant content emphases of the program.

Target Population

Generally, the most valuable source of information is the target population itself. The potential clients or students may be the best source of information, not only about their health behavior, but also about the determinants of that behavior. A useful needs assessment for an educational program to reduce drunk driving, for example, should include interviews with a sample of the target population selected to include a disproportionate number of high-risk drivers.

Staff

The professionals and other staff members who work with the target population on a regular basis are excellent sources of information for needs assessment purposes. In addition to providing information about the needs of the target population, they are very likely to reveal educational needs of their own which must be addressed if they are to have a favorable impact on the target population. Both common sense and the findings of research indicate that the actions and attitudes of health care providers influence patient outcomes. Certainly this also is the case with teachers, employers, and others. Therefore, the educational needs of supervisors, health professionals, and others should be assessed. In our hypothetical drunk driving program, the knowledge, attitudes, and behaviors of police officers, bartenders, employers, health care professionals (especially those in the emergency room), and others who might come into contact with drunk drivers, would be an important part of a comprehensive needs assessment.

Significant Others

People in the social environment who are particularly close to members of the target population comprise yet another fruitful source for needs assessment efforts. Family members, friends, community leaders, and others are important sources of information about the educational needs of a target population. The important influence of spouses, friends, and clergy on potential drunk drivers is obvious. Information gathered from this group can provide information on the target population as well as reveal the need to educate significant others and enlist their assistance.

Assessment Techniques

A wide variety of specific methods are available for surveying and assessing educational needs of the target population, only a few of which will be described here in brief form. (See Gilmore, Campbell and Becker, 1989 for a detailed treatment.) These examples will serve to introduce readers to the range of methods available and suggest the most common applications of these methods.

Forums and Group Discussions

One way to determine the needs of a target population is to get a representative sample together in a nonthreatening environment and discuss the issues. Depending on the demands of the situation and the resources available, different modes of organization and procedures must be selected to secure the best result. Consequently, a number of standard techniques have been developed among which the **nominal group process** is one of the more structured and effective examples. As described by Gilmore and associates (1989), it involves a careful selection of participants to insure proper representation, and a set of procedures designed to elicit well-reasoned opinions. In a typical application, the participants are organized into small groups with trained discussion leaders who pose a series of questions; the group members are given time to plan their responses and then asked to write brief answers. These written responses are read in turn to the group; later, following a general discussion, the various listing of problems and/or proposed solutions are voted upon to determine a consensus or majority opinion. These individual group responses are then discussed in a general session in a similar process to pool the results. This rather elaborate process is highly effective when properly implemented; however, it can be expensive in terms of time and resources. It frequently takes more than two hours to complete, thus requiring highly motivated participants; skilled leadership is also needed. In short, nominal group process is a highly elaborate procedure designed to elicit from a concerned group their collective perception of the most important problems and/or potential solutions in such a manner as to prevent or discourage a few highly vocal participants from dominating the group.

A simpler, more natural discussion format is provided by the **focus group** technique. As described by Kreuter (1988), these groups are organized in much the same way as in the nominal group discussion but the members are encouraged to comment freely on the discussion questions; no written answers are required and no votes are taken. This process can be completed in less time with fewer demands on the participants; however, the results are purely qualitative and there is more risk of domination by a vocal minority.

The **round robin** includes some elements of both preceding methods. Here the opinion of each participant is solicited in turn. Group members may respond with comments if they wish. This process insures that all members will be heard even though there is no means to rank or vote on the responses.

The **community forum**, although most commonly used by town councils, school boards, and other government agencies, can also be useful to those planning health promotion programs. As described by Gilmore and associates (1989), it takes the form of an open public meeting with all interested persons invited to participate. Depending on the number of people attending and the degree of interest, a time limit may be needed for individual contributions and sometimes persons representing groups may be given preference over individuals speaking on their own behalf. This format generally provides a means of soliciting a broad range of views and concerns; however, it may not always provide an accurate representation of the total community.

There are many other group approaches to assessing needs and several variations on the few approaches mentioned. For example, the formation of an expert advisory committee that meets regularly to discuss the educational needs of a specific target group can be invaluable to the needs assessment process. Sometimes very informal meetings of workers, community members, students, patients, providers, or teachers in their natural gathering places can be highly informative, especially prior to a more formal needs assessment. It is important to keep in mind the tendency of groups to influence participant opinion in subtle and not so subtle ways. Nevertheless, meeting with available members of the target population in these comfortable settings or on the job can be a very useful part of needs assessment. Often this process makes it easier to organize more formal assessments at a later date.

Observation

A great deal can be learned about the educational needs of a population by observation. For example, the safety practices of factory workers or the communication patterns of health care providers can be assessed by observation. Structured observation procedures have been developed to reduce the subjective bias of the observer. Simons-Morton and others (1991b), for example, developed an observational procedure for assessing the amount of physical activity children obtain during physical education classes and the instructional methods used in these classes. Once established, such observational assessments frequently take the form of checklists that eliminate the need for the observer to do anything more than check the appropriate box.

Checklists are also useful for identifying subjective training needs. First, a list of all the possible training needs is developed. Then a column is provided for knowledge, attitudes, and skills next to each item, which the participant can mark according to his/her perceived needs. This very simple method is especially useful in assessing needs quickly at the beginning of an intensive workshop or training program. This device is sometimes termed a **skills inventory**.

In **job analysis** or **task analysis** an established list of job functions or tasks is compared with an observed measure of performance. This procedure is usually employed to improve employee efficiency but can also be employed to assess education needs. Again, the observation of a health care provider in a session with a patient would be a good example of its use.

Surveys

In contrast to the rather cumbersome and expensive process of bringing representatives together in meetings, survey techniques can generally search more widely with less expense (Kettner, Moroney, and Martin, 1990). The trade-off, of course, is that there is no opportunity to interact with other community members and the responses may be more superficial than those elicited in group meetings. These disadvantages can be greatly reduced by the use of good techniques. There are a number of methods for conducting surveys; among the most common are various forms of direct interviews, telephone surveys, and mail-out questionnaires.

Structured interviews using preselected questions are very worthwhile, especially in the early stages of a needs assessment (Gilmore, Campbell, and Becker, 1989). Also, the inclusion of some open-ended questions allows the interviewee to express more wide-ranging subjective impressions and feelings. There is much literature on the advantages and disadvantages of interviews in terms of obtaining accurate information. One typical problem is the influence of the interviewer's dress, gender, and tone of voice on the subject's response to the questions. The precise wording of each question is also important in this regard. As an informal tool, interviewing is invaluable. As a formal assessment procedure it must be rigorously developed and administered to assure valid responses. With large numbers of people, interviewing may be too costly. In such cases a sample can be selected or a questionnaire can be developed, depending on the nature of the subject, the accessibility of the target population, and other concerns.

Although limited in many ways, telephone interviews can often yield information on a target group more quickly and inexpensively than any other method. A good survey requires that one make a strong effort to circumvent such obstacles as unlisted numbers, screening via answering machines, and odd working hours. This often involves special efforts to secure current, accurate phone lists; use careful sampling techniques to insure that a disproportionate number of the unemployed or elderly shut-ins are not included; provide advanced publicity; and adopt a careful approach to help improve the credibility of the interviewer.

Perhaps the most used and the most useful tools for assessing needs are the various forms of questionnaires. They are adaptable to so many problems and situations and they are relatively inexpensive to develop, administer, and evaluate. Questionnaires are especially useful for determining perceived needs, beliefs, and attitudes, as well as the demographic make-up and even the knowledge of a large group of people. Their effective use, however, requires considerable attention to both the development of the questionnaire and its administration to insure the validity and reliability of the results. Furthermore, they are subject to the same ethical constraints of informed consent and confidentiality as other forms of assessment.

Planners must take care to insure an adequate level of response. The cover letter accompanying the questionnaire should carry an impressive letterhead and, if possible, include the endorsement of influential persons and/or organizations. It should be carefully worded to impress upon the respondent the importance of the survey. The survey instrument should be as short as possible and require the least amount of writing by the respondent as is consistent with obtaining the necessary information.

Although the items within a questionnaire can take a number of forms, rating scales are perhaps the most common. For example, the following items were taken from an unpublished questionnaire that was employed in part to assess the educational needs of high blood pressure patients.

QUESTION: How much does each of the following create a problem for you?

	A big problem	Somewhat of a problem	Not much of a problem	No problem at all	Don't know
Sometimes I worry that taking high blood pressure medicine can cause health problems.	1	2	3	4	9
Taking my high blood pressure medicine disrupts my daily schedule and makes it difficult to get things done during the day.	1	2	3	4	9

Rating scales also can be used, like checklists, to establish perceived educational priorities, as in the following example.

QUESTION: Rate the following items in terms of what you would most like to learn about during this workshop. Circle the appropriate number.

	Level of Interest			
	Very High	High	Somewhat High	Not Very High
Needs Assessment	1	2	3	4
Planning Models	1	2	3	4
Budgeting	1	2	3	4
Educational Methods	1	2	3	4
Educational Designs	1	2	3	4

The **Delphi Technique** is a survey method that embodies some of the features of the nominal group process in that participants have the opportunity to react to the views of other members of the target group. As described by Green and Krueter (1991), this task is accomplished by compiling the results of an initial questionnaire that had included a very broad array of questions and then using this information as the basis for a second mailing to the original respondents. This second instrument typically includes a summary of the results and a narrower choice of responses restricted to the most widely supported items. The respondents then "vote" a second time. The process may be ended at this point or continued for a third round if the views are still quite divergent. The end result is a consensus or, at least, a short list of the more popular views.

Although more commonly used in face-to-face situations, the **traditional knowledge test** is one of the most prevalent and useful methods for assessing needs. As most students will attest, however, its use is somewhat restricted by its frequently threatening or burdensome nature. Yet, whether administered directly or by mail, knowledge tests can provide a standard measure of knowledge useful for both needs assessment and for pre/post program comparisons. The lack of specific types of health knowledge is not always a sure sign of an educational need, but it usually indicates an area that merits further attention.

Summary of Needs Assessment

Table 5.1 presents an overview of some of the general methods of needs assessment with their advantages and limitations and some suggestions for the application of each method. In general, the determination of educational needs typically involves some combination of the following components:

1. A review of existing research on the target health problem and associated behaviors with emphasis on the knowledge, attitudes, and skills of populations similar to the target population, the environmental influences, and the role and responsibility of relevant professionals and social support persons.

2. A review of existing data sources related to the nature, frequency, and circumstances surrounding the health problems, health behaviors, and education of the target population.

3. Collection by various methods of original data on the knowledge, beliefs, and attitudes of the target population, health professionals, and relevant others regarding the health problem(s) and health behaviors of interest.

Development of Program Components

Once the needs have been thoroughly assessed, the planning and implementation process can be based on a solid foundation of information. The process of forming the program plan is comprised of (1) making appropriate decisions regarding the nature and substance of the various program components and (2) describing these components in a written plan that will communicate the intentions of the planners to those who will implement the program. Both of these tasks are very important and very challenging. Many good programs that deserve wider dissemination cannot be used in other locales because they have been

Table 5.1 Comparison of Data Collection Methodologies

Method	Advantages	Disadvantages	Result Quality	Staff Requirements	Costs
Person-to-Person Interview	1. High response rate 2. Highly flexible 3. Visual aid opportunity 4. Community input and morale builder	1. High costs 2. Raises expectations 3. Travel expenses 4. Possible interviewer bias 5. Technical staff required 6. High agency effort 7. Possible computer needs 8. High call-back expenses	1. Yields detailed and high-quality results 2. Most representative results 3. Quantifiable results	1. Technical assistance for interview construction 2. Interviewer training 3. Technical assistance for data analyzation, processing, and interpretation 4. Several interviewers	High
Telephone Interview	1. Easy to administer 2. Low call-back expense 3. Community input and morale builder 4. High response rate 5. Relatively lower cost	1. Possible interviewer bias 2. Possible computer needs 3. Raises expectations 4. Representativeness and sampling problems	1. Quantifiable results 2. Relatively quality results 3. Unless corrected, some bias in results 4. Fairly detailed results	1. Interviewer training 2. Several interviewers 3. Possible technical assistance for data analyzation 4. Technical assistance for interview construction	Medium
Mail-Out Questionnaire	1. Low cost 2. Minimum staff time 3. Possible good response 4. Larger outreach 5. Community input	1. Generally low return rate 2. Possible bias and unrepresentativeness 3. Ineffective for illiterate people 4. Possible lack of question understanding 5. Possible computer needs	1. Quantifiable results 2. Low to medium quality 3. Possible major biases 4. More candid results	1. Technical assistance for questionnaire construction 2. If hand-processed, one or two untrained staff 3. Technical assistance if computer-processed	Low
Existing Records and Statistics	1. Relatively low cost 2. Minimum staff effort 3. Ongoing assessment and evaluation possible	1. No community input 2. Census data cost can be high 3. Possible agency uncooperativeness	1. Relative quality results 2. Quantifiable results 3. Relative detail in results	1. Possible technical assistance for statistical interpretation 2. One or two staff	Low to medium
Special Methodologies	1. Relative costs and staff effort 2. Possible community input	1. May require other methods for representativeness 2. Possible bias	1. Results can be quantified 2. Relative quality 3. Subjective	1. Relative—could be one staff	Low to medium, depending on scope and type
Meetings	1. Inexpensive 2. Community input and feedback 3. Flexibility 4. Opportunity for questionnaire distribution 5. Reflects aggregate community opinion	1. Hard to quantify 2. Possible result bias 3. Relatively low input for individual problems	1. Possible bias 2. Hard to quantify 3. Can be made quite representative	1. Minimal technical requirements 2. Sufficient staff to plan and organize meetings	Low monetary costs

Note: Special methodologies include systematic field observations and investigations, the action-research approach to conducting the project activity, the anthropological technique of training those who regularly collect and report data, and others.

Source: Ross, Helen S., and Paul R. Mico. *Theory and Practice in Health Education*, 1980. Reprinted with permission.

developed by planning groups who were unable or unwilling to effectively describe what they were doing; other planners with similar populations are thus forced to "reinvent the wheel" with consequent loss of time and effort. Conversely, mediocre programs based on questionable decisions are sometimes very well written and, consequently, may receive more attention than they deserve.

Good decisions regarding program content and emphasis are facilitated by the aforementioned needs assessment procedures which can identify the determinants of behavior that are the most important contributors to the target health behavior(s). It is with these determinants in mind that program planners develop or revise the components of the health education program—a highly challenging and creative task. Ideally, the development of program components is based on a melding of health behavior theory with the findings of the needs assessment and the practical circumstances of the program and the target population. The resulting program structure must also provide an opportunity for evaluating the appropriateness of the objectives and content of the program, as well as the quality of its implementation.

The general form of the written plan of most health education programs is very similar, regardless of whether it is community based and arising out of the PRECEDE framework, school based and devised according to a traditional curriculum development format, or clinically based and drafted along the lines of the "patient care plan" commonly used within the nursing profession. In almost all cases there will be (1) a set of goals or objectives indicating what the planners hope to achieve, (2) a description of behavior change strategies, media presentations, or other activities for achieving the goals, and (3) a plan for evaluating the results of the program in terms of its goals. However, despite better communication and more uniform patterns of professional training for health educators, there is frequently some confusion particularly in the use of terminology. One person's "program objectives" are likely to be someone else's "long-range goals" and yet another person's "program purposes." The situation is further complicated by the very worthwhile and more frequently occurring practice of combining health education activities with health service activities to effect a comprehensive attack on health problems. Here the ultimate purpose of the program may be expressed in health status measures, such as the "reduction of mortality by 20 percent," rather than in the learner behavior terms so familiar to school health educators. Probably the best technique for avoiding confusion is to develop the habit of examining the content and designated purpose of a particular program component while avoiding undue reliance on its label. The general form and purpose of commonly used components will be described in the following sections.

Statement of Purpose

Most written program plans begin with some sort of overview that describes its general purpose or direction and often gives at least some hint of the philosophical approach of the planning group. Such a section can be very useful to those persons responsible for implementing the program or to educators from other locales who are considering adopting of the program for their situation. For example, a plan for a high school unit on human sexuality might be directed primarily at short-term changes in behavior such as self-referral for symptoms of sexually transmitted disease (STD) or responsible use of contraceptives, or at more ambitious and positive long-range attitudes towards sexuality as a factor in human relationships. Each of these orientations would call for a different selection of program content and methods. One thing in common with many "overviews" or statements of "philosophy" is that they are difficult to formulate and thus it is not unusual, for example, for planning groups to state that their plan is based on a "positive concept of health" and proceed to focus all the learning activities on disease prevention. This is probably the result of adopting phrases that sound impressive without giving much thought to what they really mean. Planners should obviously try to avoid this mistake, while program consumers are well advised to check the various components for consistency before any adoption or implementation.

Goals and Objectives

Most program documents include a set of statements that describe in some detail the ultimate things the program is designed to accomplish. Most health education/promotion programs seek to (1) improve the learners' knowledge and/or attitudes in a way that will (2) improve their health behavior and consequently (3) improve their health status. However, as noted, modern programs are often combined with broader efforts that also seek to provide the target population with needed health services, material support—such as food supplements—and other essential items. Consequently, health education promotion planning documents may include at least five categories of goals and objectives.

Program Goal

A properly stated program goal is a single statement that clearly describes what the program is designed to accomplish. Although influenced by any needs assessments data, it is often more a function of the philosophy or mandate of the planning group. It is necessarily a broad statement and thus may or may not always be worded in a form that can be measured or tested. Consider the following examples from a K-12 school program and a community based program:

- The students will take action to protect and enhance their own health and the health of their community.
- Mortality from premature heart disease will be reduced 15 percent among the program participants within five years.

Health Objectives

A series of more specific and accountable statements, commonly termed health objectives, describe how health status is to be improved. Such objectives are also termed "outcome" objectives and represent the true "bottom line" of most programs. They refer to tasks that have intrinsic value in themselves; they are "ends" rather than "means." For example:

- Infant mortality will be reduced to 15 deaths per 1000 live births.
- Deaths from homicide among males aged 15 to 25 years will decline 50 percent.

Behavior and Learning Objectives

The assessment of educational, as distinguished from health, needs leads to two additional closely related sets of objectives, namely behavior objectives and learning objectives. Behavior objectives describe the actual things the program will encourage people in the target population to do or not do. Examples here include:

- Cigarette smoking among pregnant women will decline 50 percent.
- Arrests for weapons violations will decline 33 percent.

These behavior objectives provide guidance for the formulation of learning objectives describing the knowledge, attitude, or skill development changes the program will seek to put into effect as a means of encouraging favorable changes in behavior. Examples include:

- The clients can describe three actions that can alleviate a strong desire to smoke a cigarette.
- The clients can describe three methods of avoiding or repelling hostile attacks without the use of lethal weapons.

Both behavior objectives and learning objectives could also be termed "impact" objectives as they represent changes in the actions, capability, or feelings of the target population. They do not refer directly to health status but to the things that affect it; they are "means" not "ends."

Resource Objectives

Very often the members of the target population need more than improved behavior to care for their health. Health promotion programs seek to provide the essential services and material support. This recognition of resource needs leads naturally enough to a set of resource objectives stated in terms of what the program planners hope to provide, or hope to influence various agencies and organizations to provide for the target population. For example:

- Nicotine skin patches and related medical counseling will be provided for all clients whose smoking history and personal preference support this approach.
- The frequency of police patrols in neighborhoods that meet high risk criteria will be increased 50 percent.

Strategies

The selection of a basic strategy for the achievement of all or a portion of the program objectives represents the first operational decision for the implementation of the program. As used here, the term "strategy" refers to a general methodological approach that may encompass several learning activities, specific uses of the mass media, or other means of disseminating information or carrying out instruction. If the program objectives included the reduction of infant mortality within a particular population group, for example, the strategy selected might consist of recruiting neighborhood leaders and training them to approach and encourage the women of the community to refer themselves for prenatal care early in their pregnancies. This training process might involve the use of lecture, films, small group discussion, and role playing.

Learning Activities

The learning activities represent the heart of the program. Although many action-oriented health educators begrudge the time spent drafting goal statements or planning elaborate evaluation procedures, few quarrel with the importance of planning for instructional sessions where the actual encounter with students or clients occurs; this is recognized as the point where the "rubber meets the road." Skill in the development and application of learning activities is particularly important to the entry-level health educator who often has the help of more experienced colleagues in the planning process, but very often teaches alone. Consequently, chapter 7 treats this topic in some detail. The discussion in this chapter will be restricted to the role of learning activities within the total planning process.

There are two basic sets of decisions involved in the planning of instructional sessions: first the specific content must be selected; it most commonly takes the form of facts or concepts to be conveyed but may also include skills as with CPR classes or affective experiences such as those provided in assertiveness training; second, the learning activities must be planned in an effort to address the learning objectives and produce the best possible involvement of the learners with the subject matter. Within the broad context of an educational strategy many factors come into play in the selection or creation of learning activities. A few of the more important are:

- *Nature of the content.* For example, some content is mainly informational while others may be directed at attitudes.
- *Characteristics of learners.* Maturity and educational background make obvious differences.
- *Instructor ability.* Some instructors are far more skillful and comfortable with some techniques than others.
- *Theoretical orientation.* Some programs are committed to behaviorism, or to social learning theory and thus require techniques consistent with these approaches.
- *Available materials.* Some techniques require materials that may not be available.

Implementing the Program

The great variations in the size, scope, and specific objectives of health education programs produce parallel variations in the steps needed to get them "off the drawing board" and into action. These variations, however, tend to be ones of degree rather than of kind; generally the same tasks appear in one form or another. They include (1) the selection and training of staff; (2) acquisition of materials, equipment, and facilities; and (3) recruitment of learners into the program. A brief outline of this very complex process will be presented here.

Selecting and Training Staff

Ideally, the health education staff members who will actually conduct the educational instructional sessions will be involved in the planning process from the beginning. Unfortunately this is often not the case. Consequently, as early as possible in the program planning and development stage, staff should be hired or selected and included in the remaining planning efforts.

In the case of a small program the entire staff is often involved in the planning process; thus, orientation or special training is seldom required. But in a more typical situation, as in a large school district or city health department, the large majority of the instructors who must implement the program probably had little input into its formulation. In such circumstances, an appropriate in-service training function can serve three useful functions:

1. *Interpret the plan for instructors* (in terms of goals, objectives, methodology, and so forth) more effectively than mere reliance on written materials alone.

2. *Develop or strengthen needed competencies* in the form of subject matter (information or concepts), or teaching skills (discussion leadership or similar techniques).

3. *Generate enthusiasm and commitment to the program* by providing the stimulation inherent in the person-to-person contact of in-service sessions. This works far better than merely distributing the course guide via interoffice mail.

Acquiring Materials, Equipment, and Facilities

Health education programs typically involve the use of films, pamphlets, mannequins, textbooks, and other materials that must be purchased, rented, or in the case of free material, requested from the offering agencies. Locating, reviewing, selecting, and acquiring such materials is a time-consuming task, one that should be started as early as possible. It is very common for materials to be out of stock, for the necessary requisitions and other paper work to be out of order, for shipping delays to occur, or for borrowed or rented films to be delayed. With sufficient lead-time, delays can be managed, alternative sources can be found, or substitutions can be made with little disruption. Otherwise, program effectiveness can be seriously hampered, particularly when volunteers or inexperienced instructors are involved who tend to be more dependent on materials than full-time veteran staff members.

Similar advice applies to the arrangements for equipment and facilities. The need for sufficient space and enough chairs or desks for the classrooms or other meeting sites is obvious, yet it still takes some foresight to begin arrangements far enough in advance to handle unanticipated conflicts and problems. Also, one should make a special effort to identify any special needs in this area. If the program's methodological approach calls for small-group discussion, for example, then it is necessary to schedule meeting rooms with movable furniture. If films or videotapes are to be used, darkening curtains, along with projectors and extension cords, may be needed in some rooms.

Recruiting Participants

In many public schools, colleges, and universities, health education is mandatory; thus, the recruitment of students is not necessary. In such situations, however, the use of systematic evaluation techniques is recommended to demonstrate the merits of the program to the school board or other bodies that periodically review curriculum requirements. In some public schools and in many colleges and universities, health education is offered on an elective basis; consequently, the number of people reached by the program is dependent on its popularity with students and academic advisors. In most community settings and in many clinical and industrial settings, a similar situation prevails wherein participation is totally voluntary. Program quality no doubt merits priority concern; however, overall impact is also obviously affected by quantity—that is, by the number of people served. Attention to recruitment thus often becomes an essential part of the planning process.

In community settings, the recruitment task often requires the use of conventional publicity techniques such as press releases for newspapers, and radio and television public service announcements. It is also generally helpful to contact any cooperative service clubs, church groups, fraternal orders, or other community organizations whose members constitute part of the intended target population. This strategy is closely related to the time-honored practice of identifying and soliciting the help of indigenous community leaders who, although not bearing any formal titles, may nonetheless be highly influential. It can be particularly effective within target populations with low educational levels who tend to rely heavily on "word of mouth" communication.

Within narrower settings such as schools and corporations, publicity also is important, although lower-key methods are generally more appropriate. Information generally travels fast in these smaller organizations, and marketing techniques are of far less importance than intrinsic program quality as a factor in success. Here, the participants generally base their opinions on their perception of (1) how relevant the program seemed to be in terms of their needs and (2) how interesting it was in terms of subject matter and learning activities. It is both good marketing and good teaching to assess the learner perceptions early in the program and make adjustments if needed.

Administering the Program

In a world of limited resources, health education must maintain a high level of public and institutional support for its existence. At the same time there is a tremendous need for increased coordination of the various health education activities both between and within programs. Such coordination is also essential because the typical health education program is only one of several housed administratively in the same institution. Therefore, beyond the typical functions concerning personnel, budgets, schedules, and so forth, most health educators function to a greater or lesser extent in two basic additional administrative capacities: (1) promoting the program by preparing reports, preparing budgets and allocating funds, and participating in planning and policy development within the employing organization; and (2) coordinating the activities of the program by providing support for the staff, promoting cooperation and feedback among staff, facilitating staff activities, and assisting in the conduct of the program activities.

Promoting the Program

One of the major administrative functions health educators typically perform is promoting their programs. The ability of the administration and staff to communicate the needs, achievements, potential, and expectations of their programs is critical to the success of the programs. There is competition for every dollar, and if policymakers and others are not convinced of a program's merit, the money and attendant resources will be directed elsewhere.

One method health educators use to promote their programs is to prepare written reports and oral presentations. This function is often crucial to program acceptance. Decisions are sometimes made entirely on the basis of written reports; administrative attitudes toward a program also can be influenced by oral presentations. Not only policymakers, but health education professionals outside the program, and even the public at large, need to know about the activities of the program. The sponsoring agency might primarily be interested in how the program addresses broad health promotion goals, such as those in *Healthy People 2000* (USDHHS, 1990). Other health education professionals might be most interested in its theoretical basis, content emphasis, or specific learning activities. In any case, most of this information can be communicated in written or oral reports; these include informal memoranda, more official reports, and even scholarly presentations.

Coordinating Program Activities

Health education is often integrated into other functions and services. Most health education programs consist of a variety of subprograms aimed at different target groups, health problems, or behaviors. All of these efforts must somehow be coordinated so that there is minimal duplication and overlap, and maximum efficiency in the use of personnel and material resources.

Facilitation and Supervision

Within a health education program there are many critical coordination responsibilities. Among these are scheduling activities, assigning tasks to personnel, providing both material and emotional support to staff members, and facilitating cooperation and understanding among the various individuals and groups involved. There is seldom adequate money, facilities, or materials, and their allocation must be based on the relative benefits of the program. There is competition for learners, for prime time scheduling, and for staff time. Well-coordinated programs maximize productivity with minimum staff dissatisfaction.

In order to achieve success, the staff must work together. Conflicts and misunderstandings detract from the program. Cooperation and mutual support bolster the program's efforts. Therefore, health educators, especially those most involved with coordination, should spend considerable time working with staff members to promote cooperation and feedback, provide liaison between staff and others, and promote a broad understanding of the goals of the program and the need for everyone involved to work toward those goals.

Finally, health educators serve in supervisory capacities. Experienced health educators supervise neophyte professionals; other staff members supervise volunteers and support personnel; and administrators supervise the professional staff. Also, peer review is one form of supervision in which peers provide performance feedback to each other as a means of enhancing performances and also as a means of evaluation.

Summary

Simply stated, the task of health promotion consists of planning, implementing, and evaluating programs. This chapter focused on the planning component while viewing it in the context of the total process; it was discussed in terms of (1) assessing needs, (2) developing the components of the programs, (3) implementing the program activities, and (4) administering the program. In the abstract, the planning process appears simple and straightforward; however, once the planners address a real situation, the task soon becomes quite complex. Risk factors can be difficult to identify; when found they often involve human behavior that is complex and difficult to change; and even the ultimate goal, health status, lends itself to different interpretations. The historic struggle with these various challenges has prompted the development of a number of planning models that serve to guide the efforts of planning personnel. Currently the PRECEDE-PROCEED, MATCH, and PATCH frameworks appear as particularly useful tools. Health educators based in schools, colleges, and other highly structured situations can draw upon curriculum development technology for planning guidance. However, a good planning framework cannot take the place of good planning personnel; it can only make their work more efficient. Successful planning depends on the gathering of relevant information and on good decisions facilitated by the application of good judgment. Once the program has been developed on paper it must be implemented. Program implementation includes activities such as the selection and training of staff, the acquisition of materials and scheduling of facilities, and the recruitment of learners into the program.

The proper administration of a program is vital to its success. In addition to the obvious administrative tasks associated with personnel, budgets, and facilities, most health educators spend considerable time soliciting support for their educational activities and coordinating them with other health related programs.

Intervention Programming

Plans get you into things but you've got to work your way out.

—Will Rogers

Any time things appear to be going better, you have overlooked something.

—Anonymous

Introduction

In chapter 5 we considered general planning strategies. In this chapter we concentrate on a process for incorporating the findings from needs assessments, literature reviews, theory, and brainstorming into effective programs of intervention.

Intervention program development proceeds naturally from needs assessment. Assessment allows the planner to identify the most important target groups and select a reasonable number of objectives, giving the program focus and increasing its potential for success. Due to insufficient time and resources available to address all the possible factors influencing a health problem, the most important factors must be identified, and often only these can be addressed programmatically. Even when only a limited number of intervention objectives are addressed, awareness of the full range of important objectives allows the health educator to establish realistic expectations for the intervention and to interpret the results. Intervention effectiveness and program efficiency depend greatly on correct focus, and planning can increase substantially the likelihood that the program will have an impact on the target outcomes.

In this chapter we introduce MATCH (Multilevel Approach To Community Health), an approach to health promotion programming (Simons-Morton DG et al., 1988a). MATCH is a socioecologic planning framework that can guide the creation and implementation of effective health education and health promotion interventions when based on sound assessment and conducted within the context of planned programs. It can serve as a guide for how to get from needs assessment to effective programming. As a conceptual model, MATCH can be useful in situations where extensive local needs assessments are not possible due to the rapid pace of contemporary health education and health promotion practice. MATCH facilitates the health educator's ability to conceptualize, plan, develop, implement, and evaluate health promotion programs.

MATCH

MATCH, diagrammed in figure 6.1, is both a conceptual and practical intervention planning model. MATCH has been used for conceptualizing intervention research (Simons-Morton DG, Parcel and Brink, 1987; Parcel, Simons-Morton BG, and Kolbe, 1988), as a framework for workshops and conferences (Simons-Morton BG et al., 1988), for the development of health education and promotion graduate curricula, and as a guide for intervention (Simons-Morton BG and Simons-Morton DG, 1989). A marriage of the PRECEED and MATCH frameworks has been employed in a series of Centers for Disease Control Intervention handbooks on the prevention of smoking (Simons-Morton DG, Parcel and Brink, 1987), the promotion of physical activity (Simons-Morton DG et al., 1988b), and the prevention of alcohol-related health problems among adolescents and young adults (Simons-Morton BG et al., 1991a).

MATCH includes a set of five phases, each with several steps that can assist the planner in developing effective programs by establishing the links between health outcomes, intervention objectives, and intervention approaches. These steps are highly practical and provide a formula for creating and executing effective health promotion programming. MATCH is distinct from more general planning models in that it provides step-by-step procedures specifically created for health promotion program development. MATCH is a practical guide for developing interventions that have the greatest likelihood of achieving the intended impact on the program goals.

Ecological Conceptualization

Ecology is the study of the interrelationships among creatures and their environment. Health promotion can be thought of as a socioecologic perspective on health in that it is concerned with the range of psychosocial and environmental factors that influence health behavior and with environmental conditions that impact directly on health (Green and Johnson, 1983; Dwore and Kreuter, 1980; Minkler, 1989; Simons-Morton DG et al., 1988a; Simons-Morton BG and Simons-Morton DG, 1989).

Like other modern conceptualizations of health promotion (McLeroy et al., 1988), MATCH provides a socioecologic perspective and a basis for developing multiple interventions addressing both personal health behaviors and environmental conditions. MATCH is ecological in that it is an integrated whole, recognizing that the factors that influence health and health behavior are interrelated and occur at multiple societal levels. MATCH challenges the planner to **think globally** by taking into account the many behavioral and environmental determinants of health, but **act locally** by focusing on specific local actions. MATCH is ecological also in its emphasis on matching intervention objectives with the targets of the intervention and intervention approach.

Figure 6.1 MATCH: Multilevel Approach to Community Health

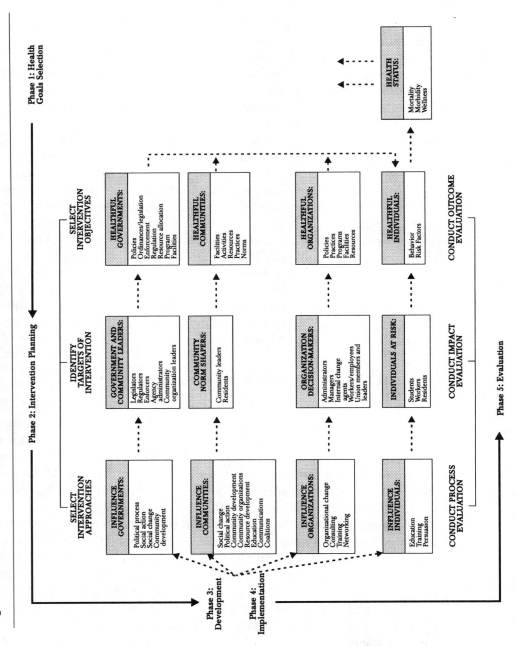

MATCH is designed to be applied when behavioral and environmental risk and protective factors for disease or injury are generally known and when general priorities for action have been determined, thus providing a convenient way to turn the corner from needs assessment and priority setting to the development of effective programs.

Intervention Planning

Health promotion planning starts by identifying a target population, health status goals, and personal health behavior and/or environmental factors related to these goals. To achieve the health status goals, intervention objectives can be targeted at the governmental, organizational, societal, interpersonal, or individual level or some combination of these. A range of intervention approaches can be employed at each societal level to achieve the intervention objectives, leading to improvements in the targeted health status goals.

Societal Level and Practice Settings

MATCH recognizes that intervention can be directed at five societal levels (e.g., individual, interpersonal, organizational, societal, governmental) and four practice settings (e.g., school, worksite, health care, and community). Objectives may be specific to any of the societal levels and applied to any of the practice settings.

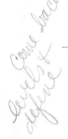

Individual-level health behaviors are substantially under the control of the individual. These include most personal health behaviors such as diet, exercise, and personal hygiene. However, owing to the influence of environmental factors on health behavior and on health itself (e.g. air pollution), objectives other than those mainly under the control of the target population are also important in health promotion.

The interpersonal level recognizes the influence of family, friends, and providers on health and health behavior. At the interpersonal level, we are concerned with the people who are known to the target population and with whom they have direct contact.

Organizational factors such as policies, resources, and programs influence health and behavior. Organizations include schools, churches, businesses, and industry. Most people belong to a number of different organizations and each organization may exert a different type of influence on its members. Many organizations, churches and schools for example, have the potential to be tremendous influences on health behavior.

Societal perspectives, trends, and support for health promoting programs, practices, and policies also are important. The societal level refers to groups of people to whom the target population relates. Members of such groups are not personally known to the target audience, but nonetheless are influential. Hence, one's friends and relatives belong to the interpersonal level, while one's general peer group, people who share some characteristics or beliefs, belong to the societal level. This peer group may be fairly local, for example seventh graders in a school, middle school students in a community, middle school students who smoke cigarettes, blue collar workers at a factory, blue collar workers who go to soccer games, or blue collar workers in general. Each person relates to many different societal groups, some of which are local and others that may be national or even international.

Government factors such as resources, programs, policies, legislation, and environmental controls are important influences on health and behavior. Some local, state, and national agencies are specifically concerned with health—for example, the environmental protection and child welfare agencies. Other agencies whose primary responsibilities lie outside the realm of health also have important health influences—for example, the U.S. Department of Transportation or U.S. Department of Agriculture. Because of their widespread influence, the policies and programs of these agencies are important targets for health promotion interventions.

Hence, a range of possible objectives at the individual, interpersonal, organizational, societal, or governmental levels may be targeted for programmatic attention, depending on the goals of the program.

Intervention objectives for any health problem can be organized according to practice settings. Four settings—school, worksite, health care, and community—have been identified as being especially appropriate for health promotion and disease prevention efforts (USDHHS, 1980). Each setting can help promote the health of the individuals who work or reside there. Because each setting is unique in certain ways, the features of effective programs also may vary by setting. Health promotion in the four practice settings is described in greater detail in chapter 15.

Intervention Targets

A unique feature of health promotion practice is that it focuses not only on the target population whose health is the concern of the program, but on other individuals who exert influence or control over the personal or environmental conditions that are related to the target health and behavior goals. In MATCH each intervention objective is identified as being controlled or controllable by the target(s) of the intervention. At the individual level, the target of the intervention frequently is the same as the target population. However, because health behavior is so often socially mediated, significant others—family members, peers, and friends—who exert a measure of influence over the target population also are possible targets of intervention at this level. At the organizational level, where the objectives focus on changes in organizational programming, policies, practices, or resources, the targets of the intervention are usually decision makers or program implementers. At the community level, where public knowledge, awareness, and attitudes are the objectives, the general population is the target of the intervention. At the governmental level the targets are decision makers, regulators, and enforcers.

Match Intervention Phases and Steps

As a practical program-planning guide, MATCH consists of five phases, each with several steps, as shown in table 6.1. The phases include:

- Phase I: Goals Selection
- Phase II: Intervention Planning
- Phase III: Program Development
- Phase IV: Implementation Preparations
- Phase V: Evaluation

Each phase represents one of the essential responsibilities of health educators and is an integral part of developing an effective program. The first four phases are described fully in this chapter. Phase V is briefly discussed here and described in detail in chapter 8.

Table 6.1 MATCH Phases and Steps

Phase 1: Goals Selection
    Step 1: Select health status goals
    Step 2: Select high-priority target population(s)
    Step 3: Identify health behavior goals
    Step 4: Identify environmental factor goals

Phase II: Intervention Planning
    Step 1: Identify the targets of the intervention
    Step 2: Select intervention objectives
    Step 3: Identify mediators of the intervention objectives
    Step 4: Select intervention approaches

Phase III: Program Development
    Step 1: Create program units or components
    Step 2: Select or develop curricula and create intervention guides
    Step 3: Develop session plans
    Step 4: Create or acquire instructional materials, products, and resources

Phase IV: Implementation Preparations
    Step 1: Facilitate adoption, implementation, and maintenance
    Step 2: Select and train implementors

Phase V: Evaluation
    Step 1: Conduct process evaluation
    Step 2: Measure impact
    Step 3: Monitor outcomes

Phase I: Goals Selection

Phase I includes the following four steps: (1) select health status goals, (2) select target population(s), (3) identify health behavior goals, and (4) select environmental goals. Typically, the most important health problems for a community or target population should be selected for programmatic attention and detailed intervention planning.

Each of the four steps in MATCH Phase I includes several considerations that are delineated in table 6.2 and described in the following paragraphs.

Step 1: Select Health Status Goals

Selection of health status goals should be based on the prevalence of the health problem and risk status of the target population, the perceived and actual importance of the health problem in relation to other problems facing the target population, the health problem's potential for change, and other considerations unique to the mission and priorities of the program. Usually, the health educator identifies an important health problem and then selects the target population according to age, gender, race, setting, location, or other considerations. Sometimes, however, the health educator may be interested in a particular problem, such as smoking or HIV prevention, and therefore will be concerned with the range of populations exhibiting high prevalence or risk status for that

---

Table 6.2 MATCH Phase I Steps

Step 1: Select Health Status Goals
   A. Prevalence
   B. Perceived and actual importance
   C. Changeability
   D. Mission, availability of programmatic resources

Step 2: Select High-Priority Target Population(s)
   A. Health problem prevalence
   B. Accessibility
   C. Programmatic interests

Step 3: Identify Health Behavior Goals
   A. Prevalence
   B. Association
   C. Changeability

Step 4: Identify Environmental Goals
   A. Access to services, products
   B. Availability of programs and resources
   C. Enabling policies, practices, regulations, opportunities
   D. Physical barriers, restrictions, protections

problem. Often a health educator is interested in the health problems of a particular age, gender, or racial group or a particular practice setting. In such cases the educator may be interested mainly in identifying the important health problems for that group.

Local data collection is the best way to identify the most prevalent and important health needs. Prevalence also can be established by extrapolating to the local situation from regional or national data sources and published literature reviews (the approach taken in the CDC Community Intervention Handbooks). Local needs assessments can also be developed on the basis of national data sets and published studies, thereby limiting costs.

Appropriate health goals for the target population may be derived from *Year 2000 Objectives For The Nation* (USDHHS, 1991), other national data sets, local needs assessments, and/or the health educator's professional interests and concerns. Health status goals normally provide the context for the program. Establishing the health goals gives the program focus, but it is not always essential for the program actually to have an effect upon the health goals, particularly if the population is young and the health status goals are distant. In situations where the health status goals are not immediate, risk and protective factors for the health problem become the end focus of the program. For example, chronic disease prevention goals for children will not be realized for several decades. Therefore, the goal of early education is to establish lifetime practices that will delay the onset of or prevent adulthood chronic disease.

Priority setting is not always an orderly process guided by data. Sometimes a health problem or target population is assigned priority based on the mission of the funding agency, or the whim of a powerful administrator, or in response to perceived public concern, rather than by evaluation of epidemiologic data. Nevertheless, data, whether collected locally or extrapolated from other sources, are often influential considerations in priority setting.

Logically, the range of important health goals, health behaviors, and environmental factors should be considered in terms of their importance and their potential for change (Green and Kreuter, 1991). Usually the most prevalent and severe health problems and risk factors should be given the highest priority for programmatic attention, assuming there is evidence that the problem can be addressed successfully. The changeability of a health problem can be determined by reviewing the research findings of studies on the **efficacy** and **effectiveness** of various intervention strategies. (Efficacy studies ask the question, "Does the intervention effect behavior change under optimal conditions?") (Effectiveness studies ask the question, "Under usual circumstances, to what extent does the intervention effect behavior change?") Important but not easily changed health problems merit less commitment of programmatic resources than more changeable problems.

Step 2: Select High-Priority Target Population(s)

The target population is the population group or groups about whose health the program is primarily concerned.

Prevalence. The target population may be those at high risk for the health problem or merely the population for whom the health educator is responsible or concerned. In public health it is usual to identify a major health problem first and then identify important target populations. It is not uncommon, however, to first identify a target population, such as pregnant teenagers or Hispanic women, and then to identify their important health needs.

Accessibility. The accessibility of the target population is a major consideration. The target population may be one for which the planners are normally responsible, for example teenagers or the elderly. The target population frequently is individuals who are accessible through a particular setting such as students at a school or in a school district, patients in a clinic or hospital, workers at a factory or corporation, or residents in a neighborhood or community. Target population selection may be based on comprehensive data collection and assessment or a local assessment of the needs of a particular group.

Programmatic Considerations. Programmatic considerations are important in the selection or identification of the target population. After all, the funding agent and the practice site have vested interests in certain target populations and health goals. Programs tend to reflect the mission and goals of the organizations in which they are located or which fund them. If the organization is concerned with aging then target populations may be limited to various elderly populations. Similarly, in public health departments, target populations often are established by public demand, political factors, or the availability of outside funding.

Step 3: Identify Health Behavior Goals

Those health behaviors that are most prevalent, most closely associated with the health goals in the target population, and changeable should be the highest priority for programmatic attention. Smoking, for example, is a prevalent health behavior that is known to cause lung cancer, heart disease, and other health problems, and research has established that it is possible to prevent smoking initiation and foster smoking cessation (Schinke, Botvin, and Orlandi, 1991). Hence, smoking is one of the highest priority behaviors for preventing these prevalent chronic diseases. Similarly, alcohol-related automobile accidents are a leading cause of injury and death among adolescents and numerous intervention methods are available to reduce the frequency of drinking and driving (Simons-Morton BG et al., 1989). Therefore, in adolescent health programs drinking and driving is a high priority.

Health behavior goals can be specified in a variety of measurable ways, as the examples show in table 6.3, thus giving direction and specificity to the program. Sometimes only the direction of change is specified, but when baseline prevalence and the efficacy of intervention is known, greater specificity can be provided.

If the health goal is to prevent lung cancer, and the target population is adolescents, specific health behavior goals might be to reduce the percentage

---

Table 6.3 Health Behavior Goals for Smoking, HIV/AIDS, Alcohol-Related Health Problems

---

Smoking

1. Delay onset: Reduce the increase over time in the percent of students who report smoking in the last 30 days.
2. Reduce prevalence: Reduce the percent of (pipeline) workers who smoke.
3. Increase prevalence: Increase the percent of smokers who practice halfway measures, limiting the number of cigarettes to less than (10, 5) per day, smoking no more than 1/2 of each cigarette, not smoking indoors . . .
4. Reduce magnitude: Reduce the average number of cigarettes smoked by the target population over the last week or month.

Alcohol

1. Delay onset: Reduce the percentage of 9th grade students who report consuming alcohol in the last 30 days.
2. Reduce prevalence: Reduce the percent of the target population who report driving after drinking in the last year and reduce the average number of reported drink/drive events.
3. Increase prevalence: Increase the use of designated drivers in situations where driving after drinking is likely.

HIV/AIDS

1. Reduce prevalence and frequency: Reduce the percent of IV drug users who shared unclean needles during the last month and reduce the average number of events.
2. Reduce prevalence and frequency: Reduce the proportion of the target population who had unprotected intercourse during the last month or year and the average number of such events.
3. Increase prevalence and frequency: Increase the proportion of the target population who regularly use condoms during intercourse.

---

of adolescents who had smoked ever in their lifetime, in the last thirty days, or in the last week. In a program focusing on adolescent drinking, the target risk factor goals might focus on age of initiation or the amounts and contexts of drinking. Examples of health behaviors to prevent alcohol-related health problems are "not drinking alcohol," "not drinking and driving," and "preventing friends from drinking and driving." A quantified health behavior objective might be "Within three years the percent of high school seniors (in the program, at a school) who report not drinking alcohol during the last thirty days will increase from 15 percent to 50 percent."

Step 4: Select Environmental Goals

Environmental factors may place the target population at risk, protect them from the health problem or from health-damaging behaviors, or promote healthful behaviors. A number of environmental factors may be related to the health and behavior goals. Of the many possible environmental factors, usually only a few high priority ones will eventually be selected as goals for programmatic attention. However, at this point in the process the idea is to list all relevant environmental factors that might be targeted for programmatic attention. Examples of selected behavioral and environmental risk factors for cancer, CVD, HIV/AIDs, and the prevention of injuries due to drinking and driving are included in table 6.4. Many of these factors could be expressed as protective factors; for example, unsafe roads are a risk factor while safe roads are protective; tobacco marketing is a risk factor while tobacco restrictions are protective.

Table 6.4 Examples of Behavioral and Environmental Risk Factors for Four Health Problems

Health Problems	Behavioral Risk Factors	Environmental Risk Factors
Cancer	Eating fewer than five fruits and vegetables daily	Marketing of foods that compete with fruits and vegetables
	Physical inactivity	Unavailability of facilities, programs
	Smoking	Tobacco product availability
Cardiovascular Disease	High-fat diets	Food marketing
	Physical inactivity	Unavailability of facilities, programs
	Smoking	Tobacco product availability
HIV/AIDS	IV drug use	Unavailability of clean needles; Drug availability; Unavailability of drug treatment programs
	unprotected intercourse	Condom unavailability; Lack of adult supervision
Injuries	Alcohol	Availability of alcohol
	Driving	Unsafe roads, vehicles
	Safety belt/harness use	Lack of passive safety devices

The presence of a particular risk factor is associated with an increased risk for a specific health problem. The presence of a protective factor is associated with a decrease in the risk for a specific health problem. Risk and protective factors are identified in epidemiologic investigations and their prevalence can be obtained for a target population by local data collection or extrapolation from regional or national surveys.

establish

The baseline rate or frequency of the risk or protective factor should be established and the goals quantified so that the amount of change desired or expected in a limited time frame is specified. A specified environmental goal for tobacco control might be "Within three years the proportion of local retail sales outlets that routinely sell cigarettes to minors will be reduced to 10 percent." Other examples include:

1. Within two years increase the availability of clean needles for IV drug users from 12 uses and 3 users per needle to 4 uses and one user per needle.

2. Within two years increase the availability of drug treatment programs from 1 space/100 needed spaces to 1 space/25 needed spaces.

3. Increase from 50 percent to 75 percent the users reporting that availability of condoms is not a barrier to regular use.

MATCH Phase I Example

In Phase I we *match* the target population with the health, health behavior, and environment goals to provide focus for intervention planning. An example of MATCH Phase I goals for a school-based health promotion program is included in table 6.5. The goal of the "Go For Health" program was to reduce the risk of cardiovascular disease among third and fourth grade students. The target population of preadolescent children was selected so that lifetime healthful diet and physical activity habits could be established just prior to the challenges of early adolescence when such habits are known to decay. Note that the health goals include both long-term (e.g., reductions in cardiovascular disease) and short-term (e.g., decreases in blood pressure and prevalence of obesity) objectives. Change in the health behaviors of the target population is targeted, as well as change in supportive behaviors of parents and change in environmental conditions, such as the food offerings of the school lunch program and the curriculum of school physical education.

Phase II: Intervention Planning

In MATCH Phase II, the health educator matches intervention objectives with the intervention targets and intervention actions. Phase II includes four steps: (1) identify the targets of the intervention actions, (2) select intervention objectives, (3) identify the mediators of the intervention objectives, and (4) select the intervention approach. Considerations for each step are included in table 6.6, and illustrated in table 6.7. As steps 1 and 2 are linked, either can come first.

Table 6.5 MATCH Phase I Applied to "Go For Health" Diet and Physical Activity Program

1. Health Goals
   A. Prevent cardiovascular disease in the future
   B. Prevent increases in cholesterol
   C. Prevent increases in blood pressure
   D. Prevent increases in obesity, fatness
   E. Prevent reductions in fitness

2. Target Population: 3rd-4th grade students

3. Personal Health Behavior and Interpersonal Factors
   A. Health behaviors
      1. Increase daily physical activity to 60 minutes
      2. Reduce calories from fat to 30%
      3. Reduce calories from saturated fat to 10%
   B. Interpersonal factors
      1. Parent factors
         a) Reinforce and support diet and activity
         b) Model and participate in healthful diet and physical activity
         c) Provide opportunities for healthful diet and physical activity
      2. Peer factors
         a) Social norms favoring healthful diet and physical activity
         b) Peer supportive actions regarding healthful diet and physical activity

4. Environmental Factors
   A. School lunch: Reduce fat and sodium
   B. Physical education: Increase amount of moderate to vigorous physical activity
   C. Classroom: Implement heart-healthy curriculum

Step 1: Identify the Targets of the Intervention Actions (TIAs)

TIAs are those who control or have influence over the intervention objective with which they are matched. For each intervention objective there can be one or several TIAs. TIAs may be identified at multiple societal levels as shown in table 6.7.

— *Societal level.* At the individual level the target population and the TIA are often the same. At the interpersonal level, those with potential to exert influence over the health behavior of the target population are targeted. Hence, persons close to the target of the intervention (family members, coworkers, friends, or teachers) and who influence target health behaviors or environmental factors are appropriate TIAs. At the organizational level the TIA may be an administrator or a teacher, day care worker, or nurse, depending on whether the

---

Table 6.6 MATCH Phase II Steps

Step 1: Identify the Targets of the Intervention
   A. Societal level
   B. Intervention objectives

Step 2: Select Intervention Objectives
   A. Prevalence, association, changeability
   B. Social level and target of the intervention
   C. Practice setting

Step 3: Identify Mediators of the Intervention Objectives
   A. Knowledge and skills
   B. Attitudes
   C. Practices

Step 4: Select Intervention Approaches
   A. Theory
   B. Objective, target, societal level
   C. Setting, channel
   D. Intervenor

---

objective is to have a program or policy adopted or implemented. At the societal level the TIA might be community leaders, and at the government level the TIA may be bureaucrats or policymakers.

Intervention objectives.   Selection of the TIA depends greatly upon the intervention objectives. In a program where the target population is adolescents and the health problem is an alcohol-related one such as injury caused by drunk driving, individual-level intervention objectives might include reducing the prevalence of alcohol use and the frequency of driving after drinking. At the interpersonal level, the TIAs might be the target population's friends or parents and the objectives might include peer protective behaviors and parental monitoring. Another intervention objective might be to implement an alcohol-use prevention curriculum, in which case the organization-level TIA would be the school administrators who approve curricula and the teachers who would implement it.

The concept of the TIAs is an important one because there are many influences on health and health behavior that are beyond the control of the target population. And while the health behavior of the target population is usually an important focus of health promotion programs, other objectives and therefore other TIAs are also important targets. Hence, each TIA is targeted for the intervention objectives over which they exercise some measure of control.

Often in health promotion the target of the intervention is another professional, such as a teacher, health worker, legislator, regulator, or enforcer who we want to adopt an innovation, take consistent action, better implement an existing program, or make available a certain resource. One intervention objective in a program to prevent drinking and driving related injuries among youth might be to implement a behaviorally based curriculum in middle school. Students would be the targets of the curriculum, which would focus on their health behavior and the mediators of their personal health behavior. But students would not be the only TIAs. At the organizational level the TIAs would include the school administrators who have authority to adopt such a curriculum and the teachers who have responsibility for implementing and teaching the curriculum.

It is crucial to identify those who can influence the intervention objective so that appropriate actions can be taken to facilitate its achievement. Intervening with those who are not in a position to influence the objective is ineffectual, and perhaps, unethical because it *blames the victim*. One aspect of blaming the victim is asking the target population to change something that is essentially out of their control; for example, encouraging sexually active youths to use condoms when they may not have access to condoms. Similarly, it is unfair to expect adolescents not to drink alcohol without also restricting their access to alcohol, providing more social alternatives to drinking, or altering adult drinking practices (Simons-Morton BG et al., 1989).

Of course, it is not uncommon that changes in health behavior or environmental goals require action on the part of a number of people. Therefore, as shown in table 6.7, a number of intervention objectives and TIAs may be targeted in a comprehensive program of intervention.

Step 2: Select Intervention Objectives

Intervention objectives are directed toward changing the target health behavior and environmental factors (selected from the list developed as part of MATCH Phase I, Steps 3 and 4).

Program success depends greatly on the selection and specificity of intervention objectives. For any health problem we can identify several possible intervention objectives from theoretical and logical considerations, literature reviews, and empirical needs assessments. Generally, programs that target multiple objectives at one or more societal levels are more likely to be successful. Because the intervention objectives provide the focus for programmatic activities, great attention should be given to their selection.

The criteria for making a behavioral or environmental risk or protective factor an intervention objective include (1) the prevalence of the factor, the strength of its association with the health goal, and its potential for change, (2) the societal level and TIA, (3) the practice setting, and (4) programmatic considerations. Of course, changing a risk or protective factor by itself may not assure a corresponding change in health or risk status, but it would be consistent with favorable changes. Identifying intervention objectives can be accomplished

Table 6.7 MATCH Phase II Objectives, Mediators, Intervention Approaches by Societal Level

Step 1	Step 2	Step 3	Step 4
Targets of the Intervention	**Objectives**	**Mediators**	**Intervention Approaches**
INDIVIDUAL - Students - Workers - Patients - Residents	Health behaviors	Knowledge Attitudes Skills Practices	EDUCATIONAL - teaching - reinforcement - counseling
INTERPERSONAL - friends - family - providers - important others	Practices Support Reinforcement	Knowledge Attitudes Skills Practices	TRAINING
SOCIETAL - citizens - activists - leaders	Programs Practices Policies Resources	Knowledge Attitudes Skills Practices	SOCIAL CHANGE - social marketing - resource development - social action - community organizing
ORGANIZATIONAL - decision makers - planners - implementers	Programs Practices Policies Resources	Knowledge Attitudes Skills Practices	ORGANIZATIONAL CHANGE - consulting - networking - organizational development
GOVERNMENTAL - decision makers - planners - implementers	Programs Practices Policies Resources	Knowledge Attitudes Skills Practices	POLITICAL ACTION - lobbying - policy advocacy - interest group pressure

through literature reviews and needs assessments; such a process is facilitated by the kind of understanding that comes from extensive involvement with a certain problem or population.

Prevalence, strength of association, and potential for change. The greater the prevalence of the risk factor in the target population the more important it may be as an intervention objective, particularly if the evidence linking the factor to a target health outcome is particularly strong and the potential for successful intervention is well established. Smoking, for example, is a fairly prevalent behavior that is strongly linked to cardiovascular disease, cancer, household fire injuries, and other health problems, and many successful interventions have prevented smoking initiation or helped people stop smoking. Physical inactivity is even more prevalent than smoking, with more than half the U.S. adult population basically sedentary. It is now well established that physical inactivity is an important risk factor for cardiovascular disease and other health problems. However, very little intervention research has been reported; moreover, the evidence that programmatic efforts can increase the proportion of a target population who exercise regularly is limited.

Societal level and TIA. Each intervention objective can be controlled or influenced by a certain group of people, not always the target population.

1. Individual-level intervention objectives. Objectives at this level are health behaviors of the target population. These may include all of the risk and protective factors identified in MATCH Phase I, Step 3, or more often a subset of these behaviors. Individual-level objectives may be considered appropriate for programmatic attention when they are consistent with the goals of the practice setting where the target population can be reached or where the program is located.

2. Interpersonal-level intervention objectives. Objectives at this societal level focus on the practices of people who are close to the target population and have the potential to influence health behavior or environmental factors. Objectives at this level may target peers' protective behavior, parenting style, class/student management, or coworker social support behavior, all of which involve influences on the health behavior or environment of the target population.

3. Societal-level intervention objectives. Societal objectives include the normative beliefs and practices of the general population of peers, neighbors, residents, and citizens. For example, the collective beliefs of a community about smoking and smoking control policies, or drinking and driving, have a great deal to do with the successful adoption of interventions to control these problems. The knowledge, beliefs, attitudes, and practices of the population with respect to smoking, drinking, and so on, form the prevailing social norms, and as such are potentially important intervention objectives. Of course, people are substantially influenced by local standards as well as by prevailing national standards. Hence, it may be important to develop objectives for the proximal societal level, for example, seventh grade students in a school, or blue collar workers at a particular factory, or church-goers in a community.

4. Organization-level intervention objectives. Objectives at this level include changes in or establishment of organizational policies, programs, practices, and resources that may protect against the target health problem.

5. Government-level objectives. Similarly, government-level objectives include changes in or establishment of local, state, or federal policies, programs, practices, and legislation. Such objectives include local government entities, such as the mayor's office, the city council, the school board, the housing agency, local zoning agencies, and others.

Practice setting. Intervention objectives vary by societal level and practice setting. Shown in table 6.8 are categories of intervention objectives at each

Table 6.8 Potential Intervention Objectives at Five Societal Levels and Four Practice Settings for Alcohol Misuse Prevention

	SETTING			
Level	**School**	**Worksite**	**Health Care Institution**	**Community**
Individual	abstinence; no DUI social norms for abstinence delayed initiation of alcohol use no riding with a driver who has been drinking	Abstinence, responsible drinking, no DUI social norms for responsibile drinking no riding with a driver who has been drinking	abstinence, responsible drinking, no DUI social norms for responsible drinking no riding with a driver who has been drinking	abstinence, responsible drinking, no DUI social norms for responsible drinking no riding with a driver who has been drinking
Interpersonal and Societal	conservative social norms	conservative social norms	conservative social norms	conservative social norms
Organizational	alcohol/drug curriculum policies banning alcohol at school events promotion of alcohol-free social events provision of rides to and from events alcohol-free gathering places	policies and practices: -written alcohol use policy -disciplining intoxication at work -limited alcohol at social events -required designated driver for social events programs: -worksite health promotion -employee assistance -supervisors trained in handling alcohol problems -increased health/accident insurance for DUI	policies and practices: -patient screening -counseling -education at routine and ER visits -providers educated in counseling for alcohol problems	server policies/practices: -no service to intoxicated patrons -no service to minors -designated driver policy -taxicab service sales practices: -no sales to minors -no sales to intoxicated persons
Governmental	required alcohol/drug curricula alcohol-program funding	funding for alcohol programs regulations for zero blood alcohol level for truck drivers	funding for: -provider education -service programs	enforce ban on sales to minors increase legal drinking age limit alcohol advertising laws to lower speed limits, seat belt laws legally required passive auto restraints: -airbags, safety belts warnings on alcoholic beverage containers

of the four practice settings for alcohol control. The objectives provided in this table are general and would need to be more specific for actual program design, implementation, and evaluation.

Programmatic considerations.   Naturally there are many programmatic considerations in selecting intervention objectives. Depending on the sponsoring organization, certain potential intervention objectives may be considered acceptable while others may be politically incorrect. A program to reduce drinking and driving, for example, may develop intervention objectives regarding public attitudes toward drinking and driving. However, if some of the organization's funding comes from sources loyal to merchants who depend on the current volume of beverage alcohol sales, targeting responsible drinking at local establishments may not be possible.

Step 3: Identify Mediators of the Intervention Objectives

The accomplishment of each intervention objective implies some change in the behavior of the TIA with respect to that objective, whether it is the health behavior of the target population or the implementation of a program by a health or education professional. Behavior change of all types is mediated largely by:

1. Knowledge
2. Perceptions
3. Attitudes
4. Values
5. Skills
6. Experiences
7. Reinforcement

Mediators are factors that are causally associated with the target behavior. Mediators are important objectives because altering them appropriately, all other things being equal, leads to a behavior change in the expected and desired direction. Hence, if a change in attitudes about using alcohol or exercising leads to a change in the frequency of these behaviors, such attitudes are mediators of that behavior. Because behavior is complex and influenced simultaneously by many variables, it is difficult to be certain that a particular variable is a mediator. However, on the basis of research and theory, we often have a very good idea which variables are likely to mediate change. Hence, in health promotion we normally work with hypothesized mediators. Mediators are best identified and specified by direct needs assessment, although literature reviews and theory sources are invaluable.

This discussion relates not only to individual-level personal behavior change, but also to interpersonal influence, organizational behavior regarding the adoption and implementation of policies and practices, community practice, and government-level behavior regarding the passage of legislation or the implementation of a policy or regulation. The TIA generally behaves toward the target objective in a manner that is consistent with their knowledge, beliefs, attitudes, and experiences. Hence, successful interventions affect the appropriate mediating variables sufficiently to produce behavior change. This is just as true at the interpersonal, organizational, community, and governmental levels as it is at the individual level, although the nature of the objectives is somewhat different.

Although the precise mechanisms are not fully understood at present, changes in behavior are mediated by changes in cognition and affect. Effective intervention is best guided by an understanding of the role of mediators in this process.

Knowledge and skills. Without knowledge, intentional behavior change is not possible. Knowledge alone may be insufficient to change behavior, but knowledge can be highly motivating and is an essential prerequisite to skill. Skills are important because they enable the learner to accomplish the behavior, should they be sufficiently motivated to try. Without skills the target population cannot overcome barriers to the target behavior.

Attitudes. Because attitudes are so important in motivation, they are frequently targeted in health promotion programs. Without favorable attitudes the target population is unlikely to be sufficiently motivated to take action. Changes in attitudes often precede a change in behavior, particularly when accompanied by changes in skills and environmental support for the target behavior.

Practices. Behavioral practices are important mediators because people learn by doing. People can know all about exercising, have favorable attitudes about exercising, and have some exercise skills, but they need to actually *practice* them for the learning to be effective. Similarly, teachers, health providers, and other health practitioners who may be the targets of health promotion interventions must be trained in relation to their daily practices, or the learning is unlikely to be inculcated. Indeed, only as these professionals attempt to implement aspects of health education into their daily practices can they fully understand the implications and potential of the intervention.

Mediators are changeable through usual educational processes. Educational programs are generally known for their ability to improve knowledge, change beliefs and attitudes, and alter practices. This is just as true for practices such as program implementation or policy adoption as it is for personal health behavior. Although examples of this relationship are better established for personal health behavior, there are ample examples of educational programs leading to changes in organizational, community, and government-level practices (Simons-Morton BG et al., 1991b; McLeroy et al., 1988).

Of course changes in mediators do not guarantee changes in behavior because the mediators are not the only determinants of behavior and not all mediators can be accessed by intervention. For example, many health behavior determinants are precursors rather than mediators. **Precursors** are factors associated with behavior, but which cannot be altered by usual intervention methods because they occurred in the past, are biological (e.g., genetics or natural ability), or otherwise are not mutable. Examples of precursors to behavior include socioeconomic status, race, age, personality, and previous experiences.

Extensive discussions of mediators are included in chapters 9 through 13. Educational objectives, which are more narrow than intervention objectives in their definition and scope, are based mainly on the mediational objectives and are the basis for specific learning activities, as discussed later in this chapter.

Step 4: Select Intervention Approaches

Intervention is an approach, process, or set of actions designed to encourage the TIAs to respond to or act upon the intervention objective by learning, deciding, or behaving. Hence, the intervention approach should stimulate the TIAs mainly by addressing the mediational variables of knowledge, beliefs, attitudes, skills, experiences, reinforcement, and the like.

Intervention approaches are conceptual—based on or adapted from theory or practice models or guidelines for change, as shown in table 6.9. The most commonly employed approaches are teaching, training, counseling, policy advocacy, consulting, organizational change, community organization, social marketing, lobbying, and social action (discussed in chapter 7). Some approaches are more appropriate for one level than another; for example, education at the individual level, organizational change at the organizational level, mass media at the societal level, and lobbying at the governmental level.

The art and craft of intervening is the single most important health education and health promotion activity. Health educators are known for their ability to organize and conduct a variety of intervention approaches, including education, training, mass media, and organizational change. The modern health

Table 6.9 Intervention Approaches at Four Levels

Individual (Education)	Organizational (Organizational Change)	Interpersonal/ Societal (Social Change)	Governmental (Political Action)
Teaching	Training	Media	Lobbying
Counseling	Consulting	Marketing	Policy advocacy
Reinforcing	Networking	Resource development	Interest groups
		Community organizing	

educator must be capable of employing and supervising the conduct of a wide range of intervention actions with a variety of TIAs.

Selecting an intervention approach depends on the specific intervention objectives. Each approach consists of a series of general processes for engaging the TIA. The approach is operationalized in the form of educational objectives and a series of learning activities or specific actions that the health educator can take to influence the TIA, thereby fostering the likelihood that the intervention objective will be achieved.

Theory. Each intervention approach is a series of methods and actions derived from theories and models of behavior change and applied to a specific health education situation. The health educator adapts the approach for the specific objective, target, channel, setting, and situation.

Because health promotion addresses a range of intervention objectives and TIAs, no one approach is appropriate for every intervention. For example, operant conditioning (reinforcement theory) is an important behavior change process that health promotion specialists employ frequently. It would not, however, be an appropriate approach to use with legislators when attempting to gain passage of a law requiring safety belt use, although elements of reinforcement are commonly employed in virtually all approaches to change.

Approaches such as teaching, training, organizational change, or policy development are general processes by which the health promoter engages the TIA. Theories describe the mechanisms by which change occurs, explaining behavior under a broad range of conditions. Each approach, theory, model, or guideline can be adapted for a limited range of applications. Some theories or models may be more appropriate for personal behavior change, others for obtaining quality implementation, engendering corporate decision making, or empowering citizens. The successful health educator is adept with a variety of change processes.

Intervention objective, TIA, and societal level. Selection of an intervention approach depends on the societal level, the intervention objective and mediators, and the target of the intervention. For example, at the individual and interpersonal levels, intervention approaches include teaching and counseling. At the societal level mass media and social marketing are appropriate. At the organizational level intervention approaches may include consulting, networking, organizing for change, and training. At the government level, intervention approaches may include lobbying, testimony, position papers, consultation, and social action.

The appropriateness of the intervention approach depends on the intervention objectives and TIAs. To promote the adoption of a curriculum by a school or school district, the health educator would raise the school administrators' awareness of the curriculum's effectiveness, ease of implementation, and low cost. To facilitate the implementation of a curriculum, teacher training and consulting is appropriate. Creating an environment that supports the objectives of the program and the curriculum requires parent training and organizational changes.

Setting and channel.   The approach to intervention may be influenced by the available practice setting or channel of communication (**communication channels** are the routes by which messages get to people, including print materials, interpersonally, or mass media), taking into account the unique characteristics of the TIA and the intervention objectives. Education, training, and counseling are possible only when the opportunity exists for multiple direct contacts with the target population, occurring usually in such formal settings as schools or health care facilities. Training is a common approach to facilitating practitioners' implementation of new programs or professional practices. When interpersonal intervention is not possible, less direct approaches can be employed.

Intervenor.   The experience, time, interests, and abilities of the intervenors are important considerations for the selection of an intervention approach. Each approach presents a framework within which behavior change might occur and specific intervention actions are chosen or created within that framework. Different health educators might develop an intervention approach somewhat differently. For example, there are a range of ways to teach adolescents how to resist peer pressures. This is because approaches, theories, and models of change provide the explanation of how change can occur and suggest some methods, but the health educator must fashion the actual intervention approach, develop specific methods, and carry out the learning activities (more about this in chapter 7).

PHASE III: Program Development

Phase III is concerned with program development, including the conceptualization and creation of program components, the development of intervention guides, and the selection or creation of materials.

Step 1: Create Program Units or Components

Many health promotion programs have several program components. All components of a program have in common the same health status goals, but may focus on different health behavior or environment goals, intervention targets, settings, intervention approaches, and in some cases different target populations. The considerations for component development are shown in table 6.10.

Under the best of circumstances, intervention programming is comprehensive, involving several or all practice settings and relevant risk factors. Unfortunately, such broadly focused programs are somewhat rare due to their cost and complexity. A broad focus, nevertheless, appears desirable, based on the promising results of the few comprehensive community programs attempted (Bracht, 1990). Even comprehensive programs, however, should recognize the

---

Table 6.10 MATCH Phase III Steps

Step 1: Create Program Units or Components
  A. Target population
  B. Targets of the interventions, intervention level
  C. Intervention objectives—health behavior, environment
  D. Structural unit
  E. Channel—interpersonal, mediated

Step 2: Select or Develop Curricula and Create Intervention Guides
  A. Goals and objectives
  B. Content
  C. Teaching and learning activities
  D. Materials

Step 3: Develop Session Plans
  A. Educational objectives
  B. Teaching/learning activities
  C. Materials
  D. Instructions, information, resources

Step 4: Create or Acquire Instructional Materials
  A. Review and select from available materials
  B. Develop materials
    1. conduct needs assessments
    2. pilot test
    3. produce

---

uniqueness of each practice setting. Typically, each setting, site, or unit becomes a separate program or a component of the overall program. Therefore, whether a program is devoted exclusively to one setting or several, it needs to develop interventions that are appropriate to the unique characteristics, potential, and challenges of the setting.

Each component of a multicomponent health promotion program may focus on a special part of the problem. Components are frequently organized according to target population subgroup (e.g., males, females, minority or age groups) objective (e.g., smoking, diet, physical activity), intervention target and level, setting and structural unit (e.g., classroom, food service, health services), or intervention approach or channel (e.g., interpersonal, media). Hence, separate components might be established for each of several settings.

Separate program components might be established within the same setting for different objectives, as shown by the example in table 6.11 for the "Go For Health" program (Simons-Morton BG et al., 1991b). The components employed in this school-based cardiovascular risk reduction program included

Table 6.11 Program Components of "Go for Health"

Objectives/ TIA/Approach	Classroom Instruction	School Lunch	Physical Education	Parent Education
Objectives	Improve student knowledge, skills, practices regarding physical activity and diet	Reduce fat and sodium in students' diets	Increase amount of daily physical activity	Encourage youth physical activity
TIA	Teachers	School lunch workers	PE teachers	Parents
Action	Training for curriculum adoption and implementation	Training for low-fat and low-salt menu and food preparation	Training to implement new PE curriculum	Educate parents
TIA	Administrators	Administrators	Administrators	None
Objectives	Adopt classroom curriculum	Adopt new school lunch menu, featuring low-sodium and low-fat meals	Adopt new PE curriculum	None

training physical education teachers and implementing a program of vigorous physical activity during physical education; training school lunch personnel and implementing low-fat, low-sodium school lunches; training classroom teachers to conduct a health education curriculum; and training parents to support healthful diet and physical activity. Hence, each component shared the same health status problem, target population, and health behavior goals, but the objectives, TIAs, and approaches were unique.

Step 2: Select or Develop Curricula and Create Intervention Guides for Each Component

The blueprint for each program component is a curriculum or intervention guide describing how the component is meant to work! Curricula provide outlines of each session, including the learning objectives, content, teaching/learning methods, and materials. Curricula may be written for use by the intervention target or health educator or other implementor. Intervention guides describe the purpose of the intervention, address its theoretical underpinnings, detail the content, methods, and materials, and explain implementation procedures. The intervention guide serves as the instructor's manual for the intervention.

Curriculum development is a demanding task. Curricula organize content into orderly sessions that fit the instructional period. Curricula can take a variety of organizational forms, but each is based on certain assumptions about learning derived from the approach, theory, or model employed by the curriculum developers. Examples of the curricula outline for the five components of the "Go for Health" program are shown in table 6.12.

Curricula are organized into units and sessions, which sequence certain content or behavior in an orderly manner. Usually, each contact with the TIA is a session, whether this contact occurs through an interpersonal channel (for example, counseling or teaching), or a mediated channel. For example, in the "Safety Belt Connection" program, a media campaign consisted of a series of informational leaflets and persuasive communications and several media events (Simons-Morton, Brink, and Bates, 1987). Each media event and each communication constituted a session. In an education program for high blood pressure patients, each patient could select one of six self-management sessions, each on a different topic, including medication taking, social support, and salt control (Reichgott and Simons-Morton, 1983). In a single-session burn prevention program, low-income mothers who were exposed to an informational cartoon in the waiting room of a health clinic were significantly more likely than the controls to report intentions to reduce the temperature of their tap water (Cardenas and Simons-Morton, 1993). A lobbying effort might consist of a series of letters and telephone calls to congressional representatives.

Step 3: Develop Session Plans

The session is the basic unit of a curriculum or intervention guide. Each session has educational objectives, teaching/learning activities, and learning materials (table 6.13).

Table 6.12 Curriculum/Intervention Guide for "Go for Health"

Third Grade Classroom Instructional Module Topics
    1. Healthful foods at school—10 sessions
    2. Healthful snack foods—10 sessions
    3. Healthful exercise—12 sessions

Fourth Grade Classroom Instructional Module Topics
    1. Healthful meals—10 sessions
    2. Healthful decisions—10 sessions
    3. Fitness fun—12 sessions

School Lunch—Year Long
    1. Menu planning guide
    2. Food purchasing guide
    3. Recipe selection/development guide
    4. Food preparation guide

Physical Education—Year-long Units; daily
    1. Walk-jog-run
    2. Aerobic games
    3. Aerobic sports
    4. Aerobic dance

Parent Education
    1. Parent newsletters
    2. Family fun runs at school on weekends
    3. Informational leaflets mailed home
    4. Student curriculum activities involving parents

Intervention guides for organizational, social, or political change processes cannot always be developed with as much detail as can guides for more standard personal behavior change or training curricula. Nevertheless, typically they include in some form objectives, content, materials, and learning activities.

Step 4: Create or Acquire Instructional Materials, Products, and Resources

In many cases materials or products must be developed, purchased, or modified and made available for the session. Among these are print materials (books, booklets, leaflets, brochures); mediated messages, and reminders (posters, announcements, audio tapes, etc.); and model proposals, policies, and laws.

Sometimes these materials constitute a major part or even the entire innovation for which adoption and implementation is sought. For example, in a program to prevent injuries due to drinking and driving by young persons,

Table 6.13 Session Plan for "Go for Health"

Objectives	Teaching/Learning Activities	Material
By the end of the session the learners will be able to . . .		
1. Distinguish low- and high-fat foods	On the board students list and categorize foods they eat	List of fat content of foods
2. Identify low-fat foods that are personally acceptable for breakfast, lunch, and dinner	On form provided students list acceptable low-fat foods for each meal	List of low-fat foods; form for listing acceptable foods
3. Initiate a food log	Using an overhead, describe the procedures for completing the food log; have students complete one for previous meal	Food log; instructions

one objective may be to implement a curriculum. If an appropriate curriculum exists, then the objective can be to implement that specific curriculum. If none exists, one must be created by either the staff health promotion specialist, or other capable professionals, or a collaboration of the two.

Similarly, if the intervention objective is to establish an alcohol-free senior prom, the product to be developed is a specific proposal for such an event at a specific high school. As part of the proposal's adoption process, key school and community leaders may be targeted and asked to become involved in creating, modifying, and adopting the proposal. For an intervention objective for youth group leaders to reinforce non-drinking among youth, product development would consist of creating the peer leader training and support. If the intervention objective were to provide persuasive communications to youth about drinking and driving, product development would focus on creating the specific messages. If the intervention objective was to provide protective barriers along a particularly dangerous roadway, product development may involve identifying or creating a practical plan that can be proposed to the city council or county administrators. Hence, product development is an essential step in the intervention process.

Product/materials development is a demanding task requiring a range of skills and great attention to the practical needs of the potential users. Sometimes the appropriate intervention objective is to adopt an existing intervention package or product, such as a curriculum or public service announcement (PSA). In other situations, it is necessary to create such an innovation and then seek its adoption, dissemination, or diffusion. Sometimes the appropriate intervention objective is to have others create the intervention materials.

Phase IV: Implementation Preparations

Upon completing MATCH Phases I and II, and III, the health educator is now ready to plan implementation and conduct the interventions (see table 6.14).

Step 1: Facilitate Adoption, Implementation, and Maintenance

A new program or program component, like a new business, has a high likelihood of failure. New programs rarely receive adequate resources and must justify additional resources on the basis of performance. New programs lack the benefit of the kinds of practical experience that can make them more effective and efficient and must be refined over time. New programs often do not initially have the support of other providers, professionals, and participants, which hinders recruitment and continuity. All these disadvantages serve to emphasize the importance of careful planning to establish conditions favoring adoption and implementation of the program.

To achieve effective implementation planners must (1) develop a specific proposal, (2) develop the need, readiness, and environmental supports for change, (3) provide evidence of the efficacy of the intervention, (4) identify/select change agents and opinion leaders and convince them of the need for change, and (5) establish constructive working relationships with decision makers.

Keep in mind that implementation requires the cooperation of others. Even if you are the intervener, you will need the approval of your supervisors and the decision makers at the institutions where the program is to occur. For example, if you work as a health educator for the public health department and you want to initiate a smoking cessation program for mothers attending prenatal clinics within the health department, you would need approval from your supervisor, the clinic directors, and the medical and nursing directors.

Table 6.14 MATCH Phase IV Steps

Step 1: Facilitate Adoption, Implementation, and Maintenance
  A. Develop proposal and advocate for adoption of change
  B. Develop need, readiness, environmental supports
  C. Provide evidence of efficacy
  D. Identify/select change agents and opinion leaders
  E. Establish support and constructive working relationships

Step 2: Select and Train Implementors
  A. Train, provide opportunities for observation and practice
  B. Monitor and support

— *Develop a proposal.* The basic document of the implementation plan is a proposal. This proposal may be very brief, only a few pages in some cases, or quite extensive. The purposes of the proposal are to document the need for change, describe the intervention, obtain input and approval from experts and decision makers, resolve any conflicts with institutional policies or practices, and obtain authorization for resources, such as the intervener's time, space, and materials. The proposal should include an abstract or short description of the program, justification of the need for the program, documentation of the potential effectiveness of the intervention, and a description of the resources needed. Potential effectiveness can be established by citing evidence from the literature or demonstration programs, or on theoretical grounds. Appended to the proposal should be the curriculum and protocols.

— *Develop the need, readiness and environmental supports for change.* Change in personal health behavior or adoption of a program innovation takes time. Develop a readiness to change by preparing people in advance of the program's introduction. Carefully identify and deliver the kind of messages that will build enthusiasm about the new idea or program.

   Environmental supports can be social and physical. If the TIAs believe that other people—peers, employers, important others—support the change, they are more likely also to support it. Physical conditions also can support or hinder change. Work to make the timing, location, and facilities supportive of the change.

— *Provide evidence of the efficacy of the program component.* TIAs are naturally dubious about the efficacy of new programs and must be convinced that the program can work. At the individual level this might mean providing a relevant (model) of someone who has experienced the intervention and whose behavior has happily changed for the better as a result of this exposure. At the organizational or community level, efficacy may be demonstrated by documenting the success of other similar programs or by conducting a small pilot program in which efficacy can be demonstrated.

— *Identify/select change agents and opinion leaders.* Usually, a program will only be successful if the opinion leaders within the organization or target population support the change. If the opinion leaders are for it, others are likely to follow. Opinion leaders are usually interested in constructive change, are easier to reach than others, and tend to be good communicators, hence they are the natural targets with whom to start intervening. They must be identified, convinced of the need for change, and recruited to aid the effort.

— *Establish support and constructive working relationships.* No program can succeed or persevere without the support of the participants, including organizational and population leaders, health and education professionals, and the target population itself. One of the most important conditions for effective implementation is establishing constructive working relationships with those involved or affected by the program, including those from whom you expect to receive referrals and those who control important resources, such as space needed by the program. Identify these important individuals and decide how to present the program, emphasizing its advantages to these individuals and its compatibility with their interests. It is frequently valuable to identify those who can influence their colleagues to adopt or accept the program, and work to obtain their support.

Step 2: Select and Train Implementors

The quality of program implementation depends on good training. If an experienced health educator is conducting the sessions, then practice may be the most important training activity. If less qualified individuals are to conduct the sessions, more extensive training may be necessary. The goal of training should be the mastery of relevant skills by the participants.

Quality control depends on process evaluation and feedback to the conductors. The quality of implementation tends to diminish over time, so maintenance activities are useful. These may include reminders or other reinforcing messages, observation and progress notes or other forms of feedback, and long-term goals.

Phase V: Evaluation

Phase V consists of three steps—process evaluation, impact evaluation, and outcome evaluation (table 6.15). These steps are discussed briefly in the following paragraphs and in more detail in chapter 8.

Table 6.15 MATCH Phase V Steps

Step 1: Conduct Process Evaluation
  A. Recruitment, planning
  B. Session/program implementation
  C. Quality of the learning activities
  D. Immediate outcomes

Step 2: Measure Impact
  A. Mediators
  B. Behavior and environmental outcomes
  C. Side effects

Step 3: Monitor Outcomes
  A. Health outcomes
  B. Cost effectiveness
  C. Policy recommendations

Step 1: Conduct Process Evaluation

By evaluating the intervention process, health educators can learn how to improve future implementations. The process evaluation plan is concerned with the utility of the implementation plan and procedures, the extent and quality of implementation, and the effects of implementation on immediate learning outcomes. Here we are concerned with developing procedures for evaluating the quality of the curriculum, sessions, and materials work; the utility of the recruitment and promotion activities; the quality of the facilities and equipment; and the quality of the conduct of the sessions. In short, to what extent were learners exposed to the intervention, what was the quality of that exposure, and, perhaps, to what extent were the session objectives met? Hence, the process evaluation may include procedures for measuring the immediate cognitive and affective learning outcomes that were the objectives of the sessions. Process evaluation must be planned, because the evaluation methods and procedures need to be in place before implementation.

Step 2: Measure Impact

Impact evaluation is concerned with changes in the targeted mediators, health behaviors, and environmental factors. Instruments to measure the mediators of knowledge, attitude, and practice are common. Of course, environmental changes and changes in complex behavior typically occur over time as a product of cumulative exposure to intervention. Therefore, we are interested in evaluating the impact of the educational program once the target population(s) has been sufficiently exposed. Often the measures of the target health behaviors have already been identified and the evaluation need only specify the design for measuring it.

Step 3: Monitor Outcomes

Outcome evaluation is typically concerned with health outcomes, but in some cases it focuses on long-term maintenance of changes in behavior or environmental factors. Because health outcomes are sometimes achieved in the distant future, they are not always evaluated. However, health outcomes are the best evidence of program effectiveness and the evaluation plan should include a reasonable approach to their assessment.

By evaluating the *impact* of our interventions we can learn the extent to which they achieved their immediate objectives. By evaluating the *outcomes* of our interventions we can learn the extent to which they achieved their health status goals.

Summary

MATCH is an intervention planning guide according to which information is compiled from needs assessments and used to develop an intervention plan.

In MATCH Phase I the most important health status goals, health behavior goals, and intervention objectives are selected for programmatic attention. In Phase II the intervention targets, objectives, and approaches are selected for programmatic attention. Generally, intervention objectives are controlled by certain key individuals, called the targets of the intervention actions (TIAs). They may be those whose health and health behavior are in question (the target population), or they may be important others, community leaders, organizational or governmental decision makers, or program implementors. The intervention objectives and TIAs are *matched* with an intervention approach. Intervention approaches such as teaching, training, social marketing, community organizing, and lobbying must be adapted for use in a particular program component. In Phase III the components of the program, usually including a curriculum and intervention guide with attendant materials, are developed and training is planned. In Phase IV, preparations and procedures for implementation are established. Phase V focuses on process, impact, and outcome evaluations.

Chapter 7

Intervention Actions

*I never teach my pupils. I only attempt to provide the
conditions in which they can learn.*

        —Albert Einstein

Introduction

In this chapter we describe the range of intervention actions popularly employed by health educators to promote the health of target populations. These intervention actions include the following: (1) teaching, (2) training, (3) counseling, (4) consulting, and (5) using media. Organizational change is addressed in chapter 12 and community and social change approaches are addressed in chapter 13. Some professional health educators are only teachers, or only consultants; many health educators practice a range of intervention actions. Over the period of a career, every health educator is likely to be involved to some extent with each of these intervention actions.

  Teaching is the foundation for many other intervention actions; consequently, a substantial portion of this chapter is devoted to the traditional concerns of teaching. Training is a special form of teaching, focusing on teaching health and education topics to health and education professionals and laypersons. Health counseling is a form of teaching that involves the counselor (health educator) and client (learner) in an intimate, interpersonal interaction directed toward the goal of personal growth, problem resolution, or behavior change. Consulting is a unique process, but the relationship of the consultant to the client is not wholly different from the one between the teacher and the student. The actual consulting process resembles other health education processes. Working with communications and media is typically a function integrated into health teaching, training, and consulting. Some health educators, however, are health communication specialists.

Teaching

In chapter 4 we described education as one of the foundations of health education and health promotion. In the following pages we draw heavily upon our educational foundations in discussing the process of teaching in health education. Teaching is one of the fundamental human occupations. From birth, humans encounter teacher after teacher. Parenting, for example, is the most universally practiced and certainly the most important and influential teaching role in human civilization.

Teaching is the primary responsibility and foremost professional concern for many health educators. Teaching takes place in schools, hospitals, clinics, communities, and industries, involving students, patients, residents, and workers. In most cases health educators teach a group of learners at one time, but there are many one-on-one teaching situations as well. As teacher, the health educator is interested in how students learn and how best to facilitate this learning. As with all teachers, health educators are most interested in the strategies, methods, and materials that they can put to use immediately in their teaching.

Naturally, any process as important as teaching has received the critical attention of many worthy scholars. Needless to say, a great deal is now known about how to teach because so much is now known about how people learn. However, there are many unsolved mysteries concerning learning and, accordingly, teaching remains as much an art as a science.

There are two principal actors in every educational experience—the learner and the educator. The process is necessarily an interactive one. The educator does more than just communicate what she or he knows to learners, although this is sometimes the case (as in a lecture). Sometimes the learner communicates what she or he knows or wants to know to the educator, or shares it with other learners, making the distinction between the educator and the learner less clear.

This interaction between educators and learners has been conceptualized in a number of ways. For example, the literature on persuasive communication attempts to explain how a communicator gets his or her point across to a recipient (learner). Persuasion is one of the foundations of modern health education practice in that the credibility of the messenger and the nature of the message are factors in learning.

Another major conceptualization of this process is education as a special form of group process. From this perspective, the teacher is the facilitator of the group. How well the health educator facilitates the group learning experience is a major factor in how much learning takes place. In this conceptualization the learner has the major responsibility for what is learned. The teacher is an agent, an advisor, a consultant. This way of looking at teaching probably comes close to how many health educators perceive the role of teacher.

There are many notions or models of the process of teaching. All of them make assumptions about the nature of learning and the role of the teacher. Most health educators, thrust into various learning circumstances, adapt their teaching approach to the situation. To do this well, the health educator must first learn to recognize and respect the internal capabilities of the learner and the external conditions required by the learner. Second, the health educator must learn how to employ a variety of educational methods to achieve optimal learning outcomes.

The Learner

Learners may be students, health professionals, parents, or patients. All learners, however, tend to share some common characteristics.

Motivation

Assume that those who show up for a course or enroll in a program are motivated to learn. They may not appear to be motivated and they may not be motivated in obvious ways, but most people would prefer to learn than not, and if we provide the proper environment and experiences, learning will occur.

Not surprisingly, this natural motivation asserts itself under conditions that take into account the learners' interests, needs, and experiences. Almost by definition people are motivated to learn about what they are interested in, what they feel they need to know, and what is relevant to their own personal experiences and circumstances. Moreover, success in learning is motivating, while failure defeats motivation (Bandura, 1986). Hence, education is a task of finding out how to work with learners' existing motivations and how to enhance motivation to learn.

Self-Esteem

People do not like to appear to be stupid, admit ignorance, or be put in situations that are threatening to them. Learning means admitting that you do not understand or are not able to do something and this can be threatening to the learner's self-esteem. Of course, some learners are more threatened than others, but learners generally protect their self-esteem, giving themselves over to the task of learning only when satisfied that their self-esteem is not going to be seriously threatened. Those students with low self-esteem may be especially difficult to work with because they have learned to defend against attacks to their self-esteem, often by not trying.

Learning environments that are respectful of the learner and learning experiences that provide frequent feedback for incremental accomplishment enhance esteem. In short, a supportive, safe environment oriented toward success and relatively free of stigma against failure reassures the learner and allows his or her motivation to overcome concerns about esteem.

Empty Vessel

Assume that the learner is *not* an empty vessel into which information and skills can be poured. The learner possesses a reservoir of previous learning and experience. Often in health education, the subject matter we deal with includes not only knowledge, but also beliefs, attitudes, values, and behavior. For many health-related subjects, learners may have experience with the behavior and thus may have developed beliefs, attitudes, and values toward it. Everyone is an expert on personal health because it is such an important part of each person's daily life, and learners have much to share on these subjects. But health behavior can be highly personal and learners may be reluctant to discuss their personal lives in environments that they do not perceive to be safe. Nevertheless, the personal experiences of the learners are important in the learning process.

Individual Differences

Assume that each learner is a unique human being. Substantial individual differences exist between learners, some of whom learn more quickly than others. Previous learning influences the pace of new learning. An important challenge in education is to start with each learner where he or she is at on the learning curve and take the individual from that point to mastery and excellence. It is also important to understand that people learn in different ways. Some learn best through reading, others from experience, still others by group process, or by reading and then discussing in groups. For some, audiovisual aids are essential, for others they are a hindrance. Some people need examples, others need to put it in their own words. The preference for certain learning styles is as true for adults as it is for children. Considerable evidence suggests that learners fare a lot better when teachers vary their teaching style.

Many target populations in health education have low literacy skills and have a history of mainly unsuccessful learning experiences (Doak, Doak, and Root, 1985). In addition, health education often must compete with demands on the learners' attention from illness, medical procedures, economic hardship, and so on. These unique circumstances and individual characteristics must be taken into consideration.

The Health Educator as Teacher

Teachers are responsible not only for imparting information, but for providing an environment conducive to learning. In planning and developing the curriculum and teaching sessions, the teacher establishes the conditions for learning, selects certain teaching-learning methods, and conducts the sessions.

Establishing the Conditions for Learning

A great deal of educational research has been concerned with the objective description of the conditions under which learning is likely to take place. This is a serious body of literature from which we can glean a few guidelines for use in this chapter. What is striking about this literature is how consistently certain characteristics or principles are found to influence learning. These principles are noted in virtually every textbook on education.

The list below is representative of the basic conditions for learning which organizations and educational programs should facilitate and assure.

1. The learner understands the objectives of the educational sessions.
2. Instruction proceeds from the known to the unknown and from the simple to the complex.
3. Information and skills are supported with meaningful methods, including examples, practice, and feedback.

The learner should know what he or she is expected to learn. This is best accomplished by developing learning objectives for each course and each session. Instruction should proceed logically from what the learners already know to what they need to learn. One purpose of curriculum development is to organize the content in a logical and progressive manner. Teaching methods should be appropriate for the content. Courses constructed according to these conditions should provide students excellent opportunities for learning.

Selecting Methods

Teachers influence learning by selecting teaching methods for use in developing specific learning activities to address specific learning objectives. Methods are sometimes called **teaching-learning** methods because they are selected by the teacher to achieve the educational objectives and they are engaged in by the learner. Learning activities are the application of teaching methods to specific learning objectives. Many teaching methods are useful in a range of learning situations and theoretical approaches.

Methods are the critical tools used in the teaching/communicating/ facilitating process of health education. Among health educators, discussions of methods tend to be animated and conference presentations on methods are frequently crowded. Methods are exciting to health educators who are involved in their use daily and who recognize that skilled application of methods motivates learning. The following observations provide a general background for the selection of health education methods.

Theory and methods. Methods are drawn from many theoretical approaches. Methods such as lecture, guided discovery, practice, and role play are drawn from cognitive and affective theories. Methods such as goal setting, reinforcement, and feedback are based on operant conditioning. However, methods should be selected because they are appropriate for specific learning objectives, not because they are consistent with a theory.

Learner references. Learners have unique backgrounds, abilities, and interests and prefer to learn in different ways and at different paces. Hence, it useful to utilize a variety of methods to increase the likelihood of engaging every learner at least some of the time.

Methods and objectives. Methods are useful to the extent they can be adapted to address an educational objective. The subject matter and objectives frequently suggest or require particular approaches. For example, factual information is best transmitted by lectures and printed materials; skills are best taught by demonstration, practice, and feedback. Attitudes are best influenced by visual and experiential methods.

Continuity. At least some of the same methods should be employed in each of the sessions or interventions that comprise a program component. This serves to tie the sessions together. Learners become more efficient and capable as they gain experience with a teaching-learning method.

Methods and learning activities.   Numerous and diverse methods already exist and new methods are rarely developed. However, a great deal of teaching skill is required in the process of adapting methods for specific learning strategies. When a health educator studies an area of concern the theoretical and research writings on the subject provide logical methods for use in an applied program. The work of the health educator is to digest this information and adapt the appropriate methods to his or her particular needs. The literature will usually reveal how these methods have been successfully employed in published programs.

Typically, any health education program could employ with some degree of success any of several methods. The best methods and learning activities are those that best facilitate the accomplishment of the objectives. But how can we know this before the program begins? Unfortunately, we rarely have complete confidence in the methods selected before they are converted to learning activities and tried in actual practice. However, we can improve the likelihood of success by approaching the selection of methods in a systematic manner.

For much-studied topics like smoking cessation or weight control, certain methods have been demonstrated to be more useful than others regardless of the target population or the conditions of the educational program. However, the literature on other health problems is seldom this consistent. In most cases, the literature does not account for the specific situation confronted by the health educator. Furthermore, learning activities are almost never described in detail in research articles and other literature, with the possible exception of a few textbooks. Hence, the teacher must be creative in developing learning activities to address specific methods.

Applying Methods

Every method has a range of applications, depending on the techniques used to employ the method. The same method directed toward the same objective by five different teachers will invariably be applied five somewhat different ways due to the technique employed. Even if several of the teachers jointly developed the method for the same objective, the conduct of the learning activity undoubtedly would not be the same. Techniques can be learned since they are a matter of skill. There are courses in most universities on how to conduct groups, how to be a persuasive communicator, how to provide reinforcement, how to organize community groups, and so on. Mastery of the tools—the methods of teaching—is essential to the success of the practicing health educator. Dewey (1916:212) put it this way:

> Methods of artists in every branch depend upon thorough acquaintance with materials and tools . . . Part of his learning, a very important part, consists of

becoming master of the methods which the experience of others has shown to be most efficient in like cases of getting knowledge.

The selection of methods and their adaptation into learning activities may depend on a rather complex and interrelated set of practical conditions described in the following pages under these headings: (1) set, (2) setting, and (3) situation. It is the *gestalt* or total picture of the learning circumstances that leads the health educator to the most appropriate methods.

Set.   The educational set includes the goals of the program, the nature of the behavior, and the characteristics of the target population. At the broadest level, set refers to the role of the educational program in the total scheme of life-long learning about health. For example, the program may be part of a kindergarten through twelfth grade curriculum directed at health knowledge and attitudes which is intended to build on past learning, anticipate future learning, and take into account the developmental learning needs of the students. Conversely, the program may be a one-shot public health information effort such as for flu vaccinations. Certainly, methods used would vary according to the goals of the program. For example, some of the methods selected to encourage high school students to eat healthy snacks would be different from those selected to encourage the elderly to obtain flu vaccinations.

The nature of the target health behavior is also a component of set. For example, weight control and other eating-behavior changes require behavioral methods because they are heavily influenced by environmental factors. For these behaviors, modifying stimuli and providing reinforcement has been demonstrated to be more effective than cognitive methods alone.

The learner is an important consideration because people learn in different ways. Adults have life experiences into which new knowledge can be incorporated. The elderly and the young have special learning needs which impact on the methods selected. The elderly generally prefer little time pressure. Within limits, children often like the excitement of timed games and physical activities. Cultural background must also be taken into account when developing strategies and selecting methods. Learning styles differ not only between the groups mentioned, but within these groups as well. For example, some learners prefer group activities while others do better working alone.

Setting.   The setting includes the location of the program. The environmental and cultural conditions of a school are different from those of a hospital, a public health clinic, a community organization, or a company. Settings such as a doctor's office provide an opportunity for learning that arises more or less spontaneously and should be capitalized upon to the extent possible because there is little time for structured intervention. Settings such as classrooms require or allow highly structured and elaborate instructional procedures.

Situation.   Situational considerations are practical in nature. How much time is available for the educational sessions? How frequently will the learner be exposed to the education? Can the learner read and how well? What staff, budget, and equipment are available? Is there enough lead time for adequate preparation? Do you have the experience and energy to do it? In the real world, health educators have too little money, too few staff, and too much to do. Given a health education task, the educator must select methods that are realistic and practical. It may be effective to give hypertensives sphygmomanometers to provide frequent blood pressure feedback, but is it realistic? Who will pay for them? It would be nice to demonstrate the proper use of infant car seats to new parents, but is it a justifiable use of staff time when simpler messages would reach more people? Perhaps it would be beneficial to conduct one-on-one life-style counseling with cardiac patients, but if the health education staff is not trained to do this type of counseling, another approach might be more reasonable.

Conducting the Teaching Sessions

So far we have discussed two major direct influences of the health educator/teacher on learning—setting the conditions for learning and selecting educational methods. A third direct influence is conducting the sessions. During the educational sessions, the health educator/teacher influences learning by creating a certain climate, using a certain style and technique, and by having prepared for the session.

Climate.   Climate reflects the nature of the teacher-learner relationship. Are questions encouraged? How much freedom do learners have to pursue topics of their interest? How open is the teacher to learner input? The teacher who is able to create a climate conducive to learning will not only facilitate learning but will also experience a continuing sense of job satisfaction.

Style.   The styles of teaching are often described in terms of the degree of teacher-centeredness or learner-centeredness. Teacher-learner styles are categorized as authoritarian, democratic, or laissez-faire. Authoritarian styles are highly teacher centered, the teacher making all decisions about what the students will study and how they will study it. In democratic climates, the teacher involves the learners in decisions about the content and methods. In laissez-faire climates, the learners decide the content and methods. The bias of most health educators is toward democratic styles. Authoritarian styles are decidedly out of favor, at present, but it can be argued that each style has an appropriate role in education. Any style can emphasize or ignore the conditions of learning and accommodate a range of teaching methods. The health educator/teacher should be proficient with several teaching styles.

Preparing the session.   Good teachers are constantly preparing for class. They are always seeking new content, new ideas, new methods, new ways of applying these methods, new ways of structuring or unstructuring learning sessions. Dedicated to making every minute of instruction time count, such teachers seek to minimize wasted time by preparing materials in advance, pilot testing learning activities, writing clear instructions, and developing smooth transitions from one activity to the next. One professor of education says, "If you get to class on time, you are late!" He argues that the teacher should arrive early for class to set up the audiovisuals, arrange the room, talk with students, and handle any last-minute details or problems.

Training

Training is a special case of teaching, and our discussion of teaching is entirely applicable to training situations. In the capacity of trainer, the health educator teaches other health educators, other health or education professionals, or volunteers how to accomplish health education objectives or how to employ health education methods. Typically, the emphasis is on the process of health education, as well as on health content. The learners are usually professionals or staff who have important health education functions. Examples include teachers, counselors, physicians, nurses, Peace Corps volunteers, cooperative extension agents, home health aides, parents, and others. Training, usually but not always, is conducted in seminars or short but intensive workshops or courses. Here are some examples of training situations:

- The Director of Health Education of the county public health department organizes and conducts regularly scheduled training sessions for staff health educators.
- The faculty of the health education department at the local university annually holds a training workshop on planning and evaluation for statewide health education professionals.
- In order to initiate a new system of patient education, staff health educators at the local hospital train nurses in the application of the system in a four-week series of Monday afternoon seminars.
- A team of health professionals, including one health educator, are contracted to train Peace Corps volunteers as health and nutrition specialists.

Health educators are responsible for training in numerous contexts. The need of health and education professionals for continuing education makes training a particularly vital health education service. In the case of a new health education program, those most involved in planning and developing the components of the program train others in the program's application. Training is a common function of health educators in school, hospital, occupation, and community settings. Training internal to the health educator/trainer's institution typically consists of seminars, workshops, or retreats. Training external to the institution typically includes conferences, short courses, and workshops.

The steps to developing successful training programs are listed below.

1. Identify the needs of the organization.
2. Specify job performance.

3. Identify learning needs.

4. Specify objectives.

5. Develop curriculum.

6. Select teaching-learning methods.

7. Obtain instruction resources.

8. Conduct the training sessions.

9. Evaluate training and provide feedback to the organization and the training program. (Nadler, 1982)

These steps differ little from any other educational program, except for the specification of job performance. The actual process of developing and conducting a training workshop differs little from the process of developing and conducting other health education program components. It requires advance planning. The needs assessment must take into account the actual and perceived needs of both the learner and the organization that sponsors the training. The program should be based on a theoretical approach to learning. Program components must be consistent with practical realities. Much preparation must be made in advance of the actual training sessions because training is often very intensive, and the trainer will have little time once the course or workshop begins. Process, impact, and outcome evaluation should be an integral part of even short courses and workshops, as appropriate.

Stages of Training

Training is commonly divided into pretraining, training, and posttraining stages. Pretraining includes organizational and learner needs assessments and planning functions, including the development of the curriculum. Training concerns conduct of the actual sessions, classes, or workshops. The posttraining stage includes monitoring, evaluation, and feedback. Training is successful to the extent that performance outcomes are improved. Therefore, whenever possible, posttraining consists of follow-up at the practice site to reinforce the new learning, to assure that it is applied correctly, and to reduce the problems associated with practical application.

Training Goals

Training programs are directed toward the accomplishment of the following goals:

1. Develop skills—for the purpose of training, each health education function or responsibility should be broken down into skills which can be easily understood, practiced, and evaluated.

2. Individual learning—training should be designed so that each participant has the opportunity to examine what he or she is learning in terms of his or her own context or working situation.

3. Process versus content—the purpose of training is to develop the learners' abilities. Therefore, in most cases, the process should be emphasized over subject matter content, which can be learned in other ways.

4. Shared learning experience—much of what is learned in training situations is a product of the learners' exposure to others enrolled in the program who are interested in the same problems and processes.

5. Opportunity for experimentation—training should provide opportunities for practice and experimentation that are generally not available elsewhere. Participants in any training program should come away from it with new information, ideas, methods, and skills. They should be armed or rearmed and ready to go back to the trenches of everyday professional life and do battle with the day's work.

Training Environment

Training can take place in one of several places, such as at the worksite, in a classroom or laboratory, or in the field. Each has advantages and disadvantages and each affords different strategies and methods. Many training programs use a combination of settings, each for a different strategy.

Training at the worksite or practice site offers the advantage of convenience to participants. The participants are already familiar with the location, know the routines and regulations, and know each other. On-the-job training is possible in this setting. The learner can immediately try out new learning methods and receive feedback from observers. The disadvantages include the tendency on the part of the participants to feel less free and creative in their work environment, the influence of the organization and/or its administrators, and the lack of suitable facilities.

Training also can take place in the field (if this differs from the worksite or office). The advantage of field training is that it can be very realistic. Training sometimes takes on greater meaning when the situation is "live." The only disadvantage to field training is the difficulty of conducting some training strategies in the field (for example, role playing, problem solving, and audiovisuals). The problems of moving equipment, giving instructions and getting feedback, and managing a complex training schedule are often substantial.

A classroom or laboratory away from the worksite is the most common place for training. The great advantage of this setting is the convenience to the trainer. Another advantage is that it takes the learner away from the distractions of the practice setting. The classroom or laboratory easily accommodates a variety of commonly employed methods—role playing, simulation, games, case studies, and lectures, to name a few.

The Trainee As Learner

Because of their status, experience, and high level of interest, one might correctly assume that professionals and volunteers would be rather unique learners. They are unique in that they are likely to have and express strong opinions about what and how they wish to learn. Surprisingly, in other ways, they are very much like other learners, at least in terms of the assumptions of learning described earlier in this chapter.

Motivation

People with a job to do are eager to channel their learning according to their perceived needs. Out in the field, away from classrooms and books, health educators and other health and education professionals must perform their responsibilities and duties as best they can. Given an opportunity to learn new and better ways of doing their jobs, they understandably want the training to address their specific needs, as well as to stimulate their interest and renew their enthusiasm.

For most participants, the motivation to learn extends beyond the desire to solve specific problems and improve job performance. For such people, competence and qualification are of issue. Training programs can develop or reinforce competence, add new knowledge and skills to the participant's repertoire, and provide him or her with the official qualifications necessary to gain new responsibilities, accomplish new tasks, and make career advancements. One other identifiable motivation of such learners is their desire to feel good about themselves in terms of their mastery of information or skills, and their contribution to society. Hence, the success of training programs depends on accurate needs assessment.

Self-Esteem

Participating in a training program can also be a threatening experience. There is an inevitable tendency for participants to compare themselves with others in the program. How will they measure up to the others in knowledge or competencies? Will their own inadequacies be obvious to others? How will they be evaluated? Will their employers be informed of their performance? All of these questions and concerns go through the mind of even the most competent and experienced participant. A well-developed training program will minimize these concerns by protecting the participants from unnecessary and excessive threats to their self-concepts, while at the same time challenging the participants to share what they already know, learn new information, consider new attitudes, and develop new skills.

Experience

Each learner is an important judge of his or her own training needs. Any group of health and/or education professionals represents an enormous collection of expertise and experience which can be employed to great advantage in training situations. A well-designed training program will take advantage of this resource by facilitating sharing among participants. One of the objectives of training is to encourage the participants to explore new applications of their existing expertise, and to share their knowledge and skills with other participants.

Individual Differences

The same types of differences exist between participants in a training program as exist in a classroom or other learning situation. At the outset there will be a range of experience, knowledge, and ability. Some participants will have greater experience and interest in a particular topic than others. Also there are likely to be differences in learning style. A well-designed training program will deal with these differences by emphasizing mastery learning, by having the participants teach each other, and by other methods. Furthermore, it will offer various kinds of learning experiences to allow each learner to benefit from his or her preferred way of learning.

Hence the participants in a training program are much like other learners. They are highly motivated; they are sensitive to threats to their self-esteem; they are experts regarding both their learning needs and their particular areas of interest and experience; and they represent a range in terms of ability, experience, and preferred style of learning. A well-considered training program will seek to maximize efficient learning by taking these learner characteristics into account, and even take advantage of them.

The Health Educator As Trainer

The trainer's primary responsibility is to see that the objectives of the program, based on a realistic assessment of both the participants and the sponsoring organization, are accomplished. As in any teaching situation, the educator's means of facilitating such learning is by establishing the conditions for learning, selecting appropriate methods, and skillfully conducting the sessions.

Establishing the Conditions For Learning

The conditions for learning are the same in training as in other teaching situations. Carefully planned and developed strategies and sessions that are based on learners' needs and are consistent with the conditions for learning are critical to the success of any training program.

Selecting Teaching-Learning Methods

The selection of methods depends on practical considerations of available time and space, as well as the educational set and situation. Although there are no methods unique to training, certain methods are frequently employed in training situations.

Simulation is one of the methods most frequently used in training. The learner is asked to simulate or act out a real-life situation that he or she is likely to encounter as part of his or her work. The learner experiences the situation, analyzes its components, and practices related skills. Simulation is a broad term encompassing these methods: games, dramatization, and role play. Each is a slightly different form of simulation. Examples of situations that can be simulated in a classroom are teaching, interviewing, and conducting meetings.

The case study method is also very popular in training programs. Relevant situations, either hypothetical or drawn from real life, are presented to the learners along with a list of questions. Each learner, working alone or in a small group as the situation indicates, responds to the questions in writing. Subsequently, the learners present their responses verbally for discussion and debate.

Conducting the Training Sessions

When conducting the training sessions the trainer establishes the learning climate through a combination of style and technique. The trainer's skill in doing so is a major contribution to the learning process.

Counseling

Counseling is a process of helping people to learn how to achieve personal growth, improve interpersonal relationships, resolve problems, make decisions, and change behavior. Counseling is distinct from psychological therapy in several ways: (1) it is generally of short duration, frequently only one or two appointments; (2) it is situational rather than general and chronic; (3) the client is normal, neither neurotic nor dysfunctional. Consider the following examples:

- After class one of your students approaches you about a course assignment. During the conversation it becomes clear that the student is concerned about some vocational and personal growth issues. You promptly schedule an appointment to discuss them.
- Your patient is suffering from shortness of breath and angina pain, but he is still smoking a pack of cigarettes a day. After the initial series of diagnostic questions, you help the patient fill out a balance sheet regarding his expressed desire to quit smoking.
- At a health fair where you are screening for high blood pressure, one of the local residents returns for a second blood pressure reading. This one is normal (as was the first) but something about her manner prompts you to invite her to the interview table. Quickly she reveals her acute concern about a health problem totally unrelated to high blood pressure.

Health counseling is an increasingly important activity of health educators. Nearly all helping professionals serve counseling functions and health educators are no exception. Every health provider counsels his or her patients, every health teacher counsels his or her students, and every community health educator counsels his or her clients. In this context counseling is a natural extension of the teaching/learning process, although it is frequently initiated by direct or indirect invitation of the client and conducted person-to-person. The adolescent with developmental concerns, the undergraduate with career decisions to make, the senior citizen with fears about his or her safety or health—these individuals frequently and in large numbers turn for help to available and approachable health professionals.

Because of the nature of their professional status and the regular contact they have with people, health care providers and teachers provide a great deal more counseling than professional counselors. Unfortunately, training in interviewing and counseling skills for health professionals is seldom adequate. As is teaching, counseling is an art and a science, and as such, can be taught and learned. Learning to be a good counselor begins with an introduction to the range of theories of counseling, and proceeds to practice in the techniques and methods suggested by each theory.

Three Approaches to Counseling

There are as many theories of counseling as there are theories of psychotherapy or theories of teaching. However, for the type of counseling most health educators do, three distinct theoretical orientations—client-centered, decision-making, and behavioral counseling—adequately illustrate the range of available options. Each of these theories has been highly researched and has demonstrated effectiveness in achieving improved health outcomes (Kanfer and Goldstein, 1986).

Client-centered counseling is foundational for the other counseling approaches. Its emphasis on the relationship between the counselor and the client is part of virtually all counselor training programs. Client-centered counseling is nondirective, meaning the counselor offers little advice or direction, focusing more on the process than the content of each interview. Conversely, behavioral counseling tends to be more directive, focusing on defining a specific behavior and specific interventions for change. However, in modern practice behavioral counselors also emphasize the relationship between the counselor and the client. The difference is that behavioral counselors consider a positive relationship as a prerequisite to successful counseling while client-centered counselors consider the relationship the *raison d'être* for the counseling process. Decision-making approaches also employ the fundamental client-centered interview approach, but lie somewhere between client-centered and behavioral counseling on the nondirective/directive continuum. Each theoretical orientation provides valuable insight into the process of counseling, and each is described here in terms of the process of counseling, the orientation of the client, the role of the counselor, and the counseling methods typical of the approach.

Client-Centered Counseling

Client-centered counseling grew out of Carl Rogers' belief that the subjective nature of the client-counselor interaction was the fundamental characteristic of the helping interview. He believed that what the client is thinking and feeling during the counseling session is of primary importance. The client-counselor relationship is an experience in a deep (even if brief) human relationship. Client-centered counseling strongly emphasizes personal growth and interpersonal goals as opposed to decision- or problem-oriented goals. It is more concerned with setting a direction for personal growth than with accomplishing specific behavioral tasks. The direction of this personal growth is determined by the client with the help of an attentive, nonjudgmental, and respectful counselor.

The counseling process.   The process of client-centered counseling consists primarily of interaction focusing on the stylistic and structural aspects of the client's participation. There is little effort on the part of the counselor to diagnose specific problems or causes. The counselor focuses instead on the immediate feelings of the client as revealed both verbally and nonverbally. The counselor reacts to the client's subjective feelings rather than the objective content of the interview. Thus, the client sets the tempo and direction of the interview.

The client.   In client-centered counseling the client is seen as a highly motivated individual whose natural tendencies are toward personal growth, health, socialization, self-realization, and independence. The vehicle for accomplishing growth toward these goals is a deep human relationship, the conditions for which can be provided by the counselor, at least temporarily. Within the context of their relationship the client's motivation for personal growth can be relied upon and his or her capacity for self-help will be manifest. If and when the client is vulnerable and perceives a facilitative attitude on the part of the counselor, growth is possible and likely. A counselor who has faith in the client's own basic goodness, a penchant for rational (versus instinctive) action, and the potential for self-knowledge, brings out these very characteristics in the client.

The counselor.   According to Rogers the role of the counselor is to strike an attitude of facilitation. There are three main qualities of a client-centered counselor. First, he or she must be genuine, fully present and absolutely without facade, harboring no moral or behavioral agenda for the client. Second, he or she must be empathetic. The counselor must strive to understand accurately and sensitively the client's feelings and meanings as the client reveals them. This requires that the counselor lay aside personal values and views in order to enter into the client's personal experience. Third, the counselor must like and respect the client as a person. The counselor warmly accepts the person and places no conditions upon this acceptance.

Client-centered counseling emphasizes the facilitative attitude of the helping professional. Therefore, training client-centered counselors is the same process as counseling itself. It consists, not surprisingly, of empathy training, group work such as encounters, and other personal growth experiences and exercises.

Methods.   Most of the now widely used methods practiced by client-centered counselors are designed to create an atmosphere within which the client's natural motivation and capacity for self-help will take over. Empathy training for counselors is an important foundation for achieving this goal. Consisting of a combination of active listening, role-playing, and sensitization methods, empathy training is valuable for all helping professionals who counsel people who are not like them in terms of values, experience, and perception. Empathy must be developed because without it the counselor cannot begin to share or understand the other's experience in life.

Encounter groups are perhaps more widely identified as client-centered than any other technique. Encounter groups are designed to bring the participants together in environments removed from the daily world of work and home. In such groups, largely unstructured and nondirective, the participants are able to get in touch with their experience and their feelings and learn more about themselves.

Counseling for Decision Making

Many counseling situations are of the decision-making variety: "Should I have intercourse with my boyfriend?" "What contraceptive device should I use?" "Should I go to graduate school or get a job?" "Should I stop smoking cigarettes?" "Should I go to the doctor?" "Should I have the operation recommended by my doctor?" "Should I seek a second medical opinion?" "What should I do about my aging parents?" These kinds of problems are common to the clients, patients, and students of health educators. Counseling for decision making is a process of logical reasoning through which realistic conflicts can be resolved during short-term counseling.

The counseling process.   Decision making can be very stressful. Stress obscures one's normal rational decision-making procedures, leading to indecision or bad decisions. The counselor, working with the decision maker, identifies the roadblocks to rational decision making and prescribes learning activities to help the client go through rational procedures for making a decision.

The client.   Janis and Mann have proposed a conflict theory model of decision making. They postulate that decision conflict is the result of "simultaneous opposing tendencies within the individual to accept and at the same time reject a given course of action" (1977:50). This results in hesitation, feelings of uncertainty, and other stress-induced reactions. The client, troubled by the conflict, is motivated to resolve it by any available means. Consequently, the client adopts one of five coping patterns: unconflicted adherence, unconflicted change to a new course of action, defensive avoidance, hypervigilance, and vigilance. Of these only vigilance is desirable. Vigilance is attained when the decision maker exhibits the following predecisional behavior characteristics: canvassing alternatives, canvassing objectives, careful evaluation of consequences, search for information, unbiased assimilation of new information, careful reevaluation of consequences, and planning for implementation and contingencies. Through counselor-prescribed learning activities based on the individual's coping pattern, the decision maker learns how to become vigilant regarding this decision, and perhaps regarding future conflict resolutions.

The counselor. The decision counselor is an educator concerned with the identification of the client's current decision-making procedures, and the teaching of rational procedures for resolving realistic conflicts. Janis and Mann contend that during the counseling interview the counselor (1) acquires "motivational power" by responding to the client's self-disclosure with noncontingent acceptance statements; (2) functions as a norm-sending communicator by recommending decision-making procedures; and (3) achieves termination by "offering assurance of continued positive regard and gives reminders that continue to foster the clients' sense of personal responsibility for their own decision" (1977:45).

In negotiating a partnership with the client, the counselor renounces the role of authority and makes no moral judgments or criticisms, yet is directive to the extent that he or she diagnoses and recommends learning exercises. The decision counselor is a teacher who individualizes instruction based on the client's situation and coping mode.

Methods. A structured interview is the initial method employed by the decision counselor. During the interview the client describes the dilemma and current decision-making procedures. The counselor employs a structured questionnaire to diagnose the coping pattern of the client. Based on this diagnosis, the counselor selects a prescriptive hypothesis and interventions to overcome or counteract defensive avoidance. Janis and Mann (1977) described four popular methods of intervention:

1. Undermining rationalizations involves listing rationalizations for a specific behavior or choice (e.g. "My uncle smoked two packs of cigarettes a day for fifty years and lived to be ninety") and presenting it to the client. Subsequently the rationalizations are refuted by lectures, readings, films, and similar presentations.

2. In role playing the client is confronted with a dramatic portrayal of the logical consequences of his actions. For example, a heavy smoker might play the role of a lung cancer patient who is receiving bad news from a physician. According to Janis and Mann, typical cognitive defenses ("It can't happen to me" or "It is impossible for me to change") can be undermined in this manner. Outcome psychodrama is a related method for use in situations in which the client is confronted with the type of decision that will commit him or her to a long-term fate, for example, selecting one job over another, going to graduate school versus taking a job, getting married, or having a baby. The client is asked to project himself into the future and to improvise a vivid retrospective account of what has happened since and as a result of making the decision.

3. The balance sheet procedure fosters vigilance by requiring the decision maker to answer questions about the risks and gains of particular decisions.

4. Stress inoculation for postdecisional setbacks is useful for decisions involving personal health that require immediate sacrifices for future health gains. It

involves counselors communicating to clients accurate information about (1) the consequences of the intended decision, and (2) contingency plans for dealing with inevitable temporary setbacks. For example, stress inoculation has been employed with some success in improving postoperative pain and recovery of patients who have elected painful medical treatments. It also has applications for backsliding dieters, joggers, and cigarette smokers.

Behavior Counseling

Behavior counseling differs from client-centered and decision-making counseling primarily in terms of its unrelenting focus on overt behavior. Behavior, rather than feelings, dispositions, or coping patterns, is the central issue. Behavior counseling—researched, elaborated, and popularized by Kazdin (1984) and others—is devoted to teaching people new ways of acting.

Behavioral counseling relies heavily on assessment by systematic observation and quantification (frequency, duration, intensity) of behavior. Based on these assessments, the counselor develops interventions and tailors them to the individual client's behavior pattern. Specific goals are decided upon and evaluation of goal accomplishment is undertaken for feedback and modification of the behavior change routine.

The client.   In behavioral counseling, behavior is motivated by antecedents (prior events) and consequences. People behave in response to or in anticipation of these events. Therefore, a great deal of behavioral counseling is devoted to detailing response patterns (frequency, duration, intensity), and the antecedents or stimuli and the consequences of behavioral responses for the purpose of (1) breaking the problem into small and manageable units, and (2) specifying interventions for specific environmental changes.

Because behavior is thought to be a product of social and physical environmental conditions, the work of clients is to alter either their environment or their response to environmental cues. Ultimately the client is the vital component in this person-environment interaction. It is up to the client to determine the behavioral goals and to provide the self-regulation upon which success in behavioral counseling is predicated. Of course, the client can also learn by observing his or her own behavior and the behavior of others, hence the importance of role models and modeling in general.

The counselor.   Behavior counselors generally adhere to the basic client-centered principles of humanistic relationships between counselors and clients but are more directive. The client determines the specific goals of counseling; the counselor facilitates or helps the individual learn the desired new way of acting. In order to be a useful facilitator the behavioral counselor must (1) become expert in systematic observation of behavior and in involving the client in the systematic observation of his or her own behavior; (2) prescribe specific observational and environmental change strategies; (3) facilitate specific behavioral goals; and (4) conduct careful evaluation of behavioral outcomes.

Behavioral counselors are perhaps more directive than other counselors due to their persistent focus on behavior. However, behavioral counseling, like other approaches, recognizes the salient responsibility of the individual in the process. Counseling is a teaching-learning situation in which the counselor possesses tools of observation and methods of intervention to facilitate behavior change, which the client learns to employ in achieving individual self-regulation of behavior, or in Bandura's terms, **self-efficacy**.

Methods. The methods of behavioral counseling, now widely employed in therapy, counseling, and education, include such classical behavioral techniques as stimulus control, reinforcement, punishment, extinction, generalization, shaping, and modeling. These are described in greater detail in chapters 10 and 11.

Counseling Technique

Counseling is not so very different from teaching. The most important skills are interpersonal communication and creative application of methods to specific learning objectives. Other useful skills for counselors include the following.

Listening and Responding

Health professionals can offer specific kinds of verbalizations in response to their patients' or clients' statements that will encourage them to elaborate upon their concerns. Exploratory responses are open-ended (e.g., "Can you tell me more about that?"). Listening responses are those which restate what the client just said. Feeling responses focus on the affect of the client (e.g., "What are you feeling right now?"). Honest labeling includes some interpretation of the client's attitudes or behavior (e.g., "You seem to be very angry with your boyfriend"). When carefully constructed and applied at opportune times, these responses keep the client on track and facilitate communication between the client and the counselor.

Feedback

Feedback refers to the ability to elicit input from clients about the counseling process, about their progress, and about their needs, feelings, and ideas. Obviously, the client's involvement at every stage of the counseling process is critical, and the more adept the counselor is at involving the client, the more successful the process is likely to be.

Empathy and Understanding

Understanding the client's behavior, attitudes, and attributions is critical in counseling. Since one can never fully understand another individual, the counselor is left with working hypotheses which can be explored with the client and revised as necessary.

Process As Content

This skill requires the counselor to focus on the interaction, the subjective experience of the session, rather than on the specific content of the interview. This is not to say that the content is unimportant. However, much of what goes on with the client does not get communicated in so many words to the counselor. Consequently, the counselor must look for and be receptive to nonverbal and verbal subjective clues which can be fed back to the client and/or otherwise explored. Counseling is a dynamic process that can be improved upon by analyzing one's role in it. Continuous self-study of one's interaction with clients is critical to improving performance. Except for training situations there is no "outside" person to provide feedback and suggestions for improving the interaction. The counselor must rely on his or her own ability and willingness to analyze the counseling interaction for clues on how to improve facilitation.

Creativity

Creativity in counseling is similar to creativity in teaching. It requires mastery of basic teaching and communication methods, an understanding of the learning task or objective, and the ability to create activities that allow the learner to achieve the objective. Jacobs (1992) provides a wealth of creative methods that the health counselor can select and adapt to specific situations.

Consulting

Consultation is important because it is one of the main processes by which the knowledge and experience of one person is used to help another person make better decisions, or to cope with problems more effectively. It spreads the know-how of one person to several or many others. It is the principal interpersonal process whereby current theory and information are used to improve actions in ongoing programs. Many agencies that could not afford to maintain a technical specialist on their payroll will call in a consultant for special information or analyses. Thus consultation is an economical means to increase the technical competence of an organization.

Consider the following situations:

- A colleague requests an appointment to consult with you on some specific problems concerning her current research.
- A national foundation hires you as outside consultant to help develop a family life education curriculum for pregnant teenagers.
- As education consultant to the local Heart Association you give technical and procedural advice concerning educational programs to reduce the risk of cardiovascular disease.

- As a state-level health educator one of your responsibilities is to gather, organize, and disseminate upon request health information and health education resource materials to professionals and to the public.

- An international consulting group hires you as a short-term consultant to evaluate a health education program in progress in central Africa.

Each of these examples represents an effort on the part of an organization to obtain technical and procedural expertise from a health education expert. The professional role of health education consultants has virtually exploded in the last decade. There is so much new knowledge about disease prevention and so much interest in developing health education programs that many health educators are employed as full-time consultants. However, it is more typical for a health educator to consult on a part-time basis or as a full-time job. Many academics and government health educators, for example, devote considerable portions of their work time to consulting responsibilities. Academics generally consult with their students, colleagues, and government and other agencies; government health educators consult with field professionals, academics, and the public.

Hence consulting quite simply is a process whereby knowledge and expertise are transmitted to those with a need to know. Consulting is an important direct health education service. Health educators serve as both informal and formal consultants. Health educators also are frequent users of other consultants' time and expertise.

The Consulting Process

The process of consulting in health education can be broken into two broad categories. The first, informal consulting, casts the health educator in the role of resource person, responsible to clients for providing information, interpreting data, identifying resource materials, and generally responding to requests. The second, formal consulting, casts the health educator in the role of technical or process expert.

Informal Consulting

Informal health education consulting is so named because a formal contract or written agreement between the consultant and the client(s) is not necessary. The informal consultant is a resource person whose major responsibilities are (1) organizing health education materials for easy access, and (2) responding to requests for information and for educational resource materials.

Informal consultation often occurs casually in hallways and in the offices of health educators—one colleague stops another to ask advice, a student makes an appointment with her advisor to solicit help on a project, an educator from one agency calls a health educator at another agency to ask for help in locating certain educational materials.

For some health education professionals, informal consulting is a major responsibility of their job. Public health educators, for example, are often responsible for responding to requests from the public or requests from health or education professionals for information and educational resource materials. Their functions in this capacity include answering specific questions about health, making referrals to others with greater knowledge when necessary, describing the function and services of community resources, and distributing educational resource materials. Naturally, the media for these functions is less often person-to-person than it is mail or telephone. In order to be effective in this capacity, the health educator not only must be knowledgeable, but also must be able to explain information in written and verbal terms that the client can understand. Furthermore, to function efficiently the health education consultant must be able to evaluate educational resource materials (books, films, print material, etc.) to determine their utility for various target populations and for various needs, as well as organize these resources for easy access.

Formal Consulting

Formal consulting is so named because a contract between the consultant and the client is necessary. Such a contract stipulates the services the consultant is expected to provide to the client and the details regarding time, money, and other concerns. The formal consultant is an expert, hired to share expertise regarding technical matters or processes.

The formal consulting process consists of several steps, most of which are similar to those generally taken by health educators. Steps in the consulting process, with their corresponding health education activity in parentheses, include: diagnosis (performing a needs assessment), recommendations (developing program components), taking action (implementing and delivering direct services), evaluation (evaluating), and termination.

The consulting process necessarily operates in an uncertain organizational and interpersonal environment. Therefore, it is necessary and beneficial to negotiate a contract—a written statement of the consulting task and the extent of client support, agreed upon by both (all) parties. Despite such contracts, consulting tasks have a way of changing over time, but once negotiated, the consulting process has begun. The contract stipulations may engage the consultant in one, some, or all of the consulting steps.

Diagnosis.   Diagnosis is the consultant's term for a needs assessment. The nature of the diagnosis depends greatly on the task. In many cases the consultant need only interview a few people and make some casual observations; in other cases extensive meetings, data collection, and data analysis are necessary.

Recommendations.   The consultant typically makes recommendations to the client in the form of memoranda or reports. These reports contain analyses of the problems based on the diagnosis as well as recommendations or suggested plans for action. Frequently the consultant lists the alternative courses of action and their relative benefits. She or he may more strongly recommend one or more actions. The recommendation may contain a detailed plan of action such as a formal curriculum outline, or a general outline of potential or suggested actions.

Action.   The consultant frequently carries out his or her own recommendations or those of others once they are agreed upon by the client. Thus, the consultant may teach a class or a course, create educational resources, conduct an evaluation, or take steps to resolve resource or system problems of an interpersonal or organizational nature.

Evaluation.   The health education consultant seeks to incorporate evaluation into the project when possible, providing suggestions about what kinds of evaluation are appropriate and how evaluation can be accomplished.

Termination.   Frequently a consultancy ends with a final report which includes a summary of the consulting activities and an evaluation as described above. In most cases the consultant is not around to see the eventual results of any of his or her efforts. Conversely the client frequently loses contact with the consultant once the contract responsibilities have been discharged. Ideally, a follow-up meeting is arranged so that both consultant and client can review and evaluate the process and results. This provides an opportunity for presenting constructive criticism about the process, for offering final words of advice, for sharing the results of the process, and for establishing the desirability of future consulting efforts.

The Client

In a formal consulting situation the health education consultant is hired by the client on behalf of an organization or institution to provide a service. Sometimes the contact person is not the true client but an intermediary. The true client may choose to remain in the background. In either case, the client-consultant relationship begins with the initial contact. The client holds a central position in the consultancy process, as initiator of the relationship, as negotiator of the contract, as doorkeeper to the client system and its resources. The client has both personal and professional needs that greatly influence the consulting process.

The client necessarily is part of the hiring institution—a hospital, an agency, a community organization, a business, and so on. Within this institution there exist at any point in time established loyalties, biases, parameters, systems, and other official and unofficial layers, through which the consultant must cut to get to the job at hand. The clients, as part of the system, tend to invest at the outset in either creating change or maintaining the status quo. Since the consultant is often in a position to make recommendations regarding resources, procedures, or systems, his or her position is eminently political. Only the client can guide the consultant past the most deadly political shoals.

On top of these systemic problems, clients often are ill-prepared in the use of health education consultants, especially as process experts. They may not know, or may not be able to articulate, exactly why they need a consultant. Sometimes, by not doing their part of the work, they are actually obstructive; worse, they may intentionally drag their feet, refuse to share what they know, or refuse to grant important access. The client has certain expectations for the consultant and for the consulting process. These may or may not be appropriate, useful, and realistic. Often their expectations for the consultant do not match the expectations and abilities of the consultant.

The client is critical to the success of the consulting process in three important ways. First, the client is the key to the consultant's ability to determine the exact needs for the consultancy. The client very often controls access to the information and to the individuals that the consultant needs in order to make an accurate diagnosis. Second, the client's expectations for the consulting process to a large extent determine or shape the consulting process. Third, the client usually has great potential to reduce the conflicts that arise within the institution that obstruct or distract the consultant. At the very least, the client can anticipate such conflicts so that plans can be made to reduce, negotiate, or eliminate them.

The client perceives the consultant as a resource in which the client has invested. Under the best of circumstances this investment pays off handsomely in the form of solutions to problems, new procedures or materials, or better health education program components and products. Under the worst of conditions the investment in a health education consultant is of little worth, or worse, counterproductive.

The Health Educator As Consultant

Ultimately, the role of the health educator/consultant is to share expertise with a client. This expertise may concern (1) information about health problems, health promotion, and disease prevention; (2) techniques for assessing needs, developing program components, teaching, or evaluating programs; (3) resources such as current literature or audiovisual aids; (4) processes such as how to select health problems or behaviors for educational attention, how to select appropriate educational strategies, how to improve teaching, and how to set up designs for program evaluation. The consulting process is complicated by the tenuous and constantly evolving relationship of the consultant to the client. As with any form of education, consulting requires a conducive learning environment, a facilitative teacher (consultant), and willing learners (clients). This combination is the substance of the often discussed relationship between the consultant and the client.

Consultants can be internal or external, indicating their institutional base inside the client organization or outside. Colleagues or faculty and students discussing research or program design are informally consulting within their organization; so is the health educator asked to critique a course syllabus, to observe a friend's class, or to offer advice about the strategies and methods selected for use in someone's program. This type of internal consulting occurs frequently, almost naturally, in academic departments and in other settings. The resident epidemiologist, statistician, computer expert, or health educator, asked to critique or advise on a project by colleagues within the institution, is involved in informal consulting activities; such activities also may develop into more formal internal consulting relationships. Some internal consulting relationships in large organizations such as government units and corporations may be more formal and may resemble external consulting arrangements.

Outside or external consultants frequently experience more difficulty than inside consultants with regard to the consultant-client relationship and the role of the consultant. The outside consultant must very quickly develop a working relationship with the client without sacrificing the freedom to act independently, as the task requires.

Successful consultants, internal or external, must interface with the hiring institution as well as with the principal clients. This sometimes requires the consultant to walk a tightrope between the rival agendas of the system (organization) and each of the participating clients. Ultimately the consultant's success depends upon not only his or her expertise, but also upon the personal influence that the consultant has established with the client.

Consulting Skills

Of the many skills useful to consultants there are several of particular and unique importance.

Seeking Information

Obtaining information and help from the client and from others is a crucial talent that consultants must master. Many consulting tasks require only that the consultant identify, select, and obtain the proper information or resources. This is more difficult than it sounds. Even when information about a problem exists, it may (1) need to be manipulated into a useable form, (2) be "owned" by someone who does not want to release it, (3) be coveted by participants who perceive power in its possession, or (4) for other reasons not be readily available. In many situations a consultant is brought in precisely because of this intrigue and the deviousness that is required. A skillful consultant quickly interprets the situation so that requests to each participant for information can be couched in the manner most likely to be respected and fulfilled.

Managing Meetings

Consultants are constantly requesting meetings, preparing for meetings, attending meetings, conducting meetings, or following up on the business of meetings. Skill in designing and managing meetings is vitally important. Meetings should have a specific purpose, be run efficiently, and be limited to the time scheduled.

Evaluating Educational Materials

Especially in informal health education consulting, the ability to assess the appropriateness of educational resource materials is vital. Health educators should be able to determine reading levels of printed materials, evaluate the validity of the content, and judge the quality of audiovisuals and other resource materials.

Writing Reports

Reports are sometimes intermediate products of consultation and are nearly always one of the final products. Preliminary reports detail the needs assessment or diagnosis and recommendations. Summary reports may include descriptions of the actions taken, an evaluation of the process, and recommendations for the future. Skill in the preparation of reports, as well as in the use of reports prepared by others, is essential for the health education consultant.

When preparing reports consultants must keep in mind the purpose of the report, the needs and interest of the client and other intended audiences, as well as the nature of the findings to be reported. Once on paper, information frequently is met with critical attention. Only carefully prepared reports emerge intact from this process.

An Example

One of the authors of this book was hired by a national foundation to help create a curriculum and resource manual on family life education for pregnant teenagers enrolled in public school and hospital-based programs across the nation. The whole project was coordinated by a professional employee of the organization, a journalist by training. However, the project was closely overseen by the director of the organization. The curriculum was actually created by the work of numerous outside consultants hired at different times, none with overall responsibility for the project. Naturally the product kept changing with the continual additions and modifications of so many experts.

When our author, the health education consultant, came into the project, many thousands of words had been written for contribution to the project. The initial consulting contract requested a critique of the work in progress and recommendations. He prepared a diagnosis or needs assessment, based on a review of literature, and recommendations for further development of the curriculum, based on the extent to which it was consistent with the diagnosis. For over a year the consultant was contacted periodically by the agency and asked to critique some part of the growing manuscript or to participate in a meeting called to decide what to do about the manual. At these meetings it was abundantly clear that the true client was the director of the agency. The various consultants at the meetings each tried to win the ear of the foundation director when present, or to line up support from the others for specific proposals.

The institution's goal of developing a family life curriculum was not being pursued in the most direct manner and concerted action to accomplish the goal was undermined by the vacillation of the director and shifting objectives. The outside consultants with technical and process expertise offered various diagnoses and recommendations and competed with each other for sufficient influence to move the project. When it was clear that the project was drifting from idea to idea, the author/consultant provided a written evaluation of the process and recommendations for getting the project on track. The memorandum turned out to be timely, because soon thereafter many of the recommendations in it were adopted and the curriculum was soon finalized.

Two points are served by this illustration. First, the consulting process is sometimes highly political and dynamic; it is always tenuous and uncertain. Second, the steps of the consulting process—diagnosis, recommendation, action, evaluation, and termination—tend to be overlapping and incomplete. Some recommendations are accepted and others are not. The consultant may participate in all or only one of the steps in the process. Not all the steps are necessarily completed. Nevertheless, many projects could not be completed without the assistance of a consultant.

Using Media

Health educators frequently employ media to deliver their messages. There are four types of media with which health educators frequently work: (1) print materials; (2) audiovisual aids (slides, videotapes, movies, and overhead transparencies); (3) programmed and computer-assisted instruction; and (4) mass media (radio, television, newspapers and magazines, and billboards). Each medium has unique educational uses requiring special skills on the part of the health educator. Print materials and audiovisual aids are widely used in health education. Computer-assisted instruction may be the wave of the educational future as personal computers become available to many learners. The use of mass media in health education is increasing, especially in national and local health promotion and disease prevention programs.

Using media is one of the major responsibilities of health educators. Some health educators specialize in conducting media campaigns. However, most health educators' responsibilities for using media are more modest—selecting the appropriate medium or aid, developing "teacher made" materials, and using audiovisual aids capably. The theory most central to any discussion of the use of media in health education is the attitude change theory of persuasive communications discussed in chapter 9.

Print Materials

Developing print materials is one of the most important functions of health educators, who pride themselves on their ability to make them user-friendly and effective. Many of the learners targeted by health education programs are not efficient readers, but need information about their health and behavior.

Consequently, print materials must be developed that are appropriate for the population.

Doak, Doak, and Root (1985) have been influential in promoting health education materials that are appropriate for the target population. For example, they identify several important considerations for developing print materials for learners with poor literacy skills. They recommend the use of very short sentences using simple words, few words on a page, and the liberal use of illustrations. However, most important their advice is to test the materials to make sure they are appropriate for the target population.

Print materials such as pamphlets, leaflets, and posters are ubiquitous in health education programs. Some of these items remain in high demand for years. Many others languish on shelves and bulletin boards. A great portion of health education program budgets are spent on developing, printing, and distributing information in this form.

Developing print materials is a very demanding job. Print materials are often the only form of health information that is provided, for example in physician's office. Sometimes print materials are used to provide additional detail or as reference material. Print self-instruction materials are sometimes the primary activity for an entire health education program. Hence it is important that they be developed to address specific objectives and tested to assure that they are appropriate for the target population.

Audiovisual Aids (AVAs)

Health education practitioners need to be skilled in the selection at use of AVAs and associated technology. AVAs selected should (1) address the educational objective(s), (2) be factually correct, (3) be unambiguous, and (4) be of high technical quality. Unfortunately AVAs, when available, often tend to be used in situations for which they are inappropriate.

Audiovisual aids include audiotapes, records, textbooks, posters, handouts, pamphlets, overhead projections, slides, filmstrips, and films. Each AVA is useful only for very specific educational purposes and each is used primarily as a supplement to other instruction. Intended to reach audiences of limited size, they are popular with learners who find them a relief from lectures and other traditional teaching methods. The effective health educator selects or develops appropriate AVAs to emphasize major points, to make the lesson more diverse and interesting, and to accomplish specific objectives. As such they are extremely useful aids to instruction. In particular, AVAs are valuable in health education when they provide role models and demonstrate specific skills.

Audiotapes are easily developed and useful for a limited number of educational purposes. They are particularly valuable as a means of providing feedback to those practicing interviewing, giving presentations, or conducting educational sessions. TelMed (telephone medicine), available in many communities, provides audiotaped information about a variety of health topics that can be accessed by telephone. Hospitals and other institutions purchase the tapes as a service to their patients or clients. Each tape provides basic information on specific medical or health topics such as otitis media, herpes genitalis, and breast-feeding. Individuals dial a central telephone number, request a tape by subject, title, or number, and are connected with the appropriate tape.

Slides and overheads are used for primarily the same purposes. Small amounts of information are projected by either means to enable a large group to see it. Anything that can be photographed with 35 mm film can be made into a slide; anything that can be photocopied can be made into an overhead. Slides are projected from the back of the room; overheads are projected from the front. For slides, the room must be darkened; for overheads the lights can remain on. Slides are fixed—they cannot be altered; overheads can be written on with a grease pencil. The most frequent mistake made in developing slides and overheads is presenting too much material on each.

Videotapes are very popular forms of educational instruction because videotape players and cameras are now generally available. Hence, it is possible to videotape an educational lesson and make it available elsewhere at very little cost. The great advantage of videotapes is the power of observational learning. Videotapes can show people just like the target population demonstrating the attitudes and skills that are the objectives of the program.

Effective use of AVAs requires advanced planning. The health educator should have a clear understanding of how the AVA can be used in combination with other methods to facilitate learning. It is also critical to master the equipment involved—overhead projectors, slide film projectors, tape recorders—and have them ready for easy access and use. It is very disturbing to the educational flow of a session when equipment is not ready for use and/or the educator does not know how to operate the equipment.

Programmed Instruction

Programmed instruction allows learners to advance at their own pace through carefully organized lessons, without the direct presence of a teacher. Examples include programmed texts and computer-assisted instruction. Programmed texts are frequently used in training and adult education situations. They are most useful as introductions to new subjects, or refreshers for continuing education. There are programmed-instructional texts on nutrition, fitness, statistics, epidemiology, and on many other relevant topics.

Computer-assisted instruction (CAI) is an exciting and potentially powerful new development. At a terminal the learner interacts with a computer programmed to take the learner from his or her level of understanding through a lesson. CAI is based on choice and mastery—the learner demonstrates competence at each step before moving on to the next. Programmed instruction allows learners to proceed at their own pace, provides numerous pathways for individual learners, and can keep records on the individual's responses. Perhaps its greatest use to date has been in universities, especially medical schools and other health science centers, where large numbers of students take the same courses, creating an economy of scale.

Interacting with the computer, learners master information by being taken through a series of learning exercises. In addition, computers can be used to provide simulations where the learner is presented a scenario and must make decisions in order to progress. Computers can thus provide a greater degree of interaction than other media. The rapid development of the technology for convenient integration of photographs, videotape, and other media into computer programs assures growth in the use of CAI.

Mass Media

Mass media are those channels of communication through which large numbers of people can be reached. The electronic media of radio and television hold particular fascination for many health educators. Daily the average American watches over six hours of television, listens to the radio for several more hours, and is exposed to at least one newspaper. Mass media are highly efficient in that large numbers of people can be reached for every dollar spent; however, they are also very expensive to use for educational purposes. Hence, most use of mass media in health education is modest in scope, relying mainly on public service announcements. Mass media, however, is widely credited with the potential for (1) increasing knowledge, (2) reinforcing previously held attitudes, and (3) encouraging behavioral intent.

Each mass media channel has a diverse and segmented following. Billions of dollars are spent annually by advertisers to research the characteristics of television audiences so that persuasive communications (advertisements) can be made according to specific audience tastes. Most television spots are prohibitively expensive for nonprofit purposes. However, radio provides a less expensive opportunity to air health education spots to a specific segment of the audience. Print sources are even better in this regard as the readership of most periodicals is highly specific.

Health educators need to be aware of the potential impact and use of mass media. Naturally, then, the first skill in order of importance is assessing media influences on the target audience. This information can be employed in planning and developing strategies that include mass media in conjunction with other interventions. Of course, most radio and all television spots require the professional and technical assistance of media experts. Newspapers and magazines, especially the more local ones—neighborhood, school, or institutional periodicals—are excellent channels for direct health education input in the form of advertisements, news spots, articles, and editorials. Health educators should be able to prepare appropriate contributions for publication. Indeed, the major responsibility of some health educators is to prepare newsletters for limited audiences. In addition to contributing to print sources, health educators need to learn how to get the press involved and interested in health education activities.

Summary

Health educators undertake a range of intervention actions including teaching, training, counseling, consulting, and communicating. Teaching is an interactive process between the teacher and the learner. Most learners are motivated, concerned with their self-concept, expert in regard to their own health behavior, and uniquely individual in terms of learning capability and style. The health educator/teacher facilitates learning by establishing the conditions for learning, selecting teaching methods, and conducting the teaching/learning sessions.

Training is a special case of teaching, usually conducted via seminars, workshops, and short courses. The process of health education is the usual subject and content, and those with responsibility for health education are the learners or participants. There are nine general goals of training programs. The health educator/trainer is responsible for establishing the conditions for learning, selecting appropriate methods, and conducting the learning sessions.

Health counseling is a special form of teaching that involves counselor and client in a one-to-one relationship directed toward personal growth, decision or problem resolution, or behavior change. In virtually all cases health educators participate in only short-term counseling situations, leaving more extensive counseling to professionally trained counselors and therapists. Individuals whose problems are severe, chronic, and/or life-threatening should be referred promptly to more qualified practitioners. However, in normal counseling situations, health educators should be able to conduct helping interviews in which they establish positive rapport, conduct basic behavioral assessment, and facilitate personal growth, problem resolution, decision-making, and/or behavior change. The better the counselor can communicate with the client, the more effective the counselor will be in assisting the client with the change process.

A health educator who serves as a consultant is by definition an expert with special skills, knowledge, and experience. Consulting may be informal or formal; formal consultation requires a contract, or written agreement, between the client and the consultant. The process of consulting includes five steps: diagnosis, recommendations, taking action, evaluation, termination.

Health educators frequently employ media to communicate their messages. They most often work with print materials and audiovisual aids. Increasingly, health educators are working with programmed and computer-assisted instruction and mass media. Each medium has unique educational uses. Their proper use requires special skills on the part of the health educator.

Evaluation

. . . there is no one best way to conduct an evaluation. Every evaluation situation is unique. A successful evaluation (one that is practical, ethical, useful and accurate) emerges from the special characteristics and conditions of a particular situation—a mixture of people, politics, history, context, resources, constraints, values, needs, interests, and chance.
—Michael Quinn Patton

Introduction

Health educators want to know whether their programs are being implemented according to plan and whether the objectives for change set during the planning process are being met. In this chapter we describe the process of evaluation and discuss technical aspects of design, measurement, and data analysis necessary to carry out program evaluations.

Program evaluation has been defined as "the systematic collection, analysis and interpretation of data for the purpose of determining the value of a social policy or program, to be used in decision-making about the policy or program" (Moberg, 1984). Evaluation provides a feedback loop to programs to make them more effective and yields information regarding whether a program should be modified or continued. The MATCH intervention phases and steps described in chapter 6 showed the integral relationship of program planning and evaluation, as the evaluation measures and design are built upon program objectives. Evaluation differs from basic research in its purposes. An evaluation is concerned with decisions regarding the implementation, continuation, or adoption of a program. Research is the process of proposing and testing theories to identify general laws of behavior. Both, however, share methods, add to the knowledge base, stimulate and develop theories, and contribute to the science of health education (Borich, 1993).

Why should a program be evaluated? There are a variety of answers, all of which are correct.

- A consumer wants to know if the program is effective and enjoyable.
- The manager wants to know if it is being implemented well, if the program is on schedule, and if the participants are satisfied with it. He or she is interested in how to improve the program.
- The program director wants to know whether the objectives of the program are being met, whether the program is justified from the standpoint of its cost, and whether or not the program should be continued.
- A researcher is concerned with whether it was the program itself—not some factor outside the program intervention—that was responsible for the outcome and, if so, what aspects of the program were most associated with the outcome.

Each of these concerns may be addressed in an evaluation. However, it is important to decide up-front what questions will be addressed in the evaluation and what the scope of the evaluation will be. As we will see, the questions asked have important implications for the evaluation design and measurement, and, in turn, for the feasibility and cost of the evaluation. It is generally not appropriate for health education practitioners to carry out full-blown research evaluations using experimental designs. Because of the expense and the expertise required, this should be left to well-funded university or private institute research programs. All health promotion programs, however, should be evaluated in terms of the quality of implementation and whether they met their short-term objectives.

Categories of Evaluation

The types of decisions to be made from the results of an evaluation have led to the identification of three general categories of evaluations: (1) diagnostic, (2) formative, and (3) summative (Green and Lewis, 1986). **Diagnostic evaluation** forms a part of the needs assessment process. It is commonly applied to individuals or groups to determine what they most need in the way of knowledge, attitude change, behavior change, or skill development. **Formative evaluation** is carried out partway through a program or intervention process to identify any needed "mid-course" adjustments. **Summative evaluation** takes place after the program is completed in order to determine whether the program should be continued or to identify needed modifications prior to the program's next use.

Others (c.f., Green and Kreuter, 1991) have delineated three levels of program evaluation: (1) process evaluation, (2) impact evaluation, and (3) outcome evaluation. Each asks a different question about the program or activity, addresses different aspects of the program or its effects, and considers different indicators (see figure 8.1). Although any one of the three may be used exclusively under certain conditions, two or all three are often used in combination. Because of the nature of the questions addressed, process evaluation is typically done as formative evaluation and impact and outcome evaluation as summative evaluation. However, it should be noted that knowledge and behavior may be assessed at points during the program and this information used to modify the program; in this case, the assessment would be considered formative evaluation. Table 8.1 shows the relationship between these two categorizations of evaluation. Note that summative evaluation is composed of both impact, and outcome evaluations in health promotion. Most of our programs are directed to changes in participants' knowledge, attitudes and behaviors. Behavioral risk reduction leads, in turn, to the outcome, a decrease in morbidity and mortality. Often the outcomes require a long period of time to measure; for example, the prevention of smoking among teenagers leads to a lower incidence of heart disease

Figure 8.1

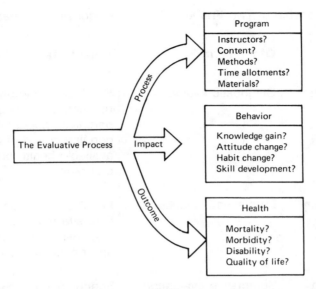

Three types of evaluation—although any one of these three may be used exclusively under certain conditions, two or all three are often used in combination.

Source: Based on Green et al., 1980.

and lung cancer several decades later. In this case, outcome data would be difficult to obtain since participants would have to be tracked for years.

We will discuss process, impact and outcome evaluation using worksheets from the Centers for Disease Control Community Intervention Handbook series (Simons-Morton BG, et al., 1991a; Simons-Morton DG, et al., 1988b; Simons-Morton DG, Parcel, and Brink, 1987). The handbooks were designed to enable a community group to plan, implement, and evaluate interventions addressing physical activity, smoking, and alcohol-related health problems. The MATCH planning approach, discussed in chapter 6, was used in the handbook design. Thus, program components directed to individuals, organizations, and governments are included in each level of evaluation (process, impact, and outcome). Refer to figure 6.1 to see the relationships of the levels of evaluation to the MATCH intervention process.

Not all evaluations will be conducted at all the societal levels included in a MATCH ecological intervention. In practice, programs vary in scope. Some evaluations will be directed to programs that primarily target individuals, such as a smoking cessation group or a health education class; others, such as a community-wide smoking control program, include multiple components directed to individuals, organizations, and government.

Table 8.1 Relationship of Two Frameworks for Categorizing Evaluations

Preferred Term	Other Term	Objectives
Needs assessment	Diagnostic evaluation	Feedback on knowledge, attitudes, risk behaviors, health status, and perceived needs of the target population and of the status of available health promotion programs
Process evaluation*	Formative evaluation	Feedback on program implementation, site response, participant response, practitioner response, and personnel competency
Impact evaluation	Summative evaluation	Feedback on knowledge, attitudes, beliefs and behavior of participants; programs and policies of organizations and governments
Outcome evaluation	Summative evaluation	Feedback on health status, morbidity and mortality

* The distinction is sometimes drawn that process evaluation is limited to monitoring of implementation during a program, and formative evaluation is a pilot study in which immediate feedback on process and impact is assessed for revision of program components, instruments and data collection procedures (Windsor et al., 1994)

Source: Adapted from McKenzie and Jurs, 1993; Green and Lewis, 1986.

Tables 8.2 to 8.5 contain process, impact, and outcome evaluation questions adapted from the CDC Handbook for Alcohol-related Health Problems (Simons-Morton BG, et al., 1991a). Refer to table 6.8 for intervention objectives for alcohol misuse prevention at the individual, organizational, societal, and governmental levels across four settings. Specific programs and policies at schools include an alcohol/drug curriculum and policies banning alcohol at school events; at worksites, a written alcohol use policy, trained employee assistance supervisors, and increased health/accident insurance for driving while intoxicated; in health care institutions, patient screening and counseling and provider education to conduct counseling for alcohol problems; and in the community, server policies/practices that prohibit sales or service to intoxicated patrons or to minors.

Our discussion of process, impact, and outcome evaluations will use the example of a multicomponent intervention designed to prevent the misuse of alcohol among college students, patterned after a program coordinated by the Student Health Center at the University of Texas at Austin. The program includes an awareness/informational component (displays on campus, articles in the newspaper, promotional events), peer educators, a designated driver program for cab rides home, individual counseling through a student assistance program, and a community/university town meeting for joint planning.

Process Evaluation

Process evaluation asks, "How well is the program being implemented?" For programs directed to individual-level behavior change, it involves a review of the program's external features in terms of the training level of the instructors; the quality of the books, pamphlets, films, or other materials used; the appropriateness and thoroughness of the written curriculum or instructional plans; time allotments in terms of the number of sessions presented and the length of each session; and the number of students, patients, or clients served by the program and the participation rate of the target population. This type of information is obtained from the records and documents routinely generated by the program, observations of class sessions, interviews and surveys of staff members and participants, and expert reviews of materials and plans to see whether they are consistent with program objectives.

Table 8.2 lists possible questions for process evaluations of individual-focused programs. These questions are generally applicable, although they were developed for the alcohol program handbook. Penetration into the target population (percent of the target population participating), the extent of implementation (percent of learning activities included), and the quality of implementation would be assessed.

Organizational-level objectives might be developed to assist an organization to change its practices or adopt a program or policy. Steps to be evaluated would include what organizational change strategies were used and how effective they were at achieving the change goal. Similarly, for influencing governments, the change strategy would be documented and evaluated and the law, ordinance, policy or program adoption would be reported. Informants would include program staff, organization staff, government representatives, legislators and their staffs, and health policy groups. Table 8.3 lists questions appropriate for process evaluations of programs to influence organizations and governments.

For a process evaluation of our college alcohol program, we would track the budget and timeline of planned activities across the year to see if activities were proceeding on schedule. For the awareness component, we would track the number and topics of newspaper articles and the number of times displays were presented on the campus, the location, and the number of students who picked up fliers or played the alcohol quiz game. For the peer educator component, we would track the number and types of students who enrolled and completed the peer educator training, their satisfaction with the training, their performance in the academic course component of training, and the

Table 8.2 Process Evaluation Questions for Individuals

Level of Intervention	Process Evaluation Questions
Programs for Individuals	1. What individuals were involved in developing and implementing the program (health department professionals, individuals from cooperating organizations, others)? 2. What were the components of the program? 3. Were some components more successfully carried out than others? Why? 4. How many participants attended the sessions or received the message? What percentage of the target population was this? 5. What percentage of the learning activities did the participants complete? 6. What educational methods were used in the program? How effective was each? How do you know? 7. What resources were expended (time, money, personnel)? 8. What were the methods and patterns of communication among the organizers? What improvements could/should be made? 9. Was the program carried out as designed? Was it modified? How? 10. What were the participants' reactions to the program? How satisfied were they with the activities, location? 11. To what extent were the program materials practical and useful? 12. Which features of the program were most appealing to the participants? Least appealing?

number, location, and attendance at the presentations they made in dormitories, sorority/fraternity meetings, and other settings, as well as the satisfaction of participants with the presentations. Similarly, for the designated driver program, in which students answer phones from 10 P.M. to 2 A.M. on weekends to connect students who are unable to get home from a club or party with a free cab ride, we would examine the number of students who called, the number of students who were picked up within 20 minutes of their call, and the satisfaction of students with the service. With individual counseling, we would be interested in the qualifications of counselors, the number of students served and the average number of sessions obtained, and student satisfaction with the services.

Table 8.3 Process Evaluation Questions for Organizations and Governments

Level of Intervention	Process Evaluation Questions
Influencing organizations	1. Who was involved in developing and conducting the program (health department professionals, individuals from the target organization, others)? 2. What individual or groups needed to adopt/support/commit to the program? 3. Who supported the innovation? Why? Why not? 4. What strategy was employed to obtain adoption? Was it effective? Why? Why not? 5. What activities, methods, materials were used to effect change? How effective were they in terms of participation, persuasiveness, feasibility, etc.? 6. What resources were expended (time, money, personnel)? 7. What were the patterns of communication among the participants, both those advocating change and those with decision-making power? 8. What individuals and levels of the organization were involved and were these the appropriate individuals and levels?
Influencing governments	1. What level(s) of government was involved? 2. What offices (departments) of the government were included? 3. Who were the key governmental decision makers? 4. What was the nature of the health department involvement? What resources and personnel were involved? 5. What materials were developed and employed? 6. What avenues of communication were employed to reach the decision makers? How effective was each channel? 7. How many contacts were made with decision makers? 8. Were the messages that were delivered to the decision makers understood? Were they effective? Would other messages have been better?

At the organizational level, we would be interested in determining the level of support from management within the student health center, student support services, and the higher administration. We would want to know who was involved in planning and coordinating the program and whether representatives from student government, the interfraternity council and other student groups, the student health center, the student counseling center, the faculty, university administration, and the community participated. In the designated driver program, we would monitor the contract with the cab company to ensure that drivers responded to calls. At the community/governmental level, the plans drafted in the town meeting would be analyzed for completeness and the change process monitored. Categories of participants in the town meeting would be described and assessed for whether or not key community members were present. For example, one activity suggested by the town meeting was limitation of local bars' happy hours during which drinks were half-price and appetizers were free. The change process to implement this recommendation would be studied and an assessment made of its effectiveness.

Process evaluation is an extremely important component of the evaluation process and should be incorporated into every program. Process measures provide feedback as to whether the program is being carried out as planned. This is basic information for management of the program. For example, if staff have not been hired or materials printed according to the project timeline, if potential clients are not signing up for the program, if participants are dissatisfied, or if instructors are not using the curriculum, the program manager must immediately take steps to get the project back on track. In addition to its management function, process evaluation also is important in interpreting the impact and outcome results of an evaluation. If a program does not meet its impact or outcome objectives, the evaluator asks, "Why?" Was it because the program was poorly conceived (i.e., the theory and its application were inappropriate to address the problem) or because a good program was not implemented well (i.e., the program was not carried out according to plan)? Process evaluation answers whether the program was carried out as planned and whether participants got a full "dose" of the program. Process evaluation also tells us whether the program is feasible. Some programs work well in highly controlled research settings, but cannot be replicated in the field. Process evaluation tells us whether a program can be implemented across different types of settings, an important question for the generalizability of programs and key to the diffusion of effective programs. For example, school-based prevention programs for smoking have been found to be effective in university-based research settings. Will these programs be effective when the typical school obtains the curriculum materials and implements them? Process evaluation of implementation by typical schools is needed to answer this question.

Impact Evaluation

The purpose of impact evaluation is to assess changes in knowledge, attitudes, beliefs, values, skills, behaviors, and practices as a result of the intervention.

Table 8.4 lists questions related to the impact of an alcohol program for each level of intervention. At the individual level, the immediate impact of the program is measured in terms of the target population's knowledge, beliefs, attitudes, and behaviors related to alcohol consumption; at the organizational level, in terms of policies, programs, and resources devoted to the prevention of alcohol misuse; at the government level, in terms of policies, plans, funding, and legislation designed to decrease the misuse of alcohol. Each of these impact variables is intermediate to the more long-range outcome of preventing morbidity and mortality related to alcohol abuse.

For the college alcohol program, we would measure students' knowledge, beliefs, attitudes, and behaviors (quantity and frequency of drinking, frequency of drinking five or more drinks at a sitting, frequency of drinking and driving) using a survey. We could also observe behaviors at campus gatherings. At the organizational level and government level, we would assess whether the university and community change objectives set at the town meeting were accomplished.

Table 8.4 Impact Evaluation Questions for an Alcohol Program

Level of Intervention	Impact Evaluation Questions
Individuals	1. Did the participants' knowledge, beliefs, and attitudes about alcohol consumption change as a result of the program? 2. What proportion of the participants decreased their use of alcohol in high-risk situations? 3. Did the consumption of alcoholic beverages by the target population decrease?
Influencing organizations	1. Was a policy adopted? How good is the new policy? 2. Was a program adopted? 3. What resources were allocated to it? 4. Rate its quality and sufficiency.
Influencing governments	1. Was legislation passed? 2. Were actions taken that decreased opportunities for the misuse of alcohol by the target population in the community? 3. Was desired funding obtained from the government entity? 4. Did the government develop a written plan to address alcohol use in the community?

Outcome Evaluation

Outcome evaluation measures improvements in health or social factors as a result of the intervention. Because decreased alcohol use affects chronic diseases such as cirrhosis of the liver and heart disease, measurable changes in morbidity and mortality may not be able to be assessed for a number of years. However, disability and death due to traumatic injury, such as motor vehicle accidents, falls, pedestrian accidents, and homicide, are more immediate. Table 8.5 lists questions assessing health outcomes of alcohol programs. Principles of epidemiology are important in the design of a health outcomes study. Because health is measured at the individual level, assessment is of the target population of individuals.

For our university alcohol program, we would track injuries and deaths among students associated with driving while intoxicated and alcohol overdose. We would collect data for the outcome evaluation from the campus and city police records, records from local emergency rooms, and a survey of students. As mentioned previously, we would not be able to set objectives and monitor changes in chronic disease incidence associated with alcohol misuse because these do not occur for many years.

Choosing a Research Design

The research design specifies when and to whom interventions will be applied and when and to whom measurements will be taken, providing the framework for the evaluation. The design chosen determines the types of conclusions the evaluator can make about the program's effect on participants. It is important that health educators be familiar with the types of evaluation designs, the strengths and weaknesses of each, and the evaluation questions they are able to answer. For most evaluation questions a general health education practitioner working in a school, worksite, health care, or community setting will encounter, a one-group pretest and posttest design is appropriate. This design answers the

Table 8.5 Outcome Evaluation Questions for an Alcohol Program

Level of Intervention	Outcome Evaluation Questions
Individuals	1. Have the morbidity rates related to consumption of alcohol decreased? 2. Have the mortality rates related to consumption of alcohol changed?

question, "Did the program meet its objectives?" Sometimes, however, it is essential that we determine whether or not specific programs (and not something else) lead to demonstrated impacts and outcomes. This requires utilization of an experimental or quasi-experimental design.

Types of Research Design

There are three major types of research design: experimental, quasi-experimental, and nonexperimental. **Experimental designs** have random assignment to experimental and control groups with measurement of both groups. Random assignment is used to make the two groups as equivalent as possible. **Quasi-experimental designs**, or nonequivalent comparison group designs, have two groups. However, there is not random assignment of subjects to the groups. It is important to select a comparison group that is as similar to the intervention group as possible. A **nonexperimental design** has only one group. Measures may be gathered before (pretest) and after (posttest) the intervention (Windsor et al., 1994).

Validity

Two types of validity, internal validity and external validity, must be considered in choosing a research design. **Internal validity** is the assurance that the program caused the change that was measured; that is, that the program, and not something else, was responsible for the impact observed. Possible rival explanations must be ruled out. A number of threats to internal validity have been identified. These confound the results and limit the inference that the program caused an effect. Three of the most frequently observed threats are instrumentation, selection, and participant attrition (Windsor et al., 1994). Instrument reliability is compromised when a change occurs in the way measures are taken at pretest and posttest, or when participants become more skilled at the measurement. For example, self-report might be used at one point and a biometric measure at another. Lack of equivalence of the treatment and comparison groups defines the selection threat to validity. For example, the treatment group might be composed of volunteers and the comparison group composed of nonvolunteers. Attrition is the loss of subjects during an intervention. Usually those who are unsuccessful in the program drop out, so that the intervention appears to be more effective than it actually is. Other threats include history, when external environmental factors cause the change rather than the intervention itself; maturation, when changes in subjects over time, such as aging, have an effect on the measures recorded; and testing, when there is an effect of being observed or tested on the outcome.

The three types of designs differ in their internal validity. Experimental designs, with random assignment into experimental and control groups, provide the strongest evidence of program effect. However, the evaluator must still be concerned with possible attrition and instrumentation differences. With quasi-experimental designs, the two groups are nonequivalent. While these designs allow the evaluator to rule out threats of maturation, history, and testing, differences between the groups, such as a volunteer bias, are a serious concern. Nonexperimental designs, without random assignment or a control group, offer little control over threats to validity. Without a control or comparison group, the effects of history and maturation cannot be addressed. The evaluator is unable to observe what changes occur in individuals not exposed to the program.

External validity is the assurance that the results of the evaluation can be generalized to other people and settings. Consider the following situation. A program to increase physical fitness using an experimental design has been shown to be effective at increasing oxygen consumption and endurance among college students. How confident are we that this program will have the same effect on employees of a large company or on senior citizens living in a retirement community? The answer to this question lies in how similar the people and setting are to those on which the experiment was conducted. College students differ from both worksite employees and senior citizens on such characteristics as age, physical capacity, previous experience with exercise, and attitudes regarding exercise. A college setting with excellent fitness facilities, organized courses for credit, and an emphasis on athletics would differ in a number of ways from a worksite and a retirement center. For example, worksites generally would have less extensive facilities, employee participation would depend on supervisor support, and fitness activities could not interfere with a full work schedule. Thus, while we would be confident that the results of a fitness program evaluation with strong internal validity would have the same effect on other college campuses, we cannot be confident that the program would have the same effect on populations different from college students or in other settings.

Randomization is an important concept for understanding external and internal validity and provides techniques to increase external and internal validity. **Randomization** means that each person in the population of potential participants has an equal chance of being selected or assigned. Randomized selection of subjects from a population allows generalization back to the population, since the subjects should not differ from the population in any systematic way. **Random selection** is the best way to achieve external validity, because the subjects are likely to be representative of the population from which they are selected. **Random assignment** of subjects to experimental and control groups is the best way to achieve internal validity. In this case each person has an equal chance of being in the different groups, so the group composition should not differ in any systematic way. (It should be noted that the use of randomization does not guarantee equivalent groups, and the evaluator should look to see whether the groups differ in any way at pretest.) Figure 8.2 illustrates random selection and random assignment.

The evaluator, knowing the strengths and weaknesses of the different designs, must then decide upon a design based on (1) the questions being asked in the evaluation and (2) the limitations of the situation. Often the situation does not allow for random assignment of individuals to treatments. For example,

Figure 8.2

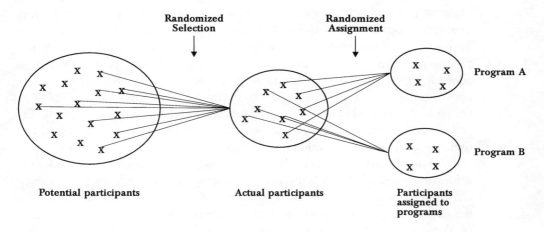

Randomized selection of participants from pool of potential participants and randomized assignment of participants to programs.

Source: Centers for Disease Control, 1988.

evaluation of new health curricula are done in intact classes, to minimize disruption of school schedules. In this case, a quasi-experimental design using classes matched on as many variables as possible (such as student age, ethnicity, gender, grade point average, major; teacher credentials and style; class curriculum and size) would be used. Most evaluations of health education programs use quasi-experimental designs.

Recent large-scale health education evaluations have randomized sites rather than individuals to programs. This recognizes the fact that programs are delivered to a unit (e.g., school or worksite) larger than the individual and that group factors (such as organizational culture, teacher rapport with students) influence all individuals within that unit. Aggregated data across individuals from the site (such as mean knowledge score of the class or prevalence of smoking at the worksite) are the measures for analysis. This addresses the problem in quasi-experimental designs that, although individuals at a site are not randomized and are subject to the group effects, the analysis is carried out on individuals as though they were randomly assigned to experimental and control groups.

Measurement Issues in Evaluation

All approaches to evaluation include the systematic gathering of evidence regarding a program's success. How does one measure program process, impact, and outcome objectives? Some of these measures are relatively straightforward, such as the percentage of employees who participate in a fitness program, the number of mammograms performed by a clinic in a six-month period, the number of participants who are not smoking six months after completion of a smoking cessation program, the number of minutes spent in vigorous physical activity during a day, or the number of hospital admissions from diabetic complications among program participants within six months of completion of a diabetic education program. The measurement of knowledge, beliefs, and attitudes using paper-and-pencil questionnaires is more prone to error than are data collected through records and observation. All measurement has limitations, reflecting reality, and the task of the evaluator is to minimize sources of error and thus increase confidence in evaluation results.

The ideal measure is both valid and reliable. A measure is **valid** when it measures exactly what it is intended to measure; it is **reliable** when it measures the object or concept consistently. Both are necessary for good evaluation, and it is important that evaluators know how to determine the validity and reliability of their measures and how to improve validity and reliability in their measurement systems.

Validity

How do you know if your instrument is valid? There are three main types of validity—content, criterion and construct validity—and there are standard procedures for assessing each. **Content validity**, also called **face validity**, is typically used in the construction of new scales and measures in health education. Experts are asked to examine the instrument to see whether it measures all relevant areas of the concept. For example, if the evaluator were developing a scale to measure perceived susceptibility to HIV infection, he or she could convene a panel of experts in the health belief model and in HIV prevention to examine whether the concept was covered appropriately.

Criterion validity is concerned with how well the measure correlates with another measure of the same phenomenon, usually already validated instruments, physiological measures, or observations. For example, one could obtain a self-report measure of smoking cessation and compare that to the measure of cotenine, a metabolite of nicotine, in the saliva. Scores on a paper-and-pencil fitness measure could be compared with direct measures of strength, flexibility, and aerobic capacity. Scores on a new measure of emotional well-being could be compared to those on an already validated hardiness measure. There are two types of criterion validity: **concurrent validity** if the two measures are taken at the same time and **predictive validity** if the measure of interest is correlated with a future measure of the same phenomenon.

Construct validity flows from the theoretical frameworks of health education. It examines whether a given instrument measures a specific concept and whether it is related to other concepts as predicted from a particular theory. For example, Eisen and colleagues used factor analysis to determine whether items from an instrument developed to measure health beliefs regarding contraceptive use loaded on separate factors for perceived susceptibility, perceived seriousness, interpersonal benefits, and barriers to contraceptive usage (Eisen, Zellman and McAlister, 1985). One can also examine whether measures are positively or negatively associated with each other as would be expected by their relationships hypothesized from theory.

Reliability

Reliability is the extent to which an instrument measures what it is measuring consistently—that it will produce the same score if applied to an object two or more times. We will consider five methods of assessing reliability that are useful in different circumstances: interobserver reliability, intraobserver reliability, test-retest reliability, internal consistency, and multiple forms reliability. The first two are used in the collection of observational data and the latter three in self-report data using questionnaires.

Various statistics are used in the process of instrument development and measure the final reliability of most instruments. Correlation coefficients, used to measure reliability, are expressed as decimal fractions on a scale with an absolute range from -1.0 to $+1.0$. A correlation of .60 is considered minimally acceptable. Commercially marketed knowledge tests are in the range of .90, which is considered very good.

Interobserver reliability is the extent to which two or more observers agree on their measures of the same subject at the same time. For example, if two persons are measuring body fat using skin fold calipers, one would assess their level of agreement on measures of the same subjects. Training and instrument calibration would be continued until consistency in measures was achieved across the observers.

Intraobserver reliability is the extent to which the same observer is consistent in measures of the same subject at different times. An example of this is the level of agreement of multiple skin fold or blood pressure measurements taken by one tester on the same subject. As before, if the measures were not consistent, training of the tester and examination of the integrity of the instrument would be carried out.

Test-retest reliability, also called stability, is the extent to which an instrument, such as a knowledge test or health beliefs scale, provides the same score at two different times. The times must be close enough that no real change in the measures would have occurred in the subjects.

Internal consistency measures the extent to which component items in an instrument are similar or measure the same concept. For example, when a knowledge test is internally consistent, persons who do well on the total score also tend to do better on each test item throughout the test than the subjects who do poorly.

Multiple-form reliability is the extent to which two equivalent forms of the instrument provide comparable results when administered to the same subjects at the same time. For example, there are two different forms to measure health locus of control, and scores from the two forms have been shown to be strongly correlated (Wallston and Wallston, 1981). **Split-half reliability** is similar conceptually to multiple-form reliability. It is obtained by randomly assigning items within an instrument to two sets of scores and examining the correlation between them.

Windsor and colleagues (1994) have identified seven general sources of unreliability: natural day-to-day variability, instructions, the instrument, the person making the measurement, the environment, the respondents, and data management problems. If the respondents do not understand the instructions, they may answer the questionnaire in different ways. The instrument items may not be clearly worded or may be at a reading level above that of the respondents. An instrument may be working poorly, for example a skin-fold caliper with a loose screw, giving different measures at different times. The person taking the measure may be sloppy in the use of the instrument. The environment for testing may be too warm or cold or too noisy. Respondents may be ill or easily distracted. Coding errors or data entry errors may compromise the data. Each of these sources of error must be minimized.

Criterion- versus Norm-Referenced Measures

With good testing instruments, it is possible to determine with reasonable assurance if students improved on some measure and, if they did improve, their approximate percentage gain. While it is useful to know whether or not students are improving, it is also important to know how they compare to some recognized standard. Two standards, norms and criteria, are used in educational assessment. **Norm-referenced measurement** provides the examinee's status in relation to the status of others being tested, while **criterion-referenced measurement** relates the performance of the examinee to a clearly defined set of behaviors, without reference to the status of others being tested. Thus, norms are relative to others being tested, while criteria are absolute and provide a clear description of what the examinee can and cannot do. Criterion-referenced measurement is preferred over norm-referenced measurement in evaluation because the results are clearly interpretable and not dependent on comparison to others who have been tested.

In norm-referenced testing, the examinee is compared to the performance of other people. Academic achievement tests in reading or mathematics, for example, are widely administered to children in all parts of the nation. It is simple to determine the average for each particular grade level and the typical distribution of scores above and below this level. When several thousand children are tested on a variable such as reading ability, the scores usually form a normal distribution, with as many children above the mean or average score as below it. In a normal distribution, the mean score (or numerical average of all scores) is the same as the median (the midpoint of all scores) and the 50th percentile. The score that places a particular child above 60 percent of the group is termed the 60th percentile, while a score that places a child above only 40 percent of the group is the 40th percentile, and so on throughout the distribution of scores. With such norms available as a reference, schools can then set standards for reading achievement. Similarly, public health agencies could examine the level of health or health behavior of the population they served and compare that experience to the norms for the nation to see whether the scores of their population were above or below average.

In criterion-referenced measurement, the individual is compared to a standard measure or criterion, not to the performance of others. Program objectives or objectives for health are set based on an absolute standard of performance, not in reference to tradition, historical experience or national norms. In contrast to norm-referenced tests, criterion referencing requires specifying in advance what score is required to meet the standard. In health promotion, behaviors or physiological measures associated with risk of disease or death might provide the standard. For example, a serum cholesterol of greater than 200 mg/dL or a blood pressure measure greater than 140/90 mm HG is associated with increased risk of heart disease. Computerized health risk appraisal provides a broad-scale criterion health measure based on the probability of death.

The criteria may be set in relationship to practical usefulness. For example, the skill level for cardiopulmonary resuscitation (CPR) must reach the level necessary to be effective in a typical first aid situation; however, fine gradations of skill beyond this level have little value. Here the standard is set by expert judgment based on knowledge of what works rather than by reference to any group performance. A shop teacher may establish five safety rules to follow when using power tools and require students to score 100 percent on a five item quiz before permitting them to use the tools.

Data Analysis

The type of data to be collected, the procedures for collecting it and putting it into usable form for analysis, and the statistical analyses to be used to answer the evaluation questions should be decided as the evaluation is planned. There are four levels of measurement: nominal, ordinal, interval, and ratio.

Levels of Measurement

Nominal and ordinal data are categorical, i.e., their units are categories with no numerical meaning. Interval and ratio data are numerical, with standard units of measurement. Interval measures can be added and subtracted. However, unlike ratio measures that have an absolute zero, they cannot be multiplied or divided. All arithmetic operations can be performed on ratio measures. Different statistics are appropriate for these levels of measurement. Table 8.6 gives the defining characteristics for each level of measurement.

Table 8.6 Levels of Measurement for Evaluation and Appropriate Measures

Type of Data: Level of Measurement	Defining Characteristic	Descriptive Measure
Categorical: Nominal	Categories; labels have no numeric meaning	Frequency counts and percentages; mode
Categorical: Ordinal	Numbers/categories imply rank order of intensity, not numeric quantity	Frequency counts and percentages; median and range
Numerical: Interval	Distances between numbers are equal (standard unit of measure)	Frequency counts and percentages; mean and standard deviation
Numerical: Ratio	Distances between numbers are equal (standard unit of measure) and there is an absolute zero point	Frequency counts and percentages; mean and standard deviation

Nominal, or name, data are often used to categorize persons in health promotion evaluations. Examples of such categories are current smoker/never smoker/ex-smoker, participant/nonparticipant, experimental group member/control group member, or ethnic group membership (e.g., non-Hispanic white, African American, Hispanic). These categories cannot be ordered. Thus, frequency measures, such as counts and percentages, are used to describe or summarize the data.

Ordinal data place categories in an order, but there is no standard unit of measure underlying the order. Examples from health promotion include light, moderate and heavy smoking; poor, fair, good, and excellent health.

In **interval scales** the distances between the numbers are equal but there is no zero. Some attitude scales are constructed to have equal intervals, and scales measuring level of agreement with belief statements (e.g., "Smoking marijuana is a good way to relax") are assumed to behave as interval scales. Systolic and diastolic blood pressure readings are also examples of interval scales.

Ratio scales have equal distances between the numbers and a zero point. These scales are common in counts of behavior such as number of months of prenatal care received, number of cigarettes smoked, number of pounds lost, and ounces of alcohol consumed, or in physiological measures such as serum cotenine.

Descriptive and Inferential Statistics

Statistics in evaluation serve several purposes. The first is to summarize and describe data. Statistics serving this purpose are called **descriptive statistics**. **Frequency counts** are totals within categories and are appropriate for all levels of measurement. For example, the number of participants at a workshop or the number of subjects with serum cholesterol over 200 mg/dL are frequency counts. The mean, the median, and the mode, three types of averages, are **measures of central tendency**. Each is a single number that represents the central tendency of a set of data. The **mean** is the arithmetic average of a set of observations. The **median** is defined as the middle observation of a group, with half of the observations occurring above and half below it. The median should be used when there are outlying data, because, in contrast to the mean, it is not affected by extreme scores. The **mode** is the most frequently occurring observation. It is the only measure appropriate for categorical data. For example, the mode could be used to point out the peak times at a fitness center.

The mean and median by themselves, however, do not provide complete information about a set of data. A **measure of spread** or **variation** is also needed. The **range** is defined as the highest value minus the lowest value in the data set and is thus influenced by extreme scores. The **variance** and **standard deviation** are measures based on the deviation of each measure from the mean score.

Measures of relationship describe whether two variables are related to each other; that is, one varies as the other varies. A **correlation** is a value between +1 (positive correlation) and -1 (negative correlation). A score of 0 indicates that there is no relationship between the variables. Suppose the correlation between perceived susceptibility for breast cancer and intention to obtain a mammogram is found by evaluators to be .75—this would indicate that these variables are positively associated; that is, if one is high, the other is likely to be too (and vice versa). A correlation is negative if a high score on one variable is associated with a low score on the other, and vice versa.

Inferential statistics answer the question of whether an observed difference between two variables could have occurred by chance alone. Inferential statistics make use of probability distributions to test the **null hypothesis** that there is no observed difference between two variables. This allows the evaluator to answer with a given degree of certainty whether the variables, such as pretest and posttest knowledge scores or quit rates from two different smoking cessation programs, are significantly different. Thus, the evaluator can answer questions such as, "Did the program work?" or "Is one program more effective than the other?" Examples of inferential statistical tests are the t-test, chi square, and analysis of variance. It should be pointed out that **statistical significance** is not the same as **practical significance**. Small differences are often statistically significant when there are large numbers of subjects; however these differences may make no practical difference to the participants' knowledge, behavior, or health status. Thus the evaluator must always use common sense in applying the evaluation findings to decisions about programs.

This section on data analysis and statistics has provided a brief overview of the subject. We suggest that all health education students take an introductory statistics class and know how to calculate and interpret frequently used statistics. Any introductory statistics book for the social sciences will provide reference information to the concepts introduced in this chapter.

Economic Analyses

Cost analysis provides important data to be used in deciding whether to begin or maintain a health education program. There are two major types of cost analysis: cost-benefit analysis and cost-effectiveness analysis. **Cost-benefit analysis** answers the question, "What financial returns am I receiving for the money spent on the program?" **Cost-effectiveness analysis** answers the question, "Of all the program options I have available, which one will provide the most efficient return on my dollar invested?" (LaRosa and Haines, 1986). Green and Lewis (1986) define these concepts as follows:

Cost Benefit: A measure of the cost of an intervention relative to the benefits it yields, usually expressed as a ratio of dollars saved or gained for every dollar spent on the program.

Cost Effectiveness: A measure of the cost of an intervention relative to its impact, usually expressed in dollars per unit of effect.

For both cost-benefit and cost-effectiveness analysis, the first step is to make a careful accounting of the costs of the program. This encompasses the costs for conducting the program, including personnel, supplies and materials, and space; and the costs to the participants or company, such as lost work time for program participation and transportation time and costs. Evaluation costs should not be included in program costs, unless they are part of the ongoing maintenance of the program. Clear specification of process objectives and definition of resources needed for program implementation are essential to computation of the dollar costs of the health promotion program. The first column of table 8.7 summarizes the categories of program costs to be considered.

In cost-benefit analysis, the benefits are also calculated and expressed in dollars. The first step is listing the benefits of the program, beginning with those benefits found through the outcome evaluation. Benefits of a health promotion program include reduced morbidity, reduced mortality, and increased quality of life. The second column of table 8.7 contains categories of health program benefits listed by Warner and Luce (1982). How does one determine the cost associated with these outcomes? For reduced morbidity, costs associated with reduced absenteeism, reduced hospitalization, and reduced physician visits could be measured. For reduced mortality, reduced rehiring and retraining costs, and future salary and productivity could be included.

While it is relatively easy to quantify some of these benefits in terms of dollars, it is very difficult to put a dollar value on others. For example, what is the dollar value of a human life? Is it measured as the value of one's life

Table 8.7 Program Costs and Benefits

Costs	Benefits
A. Personnel (e.g., administrator, health educators, nurses, clerical staff)	A. Personal health (e.g., increased life expectancy, decreased morbidity, reduced disability)
B. Supplies and materials (e.g., videotapes, print materials, screening supplies, office supplies)	B. Health care resources (e.g., savings of expensive resources such as surgery)
C. Program space (e.g., rental, equipment depreciation)	C. Work productivity (e.g., decreased absenteeism and turnover, increased morale)
D. Costs to participants (e.g., time off from work, transportation time and costs)	D. Positive social effects (e.g., access to health care or compassion)

insurance or the court awards for loss of productive life? Are the lives of homemakers, whose productivity is not measured by their salary, worth less than those of corporate employees? Recent cost-benefit analyses of prevention and health promotion have noted that the cost-benefit ratio does not favor preventive health programs. Increasing life expectancy brings with it additional costs as well as benefits. The longer a person lives, the more medical costs will be incurred and the more money an employer will have to pay in pension funds.

In a cost-benefit analysis, the dollar value of both costs and benefits are calculated. In order to compare the costs and benefits which occur at different points in time, **discounting** is used to adjust for the fact that a dollar today is worth more than a dollar in the future. The benefits are then divided by the costs to create a ratio of benefits to cost. If the ratio is 1:1, the program broke even. If the ratio is greater than 1:1, the benefits of the program exceeded the costs. A 3:1 ratio would indicate that for every $1 spent on the program, $3 were earned in benefits. If the ratio is less than 1:1, the program cost more than it earned.

Because of the problems associated with calculating the dollar value of benefits and because prevention programs lead to increased costs from pensions and health care utilization associated with a longer life, most evaluators recommend that cost-effectiveness analysis is preferable to cost-benefit analysis in making decisions about which programs to undertake. In cost-effectiveness analysis, the benefits are not required to be calculated in dollar amounts. The benefits may be long-term, such as years of life saved, or short-term, such as the number of smokers who stop or the number of pounds lost. This enables the health promotion manager to choose the most efficient program to meet the same goal. Information should be collected to show how much Program A costs to produce a given result compared to the cost of Program B to produce that result.

Brownell and colleagues (1984) compared five different weight loss programs. They found the cost per 1 percent reduction in percentage overweight to be $44.60 for a university clinic, $25.14 for professional leaders in a worksite setting, $8.28 for lay leaders in a worksite setting, $3.00 for a commercial program, and $2.93 for a worksite competition. Of the three worksite programs, the competition was clearly more cost-effective.

How to Organize the Evaluation Process

Each health education program has a number of constituents and, just as with program planning, it is important to include the different involved parties, also termed **stakeholders**, in discussions of the evaluation objectives and process. That way, the evaluation will address the different interests of the stakeholders, and the results of the evaluation will be used. Resource limitations and other constraints should be addressed and the scope of the evaluation (process, impact, outcome, cost-effectiveness) determined.

The program objectives should be identified, and a plan laid out for measuring whether or not they were met. At this time a decision is made regarding the data to be collected, and a research design is chosen. A management system for collecting, entering, cleaning, storing, and analyzing the data is set up. Process data are analyzed periodically to provide information about how well the program is being implemented for feedback to the program. Impact and outcome data are analyzed after completion of the program.

Relaying the results of the evaluation to the stakeholders requires reports tailored to their specific needs. For example, a program manager will want detailed reporting of process evaluation measures for decisions to be made as the program is being conducted. Higher level managers of the organization will be interested in how many people attended, how satisfied they were, whether the program is working, and how cost-effective it is. Program participants will have their own perspective. The format, content covered, and level of analytic sophistication will differ for different stakeholders. Memoranda, management reports, newsletter articles, professional journal articles, and annual reports may be used for reporting to different constituencies. It is important that the reports be timely, clearly understood, and disseminated to all appropriate audiences. This will enhance the utility of the evaluation results for making decisions about the program.

Summary

Evaluation is used to assess whether health education programs are being implemented according to plan, whether the objectives for change set during the planning process are being met, and whether the program itself is responsible for the change. Health educators are most likely to use nonexperimental designs when assessing whether a program met its objectives and quasi-experimental designs when evaluating the effectiveness of a program. Careful attention must be given to ensure the reliability and validity of measures used in data collection. There are four levels of measurement—nominal, ordinal, interval, and ratio—and it is important that the statistics chosen for analysis match the level of the scale. Descriptive statistics summarize the data; inferential statistics test whether differences between two variables could have occurred by chance. Economic analyses are often used to decide whether to begin or maintain a particular program, and cost-effectiveness analysis is recommended over cost-benefit analysis. The process of identifying stakeholders, the scope of the evaluation, the objectives, and the management and implementation of the evaluation was discussed. In any setting, it is essential that the evaluation address the needs of the personnel who are making decisions regarding the health promotion program and be presented to them in a form that is useful.

PART III

HEALTH BEHAVIOR CHANGE
THEORY AND METHODS

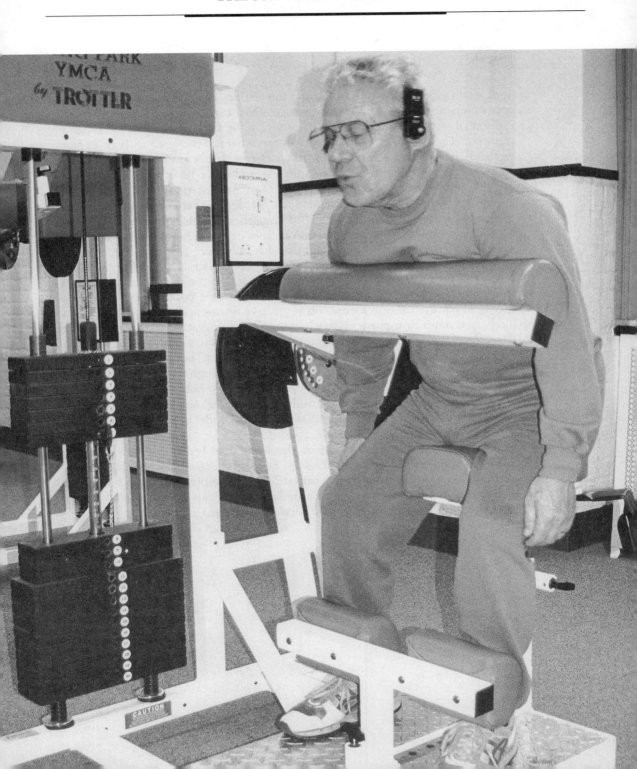

The change process is complex and interesting. Health education and health promotion are concerned about changes that can occur at the level of the individual, the organization, the community, or the government. A range of theoretical and conceptual approaches have been developed to help explain health behavior and the methods that foster health behavior change. Theory can facilitate the health educator's understanding of health behavior as well as guide the development and evaluation of programmatic activities. Cognitive aspects of behavior change include knowledge, beliefs, and attitudes, the mainstays of most health education and health promotion programs. But each cognitive theory or conceptualization focuses on a unique set of variables and provides a unique way of addressing health behavior. For example, stages of change conceptualizes the individual as being at one of four stages for any health behavior: precontemplative, contemplative, action, or maintenance. Hence, interventions should be designed based on the target population's stage. The theory of planned action focuses on subjective norms and attitudes toward the likely outcomes of a particular behavior. Social cognitive theory emphasizes the effects on learning of modeling and other social influences, and the importance of perceptions of self-efficacy or capacity to succeed. Social cognitive theory is particularly interesting because it integrates cognitive and reinforcement theories. Operant conditioning theory describes how behavior is influenced by reinforcement and even by stimuli that are associated with potential reinforcement. Behavior modification is the collection of methods and approaches stimulated by operant conditioning.

Change can occur not only at the individual level, but also at organizational, community, and societal levels. Successful organizational change starts with assessment and advances to initiation, then implementation, and finally to institutionalization. Change at broader social levels is guided by diffusion, mass communications, and community development theories.

Cognitive and Affective Learning

Nothing is so firmly believed as what we least know.
—Montaigne

Introduction

While heredity plays an important role in determining an individual's potential to learn, learning itself is the product of life experiences. Ultimately, learning is measured in terms of behavior, but knowledge, beliefs, attitudes, and values are the direct or intermediate outcomes of education and other learning experiences. The theoretical approaches reviewed in this chapter consider the importance of cognitive and affective factors in motivation and behavior change. The influence of reinforcement and social and cultural factors on learning is emphasized in other chapters.

 Health educators commonly are challenged to develop learning experiences that motivate learners to change their health behavior. In this chapter we briefly consider psychological frameworks that provide important perspectives about personality, motivation, and behavior. The bulk of the chapter provides an introduction to the cognitive and affective variables that are the primary focus of most educational interventions. Later in the chapter we describe selected conceptualizations and theories that relate cognitive and affective variables with behavior. The theories selected are those that are most appropriate to a health educator's understanding of learning and most frequently employed in health promotion research and practice.

Psychological Frameworks

One of the things that makes the study of human beings fascinating is the uniqueness of each individual. Even identical twins with the same genetic makeup and a common upbringing can be remarkably dissimilar in many ways. These differences between people in abilities, preferences, psychological states, motivation, and behavior are often striking, although it is also the case that people with similar familial and cultural backgrounds also share a great deal in common. Clearly, the influences of genetics and environment on personality development are complex and poorly understood. Nevertheless, scientists and theorists have struggled to understand the nature of personality and motivation that are defining aspects of the human condition. Here we provide an abridged discussion of three major psychological frameworks that may be important to the health educator's understanding of personality, motivation, and behavior.

A. Psychoanalytic Theory

Freud's psychoanalytic theory was an effort to explain human behavior in terms of personality. Freud theorized that there were three structures of personality. The **id** houses instincts and provides the innate source of energy or drive for psychological processes and behavior. The **ego** interacts with the demands of reality in fulfilling instinctual wishes. The **superego** represents the internalization of social standards of behavior. These structures are in constant conflict in determining whether an impulse will be expressed or controlled. According to Freud humans are challenged by the various stages of psychosexual development to which they must adjust or become neurotic and dysfunctional. Hence, according to psychoanalytic theory, **motivation** can be understood in terms of innate drives and psychosexual adjustment, moderated by socialization.

Psychoanalytic theory provides an important theoretical framework for understanding human behavior and is credited with advancing the view that behavior is determined or caused by psychological factors and, therefore, could be understood and explained. Psychoanalytic theory also advanced the notion that individual personalities are shaped by life experiences. Further, psychoanalytic theory promoted the concept of normal psychosocial development and suggested that it could be arrested by psychologic trauma or stress. Psychoanalytic theory provided important perspectives on motivation emphasizing psychosexual development and the struggle for ego gratification moderated by socialization.

Many of the specific propositions of psychoanalytic theory have been difficult to verify empirically, notably the concept of the unconscious mental states, and a number of inconsistencies within the theory have never been successfully resolved. Psychoanalytic theory has been under almost constant revision since it was developed, but, nevertheless, remains an influential psychological perspective on personality, motivation, and behavior.

B. Trait Theory

Each human being has a unique personality, but personality is made up in part by certain traits or characteristics. **Traits** are consistent and relatively enduring aspects of personality and ways of behaving that tend to distinguish one individual from another. Hence, some people may be more or less kindly, honest, hostile, rebellious, competitive, or logical. While it seems obvious that traits exist and that they vary from person to person and seem to characterize individuals, trait theory is not an entirely adequate theory of behavior. Indeed, the task of measuring traits has become a cottage industry among psychologists. Traits are not easily measured and often must be inferred from behavior. However, people are notoriously inconsistent in their behavior owing to situational and temporal variables, making the measurement of traits less reliable than desired. Some personality traits appear to be inherited and fairly immutable, for example, intelligence and aptitude. Other traits appear to be quite transient and situational, for example, certain aspects of temperament. The extent to which traits are acquired genetically or through experience and learning is not entirely clear.

Like psychoanalytic theory, trait theory is a useful way of thinking about the variability in personality, motivation, and behavior. Generally, traits are rather enduring, having derived from genetic predispositions and long-term exposure to family and other social influences. Therefore, they are not easily changeable through usual educational methods, making them generally of less interest to health educators than other variables that are more easily altered, except as indicators of risk.

Field Theory and Humanistic Psychology

Another school of psychology with important implications for health education evolved out of the work of Wolfgang Kohler, Kurt Lewin, Carl Rogers, and Abraham Maslow. Early in the twentieth century Gestalt and field theorists proposed that people typically organize the various stimuli to which they are exposed into meaningful wholes or **gestalts**. Consequently, they respond to these configurations in terms of their apparent relevance to important personal needs or goals. This perceptual gestalt is a tendency for specific events to be interpreted in terms of their context and overall effect. The components of the person's perceptual field (i.e., whatever is on one's mind at the time) are thought to interact with one another so that the character of each item is affected by the general mind set of the individual and the setting within which the stimulus is delivered and received. Accordingly, the individual interprets a single stimulus in terms of the entire field within which the stimulus is provided and the perceptual context that the individual provides from the totality of his or her previous experiences.

Field theory offers health educators a number of important lessons. One such lesson is that each person interprets stimuli from their own personal perceptual context. This helps to explain why the same stimulus (i.e., a lecture or admonishment by a teacher or parent) may be highly motivating for one individual at one point in time and not at another or for one individual but not for another. Relatedly, it is important when developing learning experiences to consider not just the content but also the context of the learning experience— who delivers it, the physical surroundings, the events that just occurred—all factors in the learner's appreciation and interpretation of the event.

Humanistic psychologists, who as a group are primarily concerned with the essential uniqueness of the individual, quickly came to understand from field theory that people not only interpret specific stimuli uniquely, but also are motivated to understand their world within the context of their unique experiences. Hence, effective counseling and education must recognize the learner's personal experience and perspective.

Humanistic psychologists, such as Carl Rogers and Abraham Maslow, recognized that people are motivated to become independent, caring, and altruistic. Further, they emphasized the powerful motivating influence of the genuinely caring human being serving as a teacher, counselor, friend, or parent. Rogers (1961) and others noted the tremendous power of interpersonal relating when freed from manipulation and offered in the context of open caring and concern. We learn from Rogers that interpersonal relations are the most powerful and motivating experiences of the human condition. Hence, an essential task for successful health educators and psychological counselors is to establish a foundation of trust by genuinely caring about and communicating with the learners and clients, thereby providing motivational influence within the context of a trusting relationship.

Learning and Behavior

Learning, generally defined as a change in behavior as a result of experience, is a fundamental characteristic of living creatures, and humans are Earth's master learners. A human's protracted development during childhood and adolescence provides an opportunity for the extensive learning that is required of our species for survival and success. Modern American life is extremely complex and dynamic, at least by historical standards, and individuals are left to resolve many health behavior dilemmas largely on their own. In the past many health behaviors, for example, sex, diet, and physical activity, were dominated by religion and culture or environmental circumstance. In modern society individual decision making about a wide range of health behaviors has become for many people a delicate balancing of influences from personal preferences, family and friends, media, school and work, religion, and culture.

A traditional way of thinking about learning and behavior is the S-O-R conceptualization, shown below, in which stimuli (S) are processed by the organism (O), thereby producing a response (R). Let's consider the S-O-R conceptualization in the context of learning about health behavior.

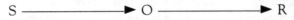

$$S \longrightarrow O \longrightarrow R$$

Learning occurs as a product of **stimuli**, which may take a variety of forms. Most of the stimuli to which people are exposed are unplanned, the product of everyday living. People learn by reading the newspaper, talking with their neighbors, perusing the grocery shelves, observing others, and having other everyday experiences. Only a small proportion of these stimuli (mostly advertisements) are actually designed to influence health behavior. Like advertisements, planned educational activities are designed to stimulate learning by providing the learner with new input, often in the form of information and experiences. Essentially, learning activities are stimuli that create new knowledge, perceptions, feelings, and experiences.

The manner in which stimuli are processed by an **organism** in part determines the response. An amoeba is a simple organism that receives stimuli through a semipermeable membrane and reacts according to genetically-coded patterns. Humans are complex organisms with a variety of senses and a complex cognitive apparatus for processing stimuli. Unlike amoebae, humans do not react uniformly to a stimulus. The existing knowledge, previous experience, current attitudes, and perhaps even the mood, personality, gender, and socialization of the individual may influence how she or he receives and processes a stimulus. This wide variation in how individuals are influenced by stimuli is partly the product of the inherent individuality of humans, partly the product of learning and partly the product of environmental circumstances and temporary states of individual readiness.

The **response** of an amoeba to a stimulus, bloating when exposed to a saline solution, for example, is quite consistent and predictable. Conversely, the consistency of human behavior is challenged by the many competing stimuli to which humans are constantly being exposed, and the complex nature of human cognitive processes, whereby they are not merely passive recipients of stimuli but active participants in processing these stimuli.

The mechanisms through which stimuli are interpreted and stored in memory are complex and poorly understood. Indeed, humans are capable of consciously considering a great number of competing stimuli, holding their impressions of them in memory, and purposefully responding or not responding to them. Hence, it is not surprising that the response of a human to any specific stimuli may be neither immediate nor completely predictable. Responses to stimuli depend not just on the stimuli, but also upon factors associated with the human organism, including its personality, capabilities, cognitive characteristics, and situational factors.

Cognitive and Affective Dimensions of Learning

Knowledge, beliefs, and attitudes are generally referred to collectively as **cognitive variables** because they are inside the mind and have to do with knowing or believing, or **psychosocial** because they are socially influenced. The term "cognitive" is also used more restrictively to describe knowledge, the factual and conceptual aspects of learning. Cognitive and affective perspectives about a particular topic are important influences on health behavior. These variables, however, do not operate independently, and are best understood within the context of the wide range of competing influences. Stated simply, healthful intentions to behave in a particular way, for example exercising, are often overcome by competing intentions and environmental circumstances. Knowledge, beliefs, attitudes, and related cognitive or psychosocial variables reside within the learner, while social and physical environment variables form the context within which learning and behavior occur.

These **intrinsic** (inside the person) psychological and **extrinsic** (outside the person) socioenvironmental variables are interactive and competitive. Indeed, it is difficult to separate psychological and social influences and often it is the perception of, rather than the actual, social influence that operates on behavior. For example, adolescents appear to be more influenced to drink alcohol by their perception that their peers will think well of them for doing so, than by what their peers actually think about adolescents who drink alcohol (Augustyn and Simons-Morton, 1995).

Although health educators generally tend to place heavy emphasis on the intermediate-term goal of facilitating specific behavioral changes, most of our more immediate educational objectives focus on knowledge and skills, beliefs (perceptions), attitudes, and social influences—factors that are thought to mediate behavior and can be influenced by education (see table 9.1). It is the task of the health educator to influence the determinants that can be influenced, and this is invariably knowledge, skills, beliefs, and attitudes.

Knowledge and skills, beliefs, attitudes, and values have both cognitive and affective components, and therefore are somewhat overlapping. Facts and concepts are generally viewed as cognitive, but carry some affective connotations to the extent people have feelings about facts and concepts. Beliefs and attitudes are affective because they are concerned with a person's feelings, but they are always about facts and concepts.

Humans learn largely from experience, some of which are planned, educational experiences, but most of which are unplanned, incidental events. People acquire cognitive attributes from structured learning experiences and from everyday life experiences, and retain this learning in their memories. While all cognitive and affective attributes are changeable, given sufficient and appropriate stimuli, some specific cognitive and affective attributes may remain essentially unchanged for years or forever, regardless of exposure to contrary stimuli.

Of course, health behavior is determined by a number of factors, learning being only one of them. **Learning**, defined as change in knowledge, skills, beliefs, and attitudes, mediates behavior, but is not the only influence on behavior. **Mediators** are factors that facilitate or help to bring about personal behavior

Table 9.1 Definitions of Major Cognitive Variables

Variable	Definition
Knowledge	An intellectual acquaintance with facts, truth, or principles gained by sight, experience, or report.
Skills	The ability to do something well, arising from talent, training, or practice.
Beliefs	Acceptance of or confidence in an alleged fact or body of facts as true or right without positive knowledge or proof; a perceived truth.
Attitudes	Manner, disposition, feeling, or position toward a person or thing.
Values	Ideas, ideals, customs that arouse an emotional response for or against them.

change. Favorable changes in cognitive and affective mediators contribute to the tendency for behavior change. Mediators may be motivational, increasing the tendency or intent to change, or enabling, making it easier to change. Other mediators of behavior include the behavior of other people—for example, social support and social norms. Mediators are changeable by usual behavior change processes. To health educators mediators are the most important category of determinants of a health behavior. Mediators are distinct from **precursors**, another important category of determinants. Precursors are rooted in previous experience—for example, traumatic events and past family, school, and community experiences; or are more or less fixed circumstances—for example, age, race, sex, income, location, personality, family composition. Of course, it can be argued that one way precursors influence behavior is through their influence on cognitive and affective variables. Nevertheless, the distinction between mediators as cognitive factors that can be changed and precursors as factors that influence behavior but are not generally changeable is important and useful in understanding and facilitating behavior change.

Practicing health educators appreciate that cognitive and affective variables mediate behavior, although achieving changes in these variables does not assure concomitant changes in health behavior because of the influence of precursors and environmental factors that cannot be modified easily. A school health educator who is teaching a group of 10-year-olds about the respiratory system does not expect to see any immediate change in overt health behavior, but hopes to build a store of knowledge, skills, and attitudes that the pupils can draw upon when needed in the future. It may be years before these pupils are challenged to refuse a cigarette or wear a protective mask in a dusty work place; meanwhile, our hypothetical educator must rely on the persistence of this early cognitive and affective learning and its possible strengthening by later experiences. Similarly, health educators who work with adolescents are committed to developing in their students the knowledge, attitudes, and skills they need to avoid unwanted pregnancies, drug and alcohol problems, and violence. However, they appreciate that while this knowledge and skill are both motivating and essential for purposeful health behavior, they may not be sufficient to overcome precursors and competing socioenvironmental influences on health behavior. Hence, we recognize the need to intervene not only with the target population but also on social influences. Further, we recognize that education has an important affect on motivation but that changes in motivation do not always lead to changes in behavior due to other factors.

Cognitive and affective variables sometimes make competing demands. A woman may take her medication because she knows that it will relieve her symptoms and because she believes her physician and her spouse may think better of her for taking it. She keeps her medical appointments because she believes in the importance of health care and has a good attitude toward physicians. She regularly uses her seat belt when driving because she knows it may protect her in the event of a crash and she wishes to provide a good example for her children. At the same time, she believes in the health benefits of exercise and even likes her after-work aerobics class, but despite her spouse's willingness to manage the children during this time she seldom attends because she more highly values the time with her children.

Knowledge, beliefs, attitudes, and values mediate behavior and these mediators can be altered by educational stimuli, leading to changes in behavior. Health education is largely a matter of developing learning experiences that lead to changes in these variables. This is not to argue that environmental factors are not important influences on behavior, because of course they are. And this is not to argue that changing environmental factors is not an important health education goal, because of course it is, as we indicated in previous chapters. Indeed, it often has been demonstrated that it is possible to alter behavior by altering the environment. Also, it is the case that cognitive and affective factors mediate the behavior of individuals who control programs, policies, practices, and other entities that influence individual-level behavior. Health education directed at the individual level seeks to facilitate responsible personal health behavior. The way people become responsible for changing and sustaining their own behavior is through changes in cognitive and affective variables, whether they are altered by environmental conditions, chance stimuli, or planned educational experiences.

One common source of confusion within health education and related fields is the overlapping nature of the cognitive and affective variables with which practitioners are primarily concerned. Within the public schools, for example, teachers and administrators frequently speak with great urgency about the importance of "attitudes" and "values"; however, it is seldom clear whether they are using these terms as synonyms or if they are referring to distinctly different entities. This confusion is often compounded by the popularity of other related terms such as self-efficacy, self-esteem, expectations, perceived norms, attributions—all of which are specific types of beliefs and attitudes that we discuss later in this chapter.

Knowledge

The adage that "knowledge is necessary, but not sufficient" is well known in health education circles. This is not to say that knowledge is not important in behavior change, only that it is not the only condition for change. Indeed, the importance of knowledge as a mediator of behavior change should not be underestimated. Without adequate knowledge, people may be unaware of and unconcerned about important health problems and unable to manage their health behavior. Knowledge objectives are included in virtually all health promotion interventions not only because information is an important mediator and knowledge is an essential aspect of intentional behavior change, but also because education professionals are ethically bound to improve the relevant knowledge of the learners they serve.

Knowledge is defined as an intellectual acquaintance with facts, truth, or principles gained by sight, experience, or report (Random House, 1990). One's knowledge of something, therefore, may include some combination of (1) a simple awareness of facts and (2) some understanding of how these facts relate to one another or to outside entities. Generally, knowledge can be viewed as a rather uncomplicated commodity—an accurate impression of some phenomenon.

Knowledge results from exposure to informational stimuli to the extent the learner pays attention to it, understands it, and retains it. Information can be delivered in a variety of forms, including structured education programs. But information also comes from unstructured sources, for example, from everyday conversations, from reading, listening to the radio, watching television, and from other life experiences.

Quite often the health educator's main task is one of helping the learner to become knowledgeable about some health topic. In addition to carefully organizing the content, the instructor also must analyze the level of complexity of the information to be developed and the level of knowledge needed by the learner. Depending on the learner's background, this education may vary from the dissemination of simple information, as in instructing new parents where and when polio immunization will be available, to relatively complex instruction, as when diabetes patients are taught how to adjust their insulin dosage to variations in their food intake and activity level. Of course, what makes health education so interesting is that different target populations need different information delivered in ways that are uniquely appropriate for them.

One key issue in health education is the kind of knowledge that is important for particular educational objectives, and therefore, the kind of information and the extent of instruction required. While the primary objective of some programs is to improve learners' knowledge and understanding about a particular health topic, increasingly, health education programs are concerned with behavior change. Relatedly, there are so many important health education topics and so much that could be taught, and generally so little time for instruction, that it is critical that decisions be made about what content should be included and what level of knowledge development is desired.

Bloom (1956) and associates developed a "Taxonomy of Educational Objectives" which provides a precise scheme for the development and classification of educational objectives in the knowledge or "cognitive domain." Bloom identified the following six increasingly complex levels of cognition: (1) knowledge, (2) comprehension, (3) application, (4) analysis, (5) synthesis, and (6) evaluation. Cognition here refers to knowledge broadly and obviously includes aspects of skill, but does not include affective components of cognition, such as attitudes and values. These six levels of cognition are essential guides for developing educational objectives and for conceptualizing and measuring knowledge.

In the development and conduct of health education programs, it is useful to keep in mind the general concept of Bloom's taxonomy and the complexity of cognitive learning (Bloom, 1956). Indeed, meticulous arrangement of educational objectives is essential for curriculum planning. For example, for a course segment on diet and nutrition, initial objectives might target an increase in knowledge about the nutrient contents of certain foods, and the students might record the foods they ate recently and look up specific nutrient values in a relevant reference manual. Comprehension objectives might focus on the student's understanding of the dynamic influences of nutrient intake on human growth, development, and regulatory functions. Application objectives might focus on the planning of meals to provide 1800 calories per day, 25-30 percent of which come from fat. Evaluation objectives might focus on the student's ability to judge the effects of a dietary pattern on his or her health and lifestyle.

As important as knowledge is in behavior change, not all knowledge is mediating. This is fortunate because in most health promotion interventions time is rarely available for all the information about why smoking is bad for health, or how the adoption of a new program or policy will lead to improved health. Besides, variables other than knowledge are also important in the change process and compete for attention in well-considered programs.

One useful way to think about knowledge is the dichotomy between knowledge "about," or awareness, and "how-to" or "essential" knowledge, which is practical and applicable. It is essential because intentional behavior change depends on it. Knowledge about a topic may be important in developing interest in the topic and may even motivate behavior. In general, however, knowledge about a problem is not as critical to behavior change as knowledge about how to perform the target behavior. This "how-to" or "essential" knowledge is a major component of skill. One may become knowledgeable about cholesterol and heart disease, but one must also learn "how to" appropriately and intentionally change dietary behavior, and thereby reduce dietary cholesterol.

Essential knowledge for lower-fat eating behavior might be knowing what foods or types of foods are high and low in fat. Knowledge about the status of one's own blood pressure and the specifics of one's medical regimen is essential to medication-taking compliance. Knowledge about the underlying causes of hypertension and the mechanisms by which medication and behavior therapies are thought to work may be a valuable part of compliance education, particularly because knowledge about underlying cause is thought to support sustained behavior, but this type of knowledge is not absolutely essential for intentional behavior change. Knowledge about the objectives and learning activities for an educational session is essential knowledge for the teacher of that session. Relatedly, knowledge about why certain activities have been included in the curriculum may be useful and even motivating for some teachers, but it is probably not essential and therefore is a lower priority than skill-oriented knowledge. Generally, it is important to identify essential knowledge and skills as intervention objectives, and to include knowledge about underlying causes as needed and as time is available.

Skills

Knowledge and skills are closely related in that skills are the practical application of essential knowledge. Once an individual understands what to do—for example, what foods to eat or what type of exercise to engage in—she or he must develop skill in performing these behaviors in a variety of settings, overcoming a variety of practical barriers.

Skill is the capability of accomplishing something with precision and certainty. Skill requires practical knowledge and ability. On many occasions an individual's inappropriate or ineffective health behavior may result from the lack of mastery of specific skills. The spouse of a heart patient might know about CPR and be very motivated to help, but fail to administer the needed procedure for lack of skill. A harried employee might allow the stress of the work day to cause unpleasant symptoms on into the evening because of a lack of skill in progressive relaxation. Teenage lovers may fail to take appropriate action to prevent an unwanted pregnancy due to the lack of interpersonal skills needed to correct the situation. As the examples suggest, health skills vary widely in their general make-up; however, they generally require a series of steps where timing, coordination, and adjustment to varying conditions become important to effective results. While knowledge about the problem is essential, how-to knowledge is also needed. Not surprisingly, instruction for skill development emphasizes how-to knowledge with substantial opportunity for practice and instructive feedback.

Some skills involve voluntary muscles, in which case the skills are termed **psychomotor**. CPR and stress management, for example, require psychomotor skills. In the realm of intellectual skills, such as problem solving or menu planning, the distinction between skill and knowledge becomes less distinct.

Interestingly, the development of knowledge and skills within the individual learner can take place without any great change in his or her attitudes. In theory, if not in practice, skills increase the competence of the learners without any "tinkering around" on the part of the educator with their personal decisions as to if, when, and where to apply these newly developed competencies. However, skill makes volitional action possible or even likely. Indeed, the process of skill or knowledge acquisition may stimulate some degree of emotional involvement on the part of the learner and emotional involvement carries the potential for attitudinal change.

The mastery of a skill that is a component of a target behavior, such as properly using condoms is to safe sex, or menu planning is to dieting, can only be assured through repeated practice, sometimes until mastery is achieved. For example, education to promote among adolescents the development skills to resist peer pressure to use alcohol involves "how-to" knowledge and classroom practice under simulated conditions. Homework may consist of practice in refusing mild peer pressure, for example, to dress a certain way or to eat certain foods. Practice under realistic conditions can be a powerful influence on behavior because these specific experiences provide the learner with new information and feedback about competence.

Beliefs

While knowledge is widely accepted to be objective truth, beliefs are what one perceives is true, correctly or not. One's store of knowledge and one's beliefs thus overlap substantially. Beliefs, of course, can be classified by external observers as true or false. But the powerful influence of beliefs on behavior is not dependent on their being correct. Indeed, a person's beliefs, even if mistaken, are a powerful guide to behavior. This is the expectancy aspect of a belief, as people come to expect certain things to occur because of the nature of their beliefs. For example, a person may know that alcohol impairs driving ability, but they may also believe that their personal driving ability will not be impaired or that no harm will come to them even if it is. Hence, beliefs are one key to understanding personal expectancies. Beliefs are thought to be important mediators of behavior, and like knowledge, beliefs are highly changeable.

Beliefs are unique from knowledge not only in that they are perceived, but also because some beliefs are held more strongly than others. A person might believe that smoking causes lung cancer, but also believe more strongly that he or she is resistant to smoking-induced lung cancer. Therefore, it is not only what people believe, but how strongly they hold these beliefs that influences behavior. Some beliefs may be intensely held but of such a nature that the occasion seldom if ever arises for their translation into overt behavior, and others may be neutralized by conflicting beliefs.

An individual's beliefs are formed into a more or less orderly structure based upon their relative importance; however, the importance of a belief is based not only upon the intensity with which it is held, but also on the number and strength of its connections with other beliefs. A belief about the certainty of life after death in a heavenly environment is likely to be connected to many other beliefs and have a broad influence on behavior. Such beliefs that directly concern "one's own existence and identity in the physical and social world" are termed **existential** and are quite central to one's belief structure. A single change here may have far-reaching effects. Beliefs concerning matters of taste, on the other hand, generally are located on the periphery of one's belief system. A person's fervent belief that chocolate ice cream is by far the best tasting flavor might be shaken by an exposure to butter pecan, but this would not be likely to have extensive affects on that person's behavior beyond the selection of ice cream.

Attitudes

Beliefs are the building blocks of attitudes. Several related beliefs usually come together to form a more general attitude toward an object or an idea (Ajzen, 1988; Ford, 1992). An **attitude** is ". . . a disposition to respond favorably or unfavorably to an object, person, institution, or event" (Ajzen, 1988:4). Attitudes are relatively enduring and consist of a series of beliefs organized in such a way that they predispose one to act or respond to some situation in a predictable manner. For example, an adolescent might have the following beliefs: (1) smoking is an adultlike behavior; (2) behaving like an adult is desirable; (3) therefore, if I smoke I might appear to be more adultlike. The first of these beliefs represents a cognitive perception or belief, while the third has a strong affective or evaluative component. Together these beliefs represent the central core of an attitude about smoking.

If many attitudes had a structure as simple as that just presented above they would not be enduring. Theoretically, if either the cognitive or affective component were not present the attitude would be lost. For example, if the individual becomes disillusioned about how adultlike smoking might be, or if such an individual were to become convinced that adultlike behavior is not desirable, then the attitude would be nullified or reshaped. Presumably, most attitudes have a peripheral array of beliefs surrounding and buttressing their central core. For example, if adultlike behavior somehow lost its appeal, the desirability of smoking might still be supported by beliefs that adolescent smoking (1) is a way of rebelling against authority; (2) will provide opportunities to affiliate with peers who smoke; (3) will give me something to do during awkward moments with peers; therefore, (4) I may want to try smoking. The individual's original beliefs that ''smoking is adultlike'' could be reinforced by tobacco advertisements that emphasized: (1) the attractiveness of young adults who smoke; (2) the material success of young adults who smoke; and (3) the fast lifestyles of young adults who smoke. Of course, many other beliefs may support not smoking— beliefs about the taste or health effects of smoking, for example. Hence, there may exist within the same individual a variety of conflicting beliefs about the same subject.

The strength of an attitude depends in part on how strongly beliefs about a subject are held and the extent to which they are consistent with each other and with various secondary belief patterns. In the case of smoking, secondary beliefs about adultlike behavior, health behavior, and peer affiliation may all contribute to attitude formation. Attitudes held over long periods of time may become part of an individual's values and go unquestioned. An attitude may become so interwoven into the person's belief structure that it becomes quite difficult to change. Nevertheless, not all attitudes are difficult to change. Going back to our adolescent cigarette smoking example, some children with quite negative attitudes toward smoking develop more favorable ones during adolescence. Similarly, adolescents and young adults are known for their tendency to experiment with smoking and their attitudes are linked to their behavior. Therefore, when people are smoking they may have more favorable attitudes toward smoking than when they are not smoking. The point is that some attitudes are held more strongly than others, but attitudes are changeable.

Values

Values refer to that which one holds in high regard or esteem. The term is traditionally reserved for relatively complex and pervasive entities which may include such abstract principles as truth, beauty, and fame; specific persons or groups such as one's spouse or family; or specific activities such as art, skiing, or working at one's craft or profession. A common quality of values is their tendency to exert strong and enduring influences on the feelings and behavior of those holding them. As Louis Raths and his associates (1978:26) describe it:

> People grow and learn through experience. Out of experiences may come certain general guides to behavior. These guides tend to give direction to life and may be called values. Our values show what we are likely to do with our limited time and energy.

As implied in this description, values are usually regarded as more complex than attitudes; they may, in fact, represent a focal point for a whole system of interrelated attitudes. A man who values his family, for example, may manifest this value in positive attitudes toward individual family members, family recreational activities, family rituals, life insurance protection, home maintenance, and a host of other family-related objects or activities. Much of this man's behavior could be readily linked to these specific attitudes; however, it might take longer to identify the value he places on his family as the underlying influence. We might see him building a patio in his backyard and consequently assume that he likes to build things. Later we might see him leaving work an hour early to attend his daughter's birthday party and thus assume that he feels birthdays are important. Upon seeing him planning a family camping trip, we might assume that he enjoys woodland recreations. As these individual observations accumulate, we reach a point where a pattern becomes apparent and the high value placed on the family is identified. Values are thus observed to exert a broad and powerful influence on behavior. Attitudes, however, are more specific, more readily discernible, and easier to change.

Information and Experience

Planned learning activities provide the learner with information and experience. Information is a type of stimulus, but information is also the product of experience. Information comes out of experiences, including formal education, watching television, playing computer games, talking with friends, and other life activities. Exposure to an experience may produce different information for different learners due to a number of factors, including how much attention they pay to the experience and how they interpret the experience. The knowledge gained from an experience might be extremely valuable if it happens to resonate with the learner's needs and perceptions.

Recognizing the importance of experience, health educators frequently develop learning experiences that extend beyond didactic information giving so that the learner can obtain the most relevant kinds of information— information that is contextual and experiential. For example, high school students might be asked to engage in a role play regarding peer pressure, and high blood pressure patients might be asked to describe in detail where they keep their medicine, when they take the medicine, and how they will overcome certain impediments to compliance. Thus the learners (and the health educator) learn a great deal from these exercises because they involve practical contexts and because the learners are participants in them, making the information personally relevant. Similarly, intense personal learning also occurs outside the classroom and clinic when the adolescent is pressured by a peer to smoke a cigarette or the patient is confronted with a problematic barrier to medication-taking compliance.

Experience is a critical behavioral mediator because it provides information that is partly contextual and partly self-generated. The more applied and less abstract this experience the more powerful a mediator it is likely to be. Simulated experiences may stimulate learners to reevaluate cognitive and affective dispositions about the relevant behaviors. Real life experiences, however, are more powerful than simulated ones, partly because success cannot be controlled and assured as it can in simulations. Unsuccessful experiences, simulated or real-life, tend to discourage behavior while successful experiences tend to encourage or reinforce the behavior. For example, a person who decides to exercise, but has difficulty overcoming practical barriers to daily exercise is likely to become discouraged and quit. A person who has developed the appropriate skills for overcoming barriers—self-monitoring and the like—should be encouraged by this success, and therefore, be more likely to continue to exercise. Similarly, a young person considering experimenting with sex can be taught in the classroom to negotiate the use of a condom with his or her partner, thus motivating the individual to use a condom in real-life situations. If an attempt to negotiate condom use in a real-life event is successful, it will reinforce condom usage, but if this negotiation is not successful, it may mitigate against subsequent attempts to negotiate the use of condoms. Health educators are constantly challenged to provide learning experiences which practically challenge the learner, offer high likelihood of success, and approximate real-life experiences.

Measurement

Because cognitive variables are psychological, they cannot be measured directly, but must be inferred from indirect measures. Knowledge and skills generally are measured by multiple-choice or true and false examinations. Knowledge assessment, relative to attitude assessment, is a relatively straightforward and precise task. It is possible in knowledge tests to achieve relatively high discrimination between those with more knowledge and those with less knowledge and acceptable levels of test-retest reliability. Naturally, while there are many important test development skills, the key to assessment of knowledge is the specification of objectives. Skill is usually measured indirectly with questions about how-to knowledge, application, analysis, and synthesis.

Beliefs, attitudes, and values are commonly measured by questionnaires. Respondents are asked how strongly they agree or disagree with carefully selected statements (see figure 9.1). A single item or an index consisting of several items may measure each belief or attitude. Values usually are assessed by asking the respondent to rank or prioritize relevant items. Although far from perfect, these

Figure 9.1   Scale for Measuring Beliefs and Attitudes

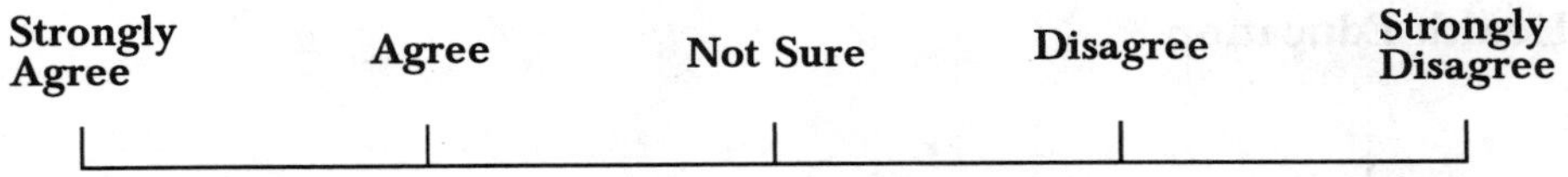

Strongly Agree	Agree	Not Sure	Disagree	Strongly Disagree

indirect questioning procedures appear to represent the best available solutions to the attitude measurement problem. It is possible with some effort to develop fairly discriminating and reliable measures of beliefs and attitudes.

Health Behavior Conceptualizations and Theories as Guides to Action

Having reviewed the basic concepts of the major cognitive and affective variables, we can now take up theories of how these variables interrelate and exert influence on motivation and behavior. In this section we discuss six important theories that deal with knowledge, beliefs, attitudes, values, and behavior.

A great many individual research studies have been conducted in an effort to understand the effects of variations in the nature and intensity of intervening variables on motivation and human behavior. However, human behavior is infinitely complex and a definitive understanding is elusive. Theorists, however, have conceptualized the possible relationships between selected variables and how they can affect behavior. The resulting models and theories have been useful in stimulating research and providing provisional guides to action.

Cognitive Consistency Theory

The cognitive consistency theory of behavior posits that people prefer to be consistent in their knowledge, attitudes, and behavior (Bettinghaus, 1986). According to this theory, new information creates dissonance between knowledge, attitudes, and behavior and this stimulates alterations in behavior consistent with knowledge and attitudes. This is an attractive theory for health educators, who as a group are proud of their ability to change knowledge and attitudes through usual educational means. According to the consistency theory, changing behavior requires only that the health educator provide information and experiences that produce knowledge consistent with the desired behavior. Logically, the knowledge gained would stimulate changes in attitudes and eventually behavior (see figure 9.2).

Figure 9.2   Cognitive Consistency

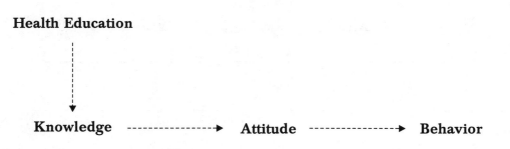

Health Education

Knowledge - - - - - - - - - -> **Attitude** - - - - - - - - - -> **Behavior**

While cognitive consistency or dissonance theory is attractive, plausible, and may properly describe some readers' health behavior, researchers have not found the theory to provide a truly satisfactory explanation of the relationships between knowledge, attitudes, and health behavior. Contrary to the theory, people appear to tolerate substantial dissonance between personal cognition and behavior. Of course, we know from our previous discussion in this chapter that information does not always lead to knowledge and that people are able to retain conflicting bits of information and interpret them according to their personal values or perspectives (gestalt). But quite apart from these problems, even when education leads to the predicted and targeted knowledge gains, consistent attitude and behavior changes do not necessarily follow. Part of the problem seems to be that people commonly filter information selectively so that they develop knowledge that is consistent with their attitudes and behavior. Also, an individual may stockpile other knowledge or have other beliefs that are inconsistent with the recently gained knowledge. Finally, knowledge can be as much a product of attitudes and behavior as attitudes and behavior are of knowledge.

Relatedly, behavior influences knowledge and attitudes just as knowledge and attitudes influence behavior. Previously we noted that personal experiences produce important personal information, information that may have more salient influence on knowledge than information provide by impersonal sources. People who do not exercise are more likely to have negative attitudes about exercising, while exercisers typically have positive attitudes about exercise. In similar fashion attitudes influence knowledge and behavior. People with favorable attitudes toward exercise are likely to be interested in exercise and therefore to exercise and become more informed about it.

Ironically, while one problem with the consistency theory is that people appear to be tolerant of a certain amount of dissonance or inconsistency, another problem is that people tend to be consistent, but not necessarily in the way suggested by the theory. That is, people may be as likely to change their knowledge and attitudes to be consistent with their behavior as they are to modify their behavior to be consistent with new information.

Of course, another major limitation of the theory of cognitive consistency is that it does not adequately take into account the effects of reinforcement and environmental factors. An individual may be cognitively and affectively predisposed toward a health behavior, but physical and social environmental factors prevent the individual from engaging in the behavior. Conversely, an individual may be cognitively and negatively predisposed against a particular behavior, but powerful environmental factors otherwise shape the behavior.

The reader may be tempted at this point to conclude that cognitive consistency theory is of little use in understanding behavior, but that would be shortsighted. A good theory of behavior orders variables logically so that they explain a phenomenon in a way that can be tested in empirical research. Research investigating the postulates of consistency theory has not validated the theory, but has led to a new understanding of behavior and the change process. One of the important things we have learned from studying dissonance and consistency is that education should target not only knowledge, but also attitudes and behavior because these variables interact in complex and dynamic ways. Rather than proceeding in a linear fashion from knowledge to attitudes to behavior, learning is the product of the simultaneous interaction of knowledge, attitudes, and behavioral experiences. Therefore, as illustrated in figure 9.3, effective health education simultaneously should target knowledge, attitudes, and behavior. Of course, this is perfectly "consistent" with what many experienced health educators have found in practice to be the best way to facilitate learning.

Figure 9.3   The Learning Process

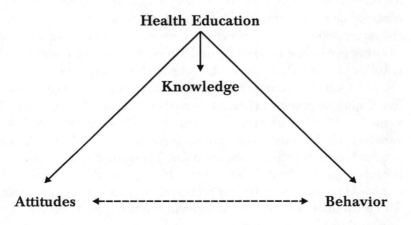

Information Processing and Persuasive Communication

Effective communication can change beliefs, attitudes, and behavior. Advertisers, politicians, and health educators, among others, are interested in methods for making their communications as believable and persuasive as possible. People are bombarded constantly with health communications, advertisements, and appeals of all sorts. They cannot possibly pay equal attention to them all. Indeed, some of these messages may be contradictory; for example, cigarette advertise- ments and admonishments to not smoke. Naturally, researchers and programmers have long been interested in how people process the information directed at them and how communications can be designed so that people will pay attention to them and be persuaded by them. What factors associated with the information, message, or cue are important in capturing people's attention and belief?

Persuasive communications may be delivered in person or via mediated means, e.g., written or videotaped. While some communications are meant primarily to inform, there are elements of persuasion in many health communications, whether they are delivered verbally by a medical provider to a patient ("I want you to take this medicine exactly according to the instructions"), or via mass media ("Use condoms and practice safe sex"). They may consist of simple presentations of facts or complex, multimedia presentations. Persuasive communications may serve different ends—creating awareness, shaping attitudes, reminding behavior. A radio spot encouraging parents to have their children immunized is one example of a persuasive communication; a print advertisement for a cigarette that is supposed to make women feel liberated is another. Any idea can be presented in a more or less persuasive way. One of the tasks of an educator is to package health-enhancing messages in ways that are persuasive, a task that has been demonstrated to be effective (Simons-Morton, Brink, and Bates, 1987).

Information processing and persuasive communications have been studied for several decades and the robust principles that have been developed can be observed daily in commercials. The goal of persuasive communication is to get the target population to believe the message. A communication that succeeds in being persuasive is not only understood by the target population, but also is believed, appreciated, valued, and therefore motivating.

McGuire (1984) has organized the study of persuasive communication into five major components: (1) source variables, (2) message variables, (3) channel variables, (4) receiver variables, and (5) destination variables. A sample of variables related to these components is presented in table 9.2. A vast literature exists relevant to each of these variables. Theoretically, if one could understand the relationships between all these variables, given sufficient time and resources, one could persuade a significant proportion of people to do just about anything. This is the approach most often taken in commercial advertising. It has worked so well that the same approach is now being employed in health promotion.

Table 9.2 The Five Components and Related Variables of Persuasive Communications

I. **Source Variables**
   A. Credibility: The more credible the source or model is perceived to be, the more believable will be the message.
   B. Attractiveness: More attractive sources are thought to be more believable and persuasive than less attractive sources.
   C. Power: More powerful sources are thought to be more believable. The power of the source may derive from position, status, or experience.

II. **Message Variables**
   A. Type of appeal: Appeals maybe humorous, attention getting, factual, emotional, or instructional. Each type of appeal may be appropriate for certain situations and populations.
   B. Content: The content of a persuasive communication is important for what is included and what is excluded. Because most persuasive communications are brief, the selection of content is critical. The order in which the information appears may be important because of the logic or emotional appeal and the tendency of people to develop impressions of the persuasive communication and to recall only parts of the message rather than the entire message.
   C. Discrepancy: Messages can be developed to be only modestly discrepant from the receiver's initial position so that the perceived extent of change is not very great or they can be portrayed as more profound or revolutionary than they really are.

III. **Channel Variables**
   A. Medium: Persuasive communications can be delivered person-to-person or via print, audiovisual, or interactive media. Often media such as videotapes are developed so that appropriate (credible, attractive, powerful) models, not available in person, can deliver the persuasive communications.
   B. Modality: Visual, auditory, and even tactile modes can be employed.

IV. **Receiver Variables**
   A. Demographics: The age, gender, race, and consumer characteristics of the target receivers are important considerations in developing persuasive communications.
   B. Psychosocial factors: Current knowledge, beliefs, attitudes, abilities, skills, practices, expectations, attributions, etc. may be important considerations in developing persuasive communications.

V. **Destination or Outcome Variables**
   A. Timing: Persuasive communications may be designed to have immediate effects, reinforce existing effects, or have latent or delayed effects.
   B. Scope: Persuasive communications may be very narrow in scope, for example focusing on a specific fact, attitude (e.g., condom use), or they may focus on general knowledge, attitudes, or practices (e.g., responsible sex).
   C. Target: Persuasive communications may attempt to create awareness while others are designed to alter comprehension (knowledge), acceptance (beliefs), affect (attitudes), or action.

Source: Based on McGuire, 1984.

1. *Source Variables.* The influence of who gives the message (Madonna or Bill Cosby), from where the message comes (the tobacco industry or the Office of the Surgeon General of the United States), or to whom the message is attributed ("authorities agree that . . . ."), depends on how acceptable that source is to the receiver. The more acceptable the source, the more effective the message. Different sources may be effective for different types of receivers (target populations) and messages.

2. *Message Variables.* The style, content, and organization of the message is an important aspect of persuasive communication. One can appeal to reason, to emotions, to fear, to images, and to associations (e.g., handsome guy surrounded by beautiful girls is drinking Ape Ale, ergo if you drank Ape Ale you would be a handsome guy surrounded by beautiful girls). One can repeat the same message over and over, or change it slightly. One can manipulate the order of the content or the relative emphasis. One can attempt to emphasize or to minimize discrepancies between the current action and the advocated one. The message may forewarn of problems that may be encountered, thereby anticipating objections and inoculating the receiver from their effects.

3. *Channel.* The choice of medium or channel is also important in persuasive communication. Printed material, posters, billboards, slides, radio, television, newspapers, journals, direct mailings, telephone calls, person-to-person contact, visual or audio aids, or a combination of these channels could be selected to deliver the message. Of course, budget, audience, message, and target behaviors are factors that must be considered in the selection of channel.

4. *Receiver Variables.* Receiver variables are concerned with characteristics of the receiver or target population. This category of variables is perhaps the single most important set of source variables for developing and delivering a persuasive communication. All the other variables depend heavily on the characteristics of the receiver. Receiver variables include the age, gender, culture, knowledge, attitudes, practices, and values of the receivers. The more programmers know about these variables the better able they are to develop and deliver communications that reach the target population, are paid attention to, are understood, and are persuasive.

5. *Destination Variables.* Persuasive communications can target a variety of destinations or outcomes including awareness, comprehension (knowledge), acceptance (beliefs), and affect (attitudes). Some outcomes are more difficult to influence than others. Awareness and knowledge outcomes require informational messages that are accessible and comprehensible to the target population. Affect-oriented outcomes require that the message have emotional impact. Finally, specific, divisible, and reversible actions are more easily targeted than more general, nondivisible, and irreversible ones. For example, it may be easier to encourage the target population to try using margarine or low-fat milk, than it would be to encourage them to become vegetarians. To be effective, messages should be created to address very specific objectives.

All of these variables must be considered together, interactively, in developing the most effective communication. An effective communication is one that attracts the attention of the receivers, one that they comprehend, and one that they accept or believe. Such a communication will achieve the outcome or destination of changing awareness, knowledge, beliefs, or attitudes.

Despite a great deal of research, the development of persuasive communications is still largely an art form rather than a science. Perhaps the only accepted truism is that the developer must understand the receiver (target population) very well. Armed with a careful needs assessment, the artist in every experienced health educator can be employed to make creative decisions about each variable.

The persuasive communication framework is useful as a reference for developing and evaluating all kinds of communications from classroom and school-wide presentations to broader mass persuasion campaigns. Persuasive communications are ubiquitous in health promotion practice. Every health promotion program seems to include an information sheet, a poster, a bumper sticker, or a videotape. While some of these persuasive communications no doubt are very clever and creative, their effectiveness depends a great deal on what else the program has to offer. Persuasive communications can alter knowledge and attitudes, and therefore are motivating. They may even improve skills and therefore may be enabling. However, they address a limited number of variables and are but one small part of a well-considered health promotion program. They may serve to inform, remind, and encourage people, but most behaviors can be altered only when people are exposed to substantial educational programs.

Advertisers are keenly aware that belief and action depend greatly on repeated exposure to persuasive communications because there is so much competition for people's limited attention span. Where the profit potential is large—for example, in selling cars—commercial interests will support massive advertising campaigns to penetrate and saturate the market according to preestablished marketing research and guidelines. Conversely, most nonprofit public health campaigns are comparatively abbreviated because they depend on free advertising and cannot hope to achieve adequate market penetration.

Commercial marketers are careful to coordinate all marketing aspects. When a new product becomes available, or when a commercial interest is attempting to increase its market share, marketers coordinate advertising in appropriate sources with point of purchase adds, price discounts, and other product inducements. Advertising alone, without an effort to make the product more attractive and available, is not likely to be very successful. Social marketing, discussed in more detail in chapter 13, is an approach to health promotion that incorporates principles of information processing into more comprehensive strategies that include a variety of marketing principles and social change approaches (Frederiksen, Solomon, and Brehony, 1984).

Health Belief Model

Among health educators the health belief model (HBM), shown in figure 9.4, is perhaps the best known of any conceptualization of health behavior. The

Figure 9.4   Basic Components of the Health Belief Model

INDIVIDUAL PERCEPTIONS   MODIFYING FACTORS   LIKELIHOOD OF ACTION

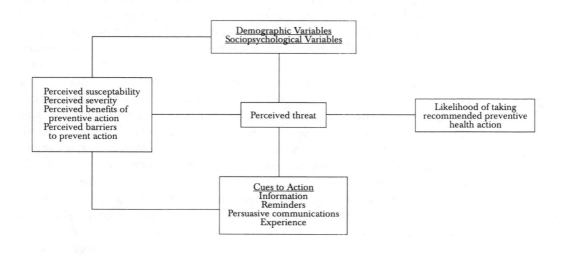

HBM was originally developed as a way of understanding preventive health behavior, specifically, to identify a few high-priority factors that might affect one's decision to comply with medical recommendations (Rosenstock, 1990).

The HBM derives from values expectancy theory, which, generally stated, refers to a view of rational decision making in situations of uncertainty. When a person fractures a leg it is clear that person needs medical attention, but if someone merely bumps his or her head, it is not so clear that medical attention is required. Similarly, chest pain could indicate indigestion, angina, or a heart attack. Decisions about when to seek care for certain symptoms, therefore, must often be based on certain assumptions about the problem and the expectations about the possible courses of action. The alternative choices—seeking care, self medicating, or waiting for further information—are in competition. Logically, individuals make decisions that are consistent with the outcomes they most value.

The HBM emphasizes the importance of **perception** in decision making. More important than objective truth is the expectation that a particular belief evokes about a certain course of behavior. That is, it is less important how effective a therapy is than how effective the patient or consumer believes it to be.

Perceptions are influenced by a variety of factors, including stimuli received by the individual; the context within which the stimuli is received; the individual's previous experience, personality, mood; and the things of which a person is consciously aware at a given point in time (gestalt or life space).

Perceptions can be quite individual. For example, several people witnessing a motor vehicle crash may have very different perceptions of the event due to factors that shade their perception, for example because they: saw it from different vantage points; became aware of the event at different times or stages of the event; were simultaneously exposed to unique influences competing for their attention; have different personalities; have had different past experiences; and were in different psychological states at the time the event occurred. All parties were exposed to the same physical event, but the perceptions that reached their brains varied considerably.

A perception is something one believes to be true, regardless of whether or not it is actually true in objective terms. Beliefs are primarily cognitive, but also contain an affective component. The cognitive component relates to the level of certainty with which the belief is held, while the affective component relates to the extent to which the belief or its consequences is valued by the individual. Hence, some beliefs are held more strongly and are more influential than other beliefs. Beliefs evoke expectations about the outcomes of a certain course of action and it is these expectations that motivate behavior.

The HBM identifies the following four categories of beliefs as paramount determinants of whether or not one will take a recommended course of preventive health behavior:

1. **Perceived seriousness** is the relative severity of the health problem. People are more likely to respond to suggestions that they obtain "flu shots" if they view influenza as a serious disease. Indeed, the elderly are concerned about influenza and are more likely than other groups to seek the vaccine.

2. **Perceived susceptibility** is the extent to which the individual believes he or she is vulnerable to the health problem. Individual perceptions of personal susceptibility to specific illnesses or accidents often vary widely from any realistic appraisal of their statistical probability. The nature and intensity of these perceptions may significantly affect their willingness to take preventive action. People who believe they are likely to get influenza, perhaps because they are frequently exposed to people with influenza, may be more likely to seek the vaccine.

3. **Perceived benefits** concern the anticipated value of the recommended course of action. Individuals generally must believe the recommended health action will actually do some good if they are to comply. Confidence in the efficacy of the flu vaccine should increase the likelihood of seeking the vaccine.

4. **Perceived barriers** include the costs involved in taking a particular action. If a person perceives that getting a flu vaccine may be time consuming, difficult, expensive, or painful that person may be unlikely to seek the vaccine.

In addition to these four salient categories, general concern with health matters, locus of control, and a variety of other potential motivational or modifying factors have been added to the HBM in recent reconceptualizations as shown in figure 9.4.

Cues are thought to mobilize or bring relevant beliefs into the receiver's consciousness and thus to bear upon a particular health decision. Cues may be incidental and unplanned, such as the untimely demise from lung cancer of a cigarette-smoking uncle; or planned, as from an advertisement or a health communication delivered via print or audiovisual media or in person by a health care provider or educator.

The HBM is frequently used as a framework for conducting needs assessments in preventive health behavior and compliance studies (Richardson and Simons-Morton, 1993). The resulting interventions almost always include cues in the form of persuasive communications directed toward increasing the salience of beliefs about the severity of and susceptibility to the health problem and the benefits of the recommended treatment or action while minimizing barriers. In some programs skills for avoiding or overcoming inherent barriers are taught.

Unfortunately, only perceived barriers are consistently associated with behavior (Janz and Becker, 1984). However, due perhaps to its intuitive appeal, the HBM continues to be used in many health promotion diagnostic studies.

Theory of Planned Behavior

The Theory of Planned Behavior (Ajzen, 1988) evolved out of the Theory of Reasoned Action (Ajzen and Fishbein, 1980). In both theories the focus is on intentions rather than behavior itself, for several important reasons. Intent is a measure of motivation or readiness to act and many studies have shown that intent is an excellent predictor of behavior. However, as we discussed previously, behaviors have a way of shaping attitudes, and environmental factors often have a powerful influence on behavior. An adolescent may intend to have sexual intercourse, but have no willing partner. A couch potato may intend to go for a bicycle ride but snowy weather prevents it. Hence, if one is concerned mainly about motivation to behave, it makes sense to measure intentions rather than behavior.

In both reasoned action and planned behavior, beliefs are viewed as the basic components of attitudes, the building blocks of attitudes (Ajzen, 1988). Both theories emphasize that attitudes toward the behavior and attitudes about what important others think they should do (subjective norms) are associated with the intention to behave in a certain way. The Theory of Planned Behavior is distinct from reasoned action mainly in that it includes a third category of variables for predicting behavioral intentions: attitudes about the ease or difficulty of performing the behavior (perceived behavioral control). The relationships between these variables are illustrated in figure 9.5 and described in the following paragraphs.

Figure 9.5   Theory of Planned Behavior

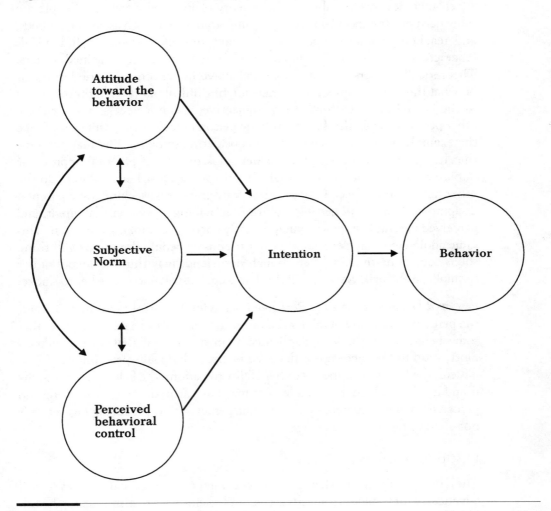

ₗₒ Behavioral Variables

ₐ*Attitudes toward the behavior.*   Attitudes toward the behavior, or more precisely, ₗattitudes toward the expected net outcome or result of the behavior, are important determinants of behavior.⌋ For example, an adolescent who is considering smoking cigarettes may have developed generally favorable attitudes about smoking, perhaps due to advertising or exposure to a kindly uncle who smokes. This same youth may believe that smoking will make her feel older or more grown up. The sum total of these attitudes toward smoking and toward the outcomes of smoking contribute toward the likelihood that she will try smoking.

Subjective norms.   One of the traditional concerns of social psychologists is the influence that other people have on a person's attitudes and behavior. Icek Ajzen includes this variable in the Theory of Planned Behavior. People are influenced by other people, particularly important others such as parents, friends, and teachers, but also peer groups, distant reference groups or individuals (characters in a book or movie, rock stars), or even imagined others. Theoretically, a person's intentions to behave in certain ways are dependent on what they believe important others might think about them if they engaged in the behavior. As with all things subjective, it is not necessary what these other people actually think, but what the person perceives they will think. Take the example of our adolescent who is considering smoking. She may perceive that her parents will disapprove of her smoking, and if parental approval is important to her, their disapproval will mitigate against her smoking. On the other hand, our adolescent may at that point in time be seeking some parental disapproval as a way of getting attention or making a personal statement, and perceived parental disapproval may actually encourage smoking initiation. This same adolescent may perceive that her friends or people she knows will think she is cool if she smokes. Even though her friends may think it uncool of her to smoke, if she believes they will think it is cool, it will encourage her to smoke.

Perceived behavioral control.   Perceived behavioral control takes into account the perceived difficulty of taking the target action. This variable recognizes that some behaviors are more complicated than others and that an individual's motivation to take action is influenced by the individual's perceptions of how difficult the behavior is and his or her ability to perform the behavior successfully (Bandura, 1986). Hence, an adolescent may have attitudes toward smoking and perceive favorable subjective norms, but perceive that procuring cigarettes is not something she can manage.

Distinct Features

The Theory of Planned Behavior provides several conceptual and methodological advances which make it an attractive and useful way to think about health behavior.

First, the theory's focus on the intermediate outcome of intentions rather than on behavior is useful in that it isolates internal motivation from extrinsic environmental influences. In many cases intentions are only modestly associated with behavior because environmental influences are also important. By focusing on intentions the role of attitudes on internal motivation can be separated from situational and environmental influences.

Second, the theory emphasizes that attitudes are made up of beliefs, which are relatively easy to measure accurately. Third, the Theory of Planned Behavior develops the idea that motivation is greatly influenced by attitudes. The importance of attitudes in motivation and behavior has long been recognized, but this theory emphasizes that it is not just how the person views the behavior (desirable or not desirable) but also perceived expectations the person has about how favorable the outcomes of their performing the behavior might be. Expectations about the outcomes of an action, realistic or not, are highly motivating. Believing that driving recklessly will have mainly favorable outcomes—for example, fun, thrills, and power—motivates teens to drive recklessly. Conversely, believing that by driving recklessly they may have a crash, alienate their friends, and lose their driving privileges, teens may be motivated to drive more cautiously.

The theory's emphasis on subjective norms is another important contribution because it recognizes the influence of other people on behavior, or more precisely the influence of one's perceptions of how other people will view the person, should he or she engage in the behavior. The idea is that each individual is more or less influenced by perceptions of how significant others evaluate the individual's behavior. This is important because people often have incorrect perceptions about how others view their behavior. Adolescents commonly believe that more of their peers smoke, drink, have sex, and approve of these behaviors than actually do. That is, social norms tend to be more conservative than they are perceived to be (Hanson, 1991). Accordingly, successful health promotion interventions can be developed to foster more realistic perceptions of social norms.

Fifth, the Theory of Planned Behavior also takes into account the influence on intentions of the difficulty of the behavior and the individual's perceived ability to undertake the behavior. Motivation is enhanced by personal confidence and diminished by a lack of personal confidence. Interventions that promote skills and provide opportunities for successful practice increase perceived competence and increase motivation to take certain actions.

Attribution Theory

Attribution theory suggests that people are motivated to explain and understand what causes things to happen, particularly in situations that are ambiguous, extraordinary, or unpredictable. They make causal attributions about a variety of situations and events and the attributions they make motivate their behavior. **Causal attributions** are beliefs about what caused something to happen. Selected types of causal attributions are listed in table 9.3. People may attribute the cause of an event to factors over which they have some measure of control or to factors over which they have no control—for example, to luck or fate. The more personal an influence or control a person perceives in a particular situation, the more motivated they are to exert that influence. An example may help to illustrate this.

To a sexually active adolescent girl pregnancy may seem like an uncertain event. This girl may know that sexual intercourse causes pregnancy, but from experience she also knows that sexual intercourse does not always cause her to get pregnant; after all she is not pregnant now. She may attribute her not getting pregnant to events that she controls or to uncontrollable events. If she attributes her successful avoidance of getting pregnant so far to her steadfast gories of Causal Attributions

Locus	Stability	Controllability	Globality
Individuals make determinations about the extent to which the information, experience, or relationship is something they can control (internal) or is beyond their control (external).	Individuals may interpret experiences or information or relationships as being stable or unstable.	Individuals may perceive that events depend on their level of effort or are not controllable regardless of their efforts.	
Internal locus: ability, aptitude, personality	*Stable:* constant, invariable	*Controllable:* depending on the amount of effort	*Global:* Related to a wide variety of outcomes
External locus: environment, luck, circumstances	*Unstable:* depends on the situation or circumstances	*Uncontrollable:* regardless of the amount of effort	*Non-global:* Specific to a single outcome or limited range of outcomes

use of birth control, then she may be likely to continue to use birth control. If she believes that getting pregnant is a matter of luck and caused by factors out of her control—for example, her partner, luck, or circumstances—she is less likely to be conscientious about birth control.

Similarly, a smoker who has attempted to quit but finds himself now begging cigarettes from co-workers may attribute his behavior to his personality ("I have never been able to control my behavior"); to fate ("No one in my family has ever been able to stop smoking"); to the situation ("I have difficulty not smoking when the people around me are smoking"); or to luck ("It was just my luck that my girlfriend and I had a fight the week I tried to stop smoking").

Attribution theory is relevant to a great many health education problems, ranging from substance use to medication taking. The implications of attribution theory for health education practice are substantial, particularly in the many cases where attributions can be altered by education. Of course, some attributes may be stable personality traits (e.g., locus of control) not easily changeable by education, but others are perceptions and therefore changeable. In many cases attributions about cause are not rooted in deep-seated psychological traits, but in more accessible and mutable beliefs. Indeed, many health behaviors appear to be motivated at least in part by incorrect attributions. For example, a teenager who drinks alcohol or smokes cigarettes may attribute his or her popularity to these practices and therefore become more habituated to these behaviors.

Once the attributions of a target population have been assessed, health education interventions can target them selectively to motivate health-protecting or health-enhancing behavior. For a more complete discussion of attribution theory the interested reader is encouraged to read Wiener (1992), who describes in detail the dimensions of causal attributions and the effects of consequences on attributions.

Stages of Change

Many health educators are aware that their target populations are heterogeneous with respect to interest in, concern about, and experience with any particular problem. A survey of adolescents shows that some of them are personally unaware of and unconcerned about tobacco, alcohol, drugs, and sex, but some of them are contemplating trying out these behaviors, others are experimenting, and a small proportion are engaging in these behaviors on a regular basis. Similarly, surveys of adult physical activity indicate that some are regular exercisers, some are occasional exercisers, some are considering starting to exercise, and some are not thinking about exercise and are not aware that regular physical activity confers substantial health benefits. Some of today's contemplators will tomorrow be occasional exercisers while some of today's occasional exercisers will eventually become regular exercisers.

Relatedly, it appears that individuals may go through a logical series of decision stages on their way to adopting a new behavior (Prochaska and DiClemente, 1984; Horn, 1976). This concept of stages of change has been applied to a variety of behaviors, including contraceptive use (Grimley et al., 1993), but has seen its greatest use in research on smoking cessation (DiClemente et al., 1991). Researchers have found that smokers who quit proceed through a series of stages of change in their efforts to quit. These stages have been labeled precontemplation, contemplation, preparation, action, and maintenance.

Precontemplators are not considering changing their health behavior. A precontemplator smoker is not thinking about quitting smoking, at least not in the near future. He may be totally unaware that smoking is a health or life-style problem or that quitting is an option. We can think of precontemplation as a lack of awareness. Awareness is a long way from behavior change, but if behavior is to change, awareness is an important early stage. Public awareness that high-fat diets pose a health problem is much greater than in the past and, combined with changes in the availability of lower-fat foods, may portend healthier eating in the future.

During **contemplation** a person begins to consider behavior change. A smoker may become aware that smoking is a problem for him and begin to think about quitting sometime in the future. Contemplation is an important stage of information acquisition. During the contemplation stage the person is predisposed to seek relevant information and to take more interest in information with which he comes into contact than he might have as a precontemplator. Perhaps more important, this new stage influences how the contemplator interprets experience. While in a contemplative mode, an event may be motivating that might not have been previously. For example, as a contemplator a person is more likely to be motivated to quit by learning about long-term smokers who have quit or even by persuasive communications. Hence, contemplation is not just a stage describing movement toward purposeful change, but it is also a stage of motivation. The potential for change is much greater among contemplators than among precontemplators because they are much more receptive to planned or incidental learning experiences.

During the **preparation** stage people prepare for and experiment with behavior change. A smoker in the preparation stage may intend to quit soon and may experiment with skipping a cigarette occasionally, with cutting back on the number of cigarettes or the amount of each cigarette that he actually smokes. He may even distance himself from other smokers or situations that prompt him to smoke. The preparation stage is a stage of psychological preparation where the individual tries on the idea of change, imagines himself behaving in the new way, even shares the idea with some other people to learn how they react, and hopefully, develops some skills that will be needed.

During the **action** stage, people try the new behavior. A smoker may cut back or quit briefly as a trial or may set a date and quit altogether. In some cases the action stage is one of experimentation and does not necessarily reflect a permanent change in behavior. Exercisers may try out different routines, activities, and time schedules. Successful experience is motivating while unsuccessful experience thwarts motivation. Hence the more prepared and skillful the individual is the more success he or she is likely to have.

Maintenance is a period when people establish the new pattern of behavior and take on the attitudinal and environmental supports that tend to sustain the behavior. For smokers maintenance has been defined as six months or more after quitting. Maintenance poses unique challenges for the target population and for intervention because for a lot of health behaviors the individual may be working against some fairly strong forces. Indeed, many changes in behavior do not survive. Smokers may continue to be attracted to cigarettes until their attitudes, values, and environment begin to support nonsmoking. Similarly, in our society it is easier to eat high-fat foods and not exercise than it is to eat and exercise appropriately. Purposeful change in these areas requires motivation, skill, successful experience, social support, and environmental supports.

For each health behavior the duration of each stage may be unique, but the same stages are likely to exist. Precontemplation may last indefinitely in that some people never consider smoking or quitting, exercising, dieting, or discontinuing their medicine. Similarly, contemplation may be a brief sustained period. Some people suddenly decide to exercise and begin doing it right away, while others think about it frequently but never get around to it. Preparation speeds the process in that people psychologically prepare for the behavior— they begin thinking about it and imagining how it will be. If preparation goes smoothly, then action is likely, but if preparation is accompanied by misgivings, perceived barriers, and lack of confidence, then action may not occur. A smoker who imagines severe withdrawal may never actually quit, while a smoker who imagines no negative effects may try quitting, but start again as soon as the side effects of withdrawal become apparent. During the action or trial stages the individual learns a lot about the behavior, how much he or she likes it, how much effort it requires, and other effects that may or may not be what was expected. If the individual evaluates the experience favorably, and stays with it for an adequate trial while learning how to manage the behavior, then long-term maintenance is likely, all other things being equal. For example, when people start exercising they are likely to experience soreness, fatigue, and increased appetite, which they may perceive as negative consequences of exercising. Similarly, they may find that adding exercise to a busy daily schedule is more difficult than they had imagined, leading to discontinuation.

Stage of change provides a simple, convenient, and effective way of categorizing a target population—segmenting the market, so to speak—for programmatic attention and for creating intervention components. Measuring each stage is usually quite simple, requiring only a few questions.

Each stage of change represents different challenges for the health educator. A health promotion program may seek to move the target population from one stage to another, for example precontemplation to contemplation only, leaving other programs or components to deal with later stages. A health promotion program may develop intervention components appropriate for each stage of change, targeting various segments of the target population according to stage. Importantly, unique knowledge, skill, belief, and attitude objectives may be appropriate for each stage of change.

Prochaska and DiClemente (1984) have proposed a transtheoretical approach to stages of change in which they attempted to integrate various behavior change theories with the stages of change. Other theorists, Baranowski (1992), for example, also have attempted to integrate motivational theories and stages of change. Consider how attitude change theories might be employed in developing interventions for target populations at each stage of change, as shown in table 9.4. At the precontemplation stage, novel information and persuasive communications may be particularly useful for capturing attention and creating awareness. At the contemplation stage, information, persuasive communications, and modeling may be useful for altering relevant beliefs, and changing attitudes, perceived social norms, and expectancies regarding the outcomes of health behavior. At the preparation stage, "how-to" knowledge and skill development may be important, along with continued attitude change. At the action and maintenance stages interventions based on reinforcement, support, self-management (skills), and attribution may foster positive experiences. At the action stage people often make inappropriate attributions about outcomes, particularly their success or failure, because they lack experience and understanding of the underlying causes. Dieters and people quitting smoking, for example, may be more likely to stay with their new habits if they are trained to attribute some backsliding to the natural process of change, rather than to their own inadequacy and failure (Hosper, Kok, and Strecher, 1990; DiClemente et al., 1991).

Table 9.4 Stages of Change and Particularly Relevant Intervention Approaches

Stage/Major Outcome	Intervention Approach
Precontemplation Awareness	Novel information, persuasive communications, experiences
Contemplation Knowledge acquisition	Information, persuasive communications, experiences
Preparation Deciding	How-to information, skill development, attitude change
Action	Skill, reinforcement, support, self-management, attitude and attribution change
Maintenance Continuation	Relapse prevention skills, self-management, social and environmental support

Theory and Practice

This chapter has dealt in some detail with knowledge, skills, beliefs, attitudes, and values. These complex variables are prominent concerns in the working health educator's everyday practice. Volumes have been written about these variables and our treatment of them has been necessarily brief. Modern health educators, however, are surprisingly sophisticated about the nature and role of cognitive and affective variables in health behavior change, due largely to their increased familiarity with the modern theories of behavior change discussed briefly in this chapter.

While there are many important theories of behavior change that focus on cognitive and affective domains, in this chapter we focused only on those that are used most frequently and appear to have the greatest application to health education and health promotion practice. Each of the theories discussed conceptualizes the influence of knowledge, beliefs, and attitudes on behavior in somewhat different ways and uses unique vocabulary to describe the salient variables and hypothesized relationships. However, these conceptualizations and theories tend to be overlapping in important ways. Perceptions play an important role in all of the theories presented. The Health Belief Model focuses on beliefs about susceptibility to and severity of disease and the benefits and barriers of preventive actions. The Theory of Planned Behavior emphasizes beliefs about the outcomes of a behavior, social norms, and behavioral control. Perceived behavioral control is a similar concept to self-efficacy expectancy, which is an important variable in social cognitive theory. Causal attributions are beliefs about why something happened and what is likely to happen in the future, which is similar to expectancy beliefs. Hence, these theories are not necessarily in opposition, but represent different aspects of cognitive variables and different ways of looking at essentially similar variables and processes. Clearly, there is much to learn from each of these theories and there are health education situations in which each may prove particularly useful.

If these theories and conceptualizations deal with essentially the same variables, or at most specialized cases of variables, what is the value of the theories? Do they really tell us very much about behavior or should we merely rely on the basic categories of knowledge, beliefs, skills, and attitudes? There are several important advantages to taking a theoretical approach to the change process. From a practical point of view there are just too many possible variables of interest. Theory allows the practitioner to focus on a limited number of cognitive and affective variables. Relatedly, theory brings coherence to a study or program, giving the practitioner and researcher a comprehensive grasp of the problem and facilitating a logical explanation of the evaluation or results.

Advances in theory have been especially influential in the area of needs assessment. As noted, a theoretical orientation provides direction to needs assessments and can reduce the number of variables that need to be measured. Sadly, the increased use of theory in health education has been predominantly in the area of measurement, and much less in the area of intervention. A quick perusal of any of the health education journals reveals a plethora of papers that use theory in needs assessments and studies identifying cognitive and affective variables that are statistically related to a particular health behavior. Many fewer articles report theory-based intervention.

Theory provides valuable suggestions for intervention approaches and methods. Theory can provide direction for needs assessments and determinants studies and fill in the gaps in these assessments, rounding out our programs and giving the practitioner a sense of consistency and comprehensiveness. There are many important variables that cannot be altered by our interventions, but understanding them helps us to interpret our results and improve our programming. Finally, it is comforting to practitioners and policy makers to understand that health behavior can be understood theoretically. It gives all parties a sense of confidence that improved efforts based on this understanding will lead to the desired outcomes.

Summary

Knowledge, beliefs, and attitudes are intermediate aspects of behavior. Many behavior change programs are primarily directed toward these cognitive outcomes because of their theoretical relationship to actual behavior. Clearly, these variables are associated with behavior, but the relationships are complex and not completely understood. Nevertheless, a number of useful theories are available that help to explain these relationships.

Knowledge alone does not determine behavior, but knowledge about a subject and knowledge that contributes to understanding and skill is extremely important in mediating health behavior. Often, however, it is not so much what a person actually knows, but what he or she believes is true that mediates behavior. Similarly, the strength of one's conviction and the extent to which one values or is emotionally committed to a belief or attitude is important. It is well established that knowledge, beliefs, and attitudes can be changed by creatively exposing learners to new information and experiential learning activities.

A number of theories are popularly employed in health promotion programs. Information processing theory provides a theoretical and practical foundation for other cognitive theories and provides guidelines for developing persuasive communications. The health belief model has been popular in health promotion programs for a number of years. The theory of planned change is gaining wide acceptance and is expected to be employed extensively in the future. The utility of stages of change is probably greatest when incorporated with other theoretical approaches.

Cognitive theory provides the researcher and the practitioner with tremendous advantages in developing needs assessments and interventions. Theory-based research and programs limit the number of variables that must be addressed, improve the focus of these efforts, and facilitate interpretation of the results.

Behaviorism

281

*What we need is a technology of behavior . . . . We can
follow the path taken by physics and biology by turning
directly to the relation between behavior and the
environment and neglecting supposed mediating states of
mind.*

—B. F. Skinner (1971)

Introduction

The traditional role of the health educator is to bring about favorable changes
in health behavior. This typically involves getting people to do things voluntarily
they otherwise would neglect, delay, or do differently. Unlike public health
officers, who often have the legal authority to coerce people into prescribed
paths of behavior in situations involving immediate threats to the community,
the health educator typically uses less direct methods. The intuitive approach
to behavior change, as described in the previous chapter, is to use persuasion
in the form of carefully selected information and appeals to the subject's logic
and reason. However, any attempt to study or refine this process soon involves
the educator with attitudes, beliefs, values, fears, misconceptions, and other
internal components of clients' personalities. At this point the task becomes
troublesome. These items, which are central to the work of educators and
cognitive psychologists, are notoriously difficult to identify and measure with
a high degree of precision. No one has ever seen or touched any of these
"hypothetical constructs"; their very existence can only be inferred indirectly
from our observations of what people say and do. The elusive quality of these
various items has prompted some psychologists to view them as an improbable
foundation for a serious study of human behavior.

In fairness, we must recognize that only the most radical behaviorists deny
the existence of internal cognitive variables and other such qualities that
commonly define human nature. The more moderate behaviorists recognize
the importance of these private events but are primarily concerned with variables
that can be represented by some visible manifestation. They insist on (1)
specificity, meaning that a single action always represents the same variable;
(2) objectivity, meaning that the behavior is so clearly defined that different
observers will make identical interpretations, and (3) observability, meaning
that the behavior is visible (Karoly and Harris, 1986).

Rationale for a More Direct Approach

The elaboration of these basic concepts of behaviorism led to a more direct
and forthright theory of behavior change pioneered by Watson and Plavov and

later refined by Guthrie, Hull, and Skinner (Bower and Hilgard, 1981). In terms of practical applications, its practitioners seem to say, "We can increase the frequency of behavior by providing reinforcement for it and we can decrease the frequency of a behavior by punishing it." In terms of theory, its advocates focus on the external, observable aspects of behavior and the circumstances that surround it. They scrupulously avoid speculating about what may be going on in the subject's (organism's) mind. This basic line of thinking has matured into a more rigorously scientific approach to behavior change which, while narrower in scope, lends itself to more systematic applications and more predictable results than do traditional cognitive strategies.

The practical methodology that subsequently arose from this theoretical approach has been commonly termed **behavior modification**. In many tightly defined situations, such as when well-motivated clients wish to lose weight or stop smoking, its various applications have produced excellent results. Its advocates view it as a much needed way to escape from the morass of abstractions involved in cognitive-based approaches and thus deal more effectively with problematic behavior at a time when the very fabric of our society is threatened by crime, family disorganization, various addictions, and other human failings. Its critics view it as mechanical and dehumanizing; they maintain that behavior modification, with its overwhelming emphasis on external actions, neglects and may damage the self-confidence, basic trust, sense of mastery, and other important internal components of the client's personality. Moreover, the critics charge that the emphasis on "bribes" and "threats" results in short-term results.

Behaviorists respond by claiming that the goal of behavior change is not coercion or the control or manipulation of behavior but self-management and self-control. Self-management is a skill that is eminently positive for mental health, with no conceivable ill effects. Relatedly, behaviorists claim that attempting to facilitate behavior change without attention to environmental conditions is an exercise in futility for both the facilitator and the learner. Incentives, rather than being bribes to get someone to do something they do not want to do, are used to increase the learner's motivation to initiate a response that is infrequent.

In modern practice, the principles of behaviorism are a common part of health education and health promotion practice. Actually, most modern behaviorists have adopted cognitive methods to enable the target population to self-manage its behavior, rather than relying on external controls. Indeed, social learning theory, discussed in the next chapter, is a theory that fully integrates cognitive, social, and reinforcement principles. However, before considering such a synthesis, it is useful to take a look at behaviorism in its unembellished form. Consider the following examples:

- A mother is concerned about her daughter's tendency to eat too much "junk food." She subsequently moves all the cookies, potato chips, and other such items to inconvenient locations. She makes sure that apples, oranges, carrot sticks, and similar nutritious snacks are readily available and then sets up an incentive system whereby she adds a bonus to her daughter's weekly allowance for every five days of "healthy" snacking.

- A man who is attempting to stop smoking finds the task much easier if he (1) takes a shower as soon as he arises in the morning and (2) leaves the dinner table as soon as he finishes for a game of chess at his computer.

- A kindergarten teacher is troubled by two boys who frequently bother each other and get into noisy arguments. She decides to ignore their troublesome behavior and make a special effort to compliment them during their rare instances of pleasant cooperation. Soon the noisy arguments cease.

In each of these examples behavior was improved without any appeals to logic or reason; there were no lectures or pleas; no significant information was provided; there was no attempt to "educate" anyone in the usual sense of the term. Instead, the persons involved dealt with (1) the **antecedents** or "triggers" of the relevant behaviors—as when the mother removed the snacks which serve as cues to undesirable responses, (2) the behavior itself—as when the shower or chess game was substituted for a smoke, and (3) the consequences—as when the kindergarten pupils found that cooperative behavior rather than noisy arguments gained them the desired attention of the teacher. This type of analysis has led some psychologists to term behaviorism the "ABC" approach involving *a*ntecedents, the *b*ehavior itself, and the pleasant or aversive *c*onsequences of the behavior (Elder et al., 1985). Karoly and Harris (1986) use the following diagram to describe the same components using more formal terminology:

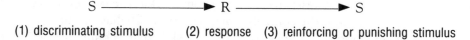

S ⟶ R ⟶ S

(1) discriminating stimulus   (2) response   (3) reinforcing or punishing stimulus

Either scheme serves to distinguish a behavioristic explanation from the cognitive theorists' S-O-R which includes the "organism," with its attitudes, values, and other illusive variables as the central feature of their framework.

Theoretical Framework

As noted, this emphasis on the manipulation of external factors that either cue or reinforce the target behavior contrasts rather sharply with the conventional approach of presenting the student or client with lectures, reading material, films, and other learning experiences directed toward such internal factors as knowledge, attitudes, values, or beliefs. This approach also differs markedly from those intervention strategies based on social support, as represented by Alcoholics Anonymous and the various weight-control and smoking-cessation programs which use the pressure and encouragement developed by group meetings to strengthen one's resolve to stay on the "straight and narrow" until the next session—an approach that is also focused on factors within the individual. But despite these differences in application, the basic principles of behaviorism tend to complement rather than conflict with the theoretical bases of the major competing approaches.

Responses

Virtually all human activity, whether it be creating a great work of art, purchasing an automobile, or scratching one's nose, consists of responding to stimuli. Various stimuli enter our nervous system through our perceptive organs, and usually reach the brain, where impulses to specific muscles or glands are sent out and eventually manifest themselves as responses which are often observable and measurable. Consider the case of a woman struggling with a weight-control problem who opens her refrigerator to get a bottle of milk and, in the next instant, finds herself impulsively snacking on yesterday's pizza. As she saw the attractive but unneeded food a dozen thoughts may have flashed through her mind, such as whether it was too stale to enjoy, how fattening it might be, how much lunch she had eaten, and so forth, but the behaviorist tends to ignore these internal reactions and focus on the visible events: she saw the pizza (stimulus) and she ate it (response).

According to Bower and Hilgard (1981), Skinner distinguished between **elicited** responses and **emitted** responses. Elicited responses are those resulting from known and definitive stimuli, such as the constriction of the pupil of the eye in response to a bright light; such responses are termed **respondents**. Many of these respondents are involved in such conditions as high blood pressure, migraine, colonitis, and similar problems centered on the autonomic nervous system and are of great interest to practitioners of biofeedback. Of more interest to health educators are the emitted responses which are not linked to any particular stimuli and thus represent personal choice behavior. Such responses, termed **operants**, have become the focus of an elaborate system of behavior change technology called **operant conditioning**.

Stimuli

Behaviorists distinguish among several different types of stimuli; however, three categories are particularly important to health educators.

Discriminative

Discriminative stimuli alert the individual's attention to a particular response but do not force the response involuntarily. A child at play may receive such a stimulus in the form of a parental call to come in for dinner; although the call may seem compelling, the child still has a choice which will presumably be based on a review of the various rewards and/or punishments that compliance or noncompliance may involve. Such stimuli are also termed **cues** to behavior and as such occupy an important role in most efforts to affect health behavior;

the call to "fight cancer with a check and check-up" and the dentist's six-month reminder cards are typical examples.

Reinforcing

Reinforcing stimuli, or reinforcers, in contrast to the prior example, occur after rather than before the target behavior. Such stimuli may involve the presentation of something pleasant such as the praise given to a child who has just taken his or her vitamin pill. Here something is *added* to the situation that supports the target behavior in a process of **positive reinforcement**. Reinforcing stimuli may also involve the *removal* of something unpleasant followed by an increase in the target behavior in a process of **negative reinforcement**. For example, the taking of aspirin may be reinforced by the removal of an unpleasant headache. Negative reinforcement should not be confused with punishment, which tends to suppress rather than reinforce the target behavior.

Aversive

Aversive stimuli, or punishments, tend to reduce the tendency to repeat a particular behavior. Although examples of such stimuli might appear to be obvious, the behaviorists caution that one should always look first to the effects on responses, rather than to the nature of the stimulus itself before deciding whether it is reinforcing or aversive. Praise to a young child for drinking his or her milk may result in better milk drinking, but the same praise heaped on an adolescent in the presence of peers may actually represent a form of punishment and inhibit such behavior in the future. Likewise, a wife who continually nags her husband to stop smoking may be reinforcing his habit; subconsciously, he may enjoy the attention and expressions of concern provoked by his unhealthy behavior.

Respondent Conditioning

Human physiological responses such as high blood pressure, nausea, or even pleasant relaxation represent natural responses to specific stimuli as do closely related emotions such as joy or fear. We do not consciously learn these behaviors; they simply happen when the appropriate pattern of eliciting stimuli occur. However, when an unnatural stimulus is presented at the same time, or nearly the same time, as the natural stimulus, then it too becomes capable of producing the response in the future according to the principles of respondent conditioning. For example, some viral infections normally cause nausea and vomiting which the victim might term stomach flu. However, if the onset of the disease occurred soon after a new food had been eaten, then this food may cause nausea on future occasions regardless of whether or not the individual realizes the association was a mere coincidence. (A similar situation is shown in figure 10.1.) Conversely, food that is regularly eaten under particularly pleasant circumstances may come to rank high on one's list of favorites.

Figure 10.1

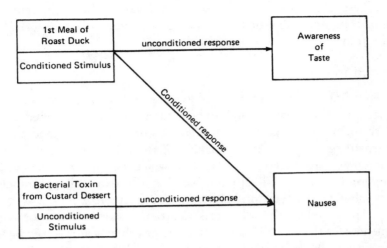

Respondent conditioning. One's first experience with a new food might be pleasant at first; but, once it has been innocently associated with the nausea of food poisoning, it may never be pleasant again.

Aversion therapy in the treatment of alcoholism represents perhaps the most dramatic example of an attempt to apply respondent conditioning to health behavior. In a hospital setting, the patient is given a drug that will soon induce nausea; then he is given an alcoholic drink just before the aversive reaction occurs. After a few such treatments, the conditioned stimulus (alcohol) will usually elicit the response (nausea) in the absence of the unconditioned stimulus (drug). Respondent conditioning also takes place spontaneously in a multitude of instances that combine to influence a person's preferences and attitudes. Children who have unpleasant experiences in their early encounters with physicians and/or hospitals may find themselves reluctant to seek medical care as adults. Even though they "understand" the value of preventive care, for example, they just do not feel comfortable; they have become conditioned to respond to such situations with fear and anxiety.

Operant Conditioning

Behaviorists believe that most of the average person's voluntary behavior results from the process of operant conditioning which, according to its formal definition, is "a type of learning in which behaviors are altered primarily by regulating the consequences that follow them" (Kazdin, 1989). According to this particular aspect of behavioral theory, the responses (behaviors) that one selects often tend to evoke some type of reaction from the physical or social environment. The nature of these reactions obviously can vary greatly, often with important consequences to the individual; also, the timing and frequency of these consequences can also vary. Each of these different aspects have important effects on the likelihood the individual will repeat the behavior and the frequency of any repeated behavior.

Reinforcement

Depending on the reinforcing or aversive nature of the consequences of these reactions, the behavior tends to be extinguished or maintained. As noted, reinforcement can be positive or negative and both types tend to encourage or perpetuate the associated behavior. If the subsequent consequences tend to discourage the behavior, then they would be deemed aversive rather than reinforcing; this classification is based, not by external appearances, but solely on subsequent effects on behavior. (See figure 10.2.)

It is a relatively simple task to arrange either pleasant or aversive consequences for the target behavior that the health educator is seeking to encourage or extinguish. More challenging, however, is the problem of stimulating the behavior in the first place since an operant, by definition, is initiated by the learner. Depending on the situation, this can be handled in a variety of ways. Sometimes incentives are used to get the process started; often the instructor/trainer must remain alert for naturally occurring stimuli in the environment that trigger the desired behavior; or sometimes precursors to the behavior have to be reinforced and gradually shaped into the target behavior. A child, for example, may be praised at first for simply getting the toothbrush in her mouth, soon she may have to do a few strokes to gain any recognition, and finally a thorough cleaning job is expected.

Another key point in the understanding of operant conditioning is the fact that it is seldom a process of a controller manipulating the behavior of a passive subject. At its best, both discriminating stimuli and reinforcers are either controlled by the learner from the beginning or shifted to the learner's control early in the process. This strategy enables the target behavior to be reinforced or discouraged regardless of where or when it occurs. Also, covert

---

Figure 10.2

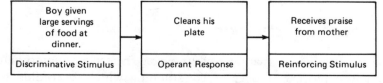

Operant conditioning. When naturally occurring responses are rewarded they tend to be repeated; changes in the nature, frequency, and time pattern of the reinforcing stimuli produce many variations in this simple pattern.

behaviors, such as depressing or anxiety provoking thoughts, can be addressed by the one person who knows when they occur. Finally, self-management of behavior modification programs greatly increase the chances of effecting permanent or long-term behavioral changes (Kazdin, 1989).

Hierarchy of Reinforcers

Although the process of reinforcement appears quite mechanical, its effectiveness is dependent on the subjective judgment of the learner who must view the reward as valuable enough to merit the desired response. Several experiments with school-aged children, for example, demonstrate that students will work hard for jelly beans or perhaps tokens that may be accumulated for a prize of some sort. But while the results are often good over the short term, the use of such incentives often is criticized as fostering a habit of working only for extrinsic rewards, rather than for the inherent value of learning to read, to behave properly in class, to complete assignments, or whatever. The behaviorists counter this argument with the concept of a hierarchy of reinforcers. According to this view, material rewards are often needed simply to get the behavior moving in the proper direction. Then, the reinforcing stimuli may be gradually upgraded from food to tokens to praise and finally may be eliminated as the learner comes to value the activity for its own sake.

MacMillan offers a continuum based on the apparent "maturity" of the reinforcers (MacMillan, 1973:113):

1. primary rewards: food and water
2. toys or trinkets
3. tokens or checks, with backup reinforcers (toys, food, etc.)
4. visual evidence of progress: graphs, letter grades, etc.
5. social approval
6. sense of mastery: "learning for the love of it"

If a higher reinforcer is presented to the learner at the same time as a lower one that has proven effective, then the learner will presumably become conditioned to respond to the higher one. This process is then repeated until the learner is working for a sense of mastery or, as a nonbehaviorist might say, until the behavior becomes internalized. MacMillan notes, however, that his continuum does not apply universally to all learners; individuals may vary in the way they respond, with some items interchanging positions on the hierarchy, for example. However, with good management this process enables the behavior modification to start with candy, tokens or other dubious "bribes" and end with the learner's good behavior driven by socially desirable and presumably enduring motives.

Scheduling

Behaviorist clinicians or researchers attach considerable importance to the process of scheduling, i.e., the frequency and timing of reinforcing stimuli. In laboratory situations scheduling has evolved into a complex process with the formulation and study of such patterns as continuous reinforcement, intermittent reinforcement, fixed ratio, variable ratio, and more. Health educators working in field situations seldom have either the opportunity or the need to maintain close control over the scheduling of reinforcing or aversive stimuli. However, a few general observations concerning this topic can be helpful in the management of basic programs.

1. Generally, newly established behavior is best maintained with continuous or frequent reinforcement during its early stages. Later, it can be maintained with only intermittent reinforcement, and ideally, extrinsic rewards can be dropped completely as the desirable behavior becomes internalized.

2. Punishment tends to become ineffective if not applied at most or all instances of the undesired behavior. This is one of several reasons it is generally better to concentrate on reinforcing alternative, desirable behaviors, rather than relying on punishment. Witness the dismal record of trying to enforce highway speed limits with an occasional citation, regardless of the size of the accompanying fine.

3. Conversely, in regard to positive reinforcement, the seductive quality of variable ratio, essentially random, reinforcement should be capitalized upon when practical. The knowledge that any given effort might achieve success has for years kept people in the hot sun pulling the cord of balky lawnmowers, or in stuffy casinos pulling the lever of "one-armed bandits" with extraordinary frequency.

Emotion and Motivation

The logical principles and research evidence which underlie behaviorism as a theoretical approach also provide the basis for a useful array of behavior change strategies and techniques that will be described in the following section. Perhaps the most appealing aspect of this general approach is its very direct, near mechanical quality; people problems become, in effect, engineering problems. Moreover, this impersonal quality reduces the risk of inducing guilt and feelings of incompetence within the clients. If their behavior is unfavorable, health educators committed to behaviorism cannot ascribe their shortcomings to laziness, insensitivity, or lack of ambition; they must instead look to the external conditions or the antecedent experiences of the clients for explanations and clues to program development. But health educators are seldom wedded to a single approach and may find themselves uncomfortable with certain features of behavior modification, particularly its practice of ignoring internal motivational states.

The concept of motivation refers to the internal drives of the individual. Although a number of competing theories exist as to the origin of and factors that affect motivation, there is general agreement that the eventual result is an arousal to action that involves physiological mechanisms. The hunger drive represents perhaps the clearest example; after a few hours of food deprivation internal balances are disturbed; these imbalances are experienced as tension and discomfort which tends to energize the individual toward behavior to restore the physiological balance. Obviously, hunger as an internal state can motivate food-seeking behavior; however, the concept becomes more complicated when acquired, rather than innate, needs become involved. Under different circumstances we might find the same subject on a "hunger strike," rigorously avoiding food to protest some perceived injustice.

Behaviorists do not accord motivation any special place in their theoretical framework. Skinner, for example, viewed internal drives as "relatively useless explanatory constructs" and preferred to change internal variables such as "hunger" into externally measurable components such as "hours of food deprivation" (Bower and Hilgard, 1981:199). In other situations, quantification may be achieved by measuring the effort that a person will make, or perhaps the money or tokens he/she is willing to pay, to engage in the desired behavior. The flip-side of the equation occurs when the learner perceives the target behavior as aversive because of its tedious or burdensome quality. In such cases the negative drive, or resistance, can be quantified in terms of the size of the reward that is required to increase the frequency of the behavior. For difficult, complex, or unvalued behaviors relatively large incentives may be needed early in the program to overcome inertia or active dislike for the activity—such as many people seem to have for flossing teeth or exercising, for example. Once the target behavior is initiated, then an intermittent or diminishing schedule may be used until the behavior become self-reinforcing or habitual. Again, these various strategies neither recognize nor deny the existence of internal drive states, but place motivation in a context where it can be measured and dealt with in a systematic fashion.

Clearly, these procedures work better in some situations than others. Sometimes the major factors influencing internal drive states are readily identifiable and easy to measure. In other instances the roots of motivation extend back into years of individual life experiences. Also, genetically based factors, such as tolerance to pain, metabolic levels, and minor organic defects can affect a particular individual's response to a specific health appeal. In fairness, we must recognize that no approach enables us to completely understand and modify human behavior. This failure is undoubtedly more a blessing than a problem and should serve to remind us that our responsibility is to make our best effort.

The Technology of Behavior Modification

Within the field of health education/promotion, behavior modification techniques have proven particularly useful in the management of addictive type problems such as smoking cessation, weight reduction, and various types of drug abuse. In many of these cases the individuals seek out classes or counseling because they have already decided that their habits should be changed. They do not need persuasion; they need help in managing their own behavior. In such instances behavior modification is very appropriate and enjoys its best record of success. The use of behavior modification on individuals without their knowledge or consent is more hazardous and often poses the risk of ethical, legal, or philosophical problems. However, in situations wherein the educator's responsibility is clear and the behavior change sought is undeniably beneficial, there are useful and legitimate applications on unknowing subjects. Parents and teachers have clear responsibility to train children in socially acceptable ways of behaving. Likewise employers frequently have both a mandate and a legal responsibility to foster safe and healthful behavior patterns in the workplace. In these situations the application of behavior modification principles can increase the effectiveness of penalties, incentives, cues, and other such traditional devices.

Program Development

The application of behavior modification in its pure form requires that (1) the behavior to be changed is one that can be clearly defined, (2) the health educator has a clear ethical mandate to facilitate the change, and (3) the health educator can exert reasonable control over certain factors and contingencies in the learner's environment. Once these conditions are met, the program can often proceed in a very precise and methodical manner. Kazdin (1989:4) provides a general framework for program development and describes measurement and evaluation as central to the total process:

> First, the behaviors to be altered are carefully assessed. The assessment may consist of several ways of measuring the problem or desired behavior, including direct observation of how the person performs at school or at work, evaluations by significant others (parents, spouses, peers), and, of course, evaluations by the clients themselves. The assessment is central to identifying the extent and nature of the problem.

> Second, the goals and means for reaching them are usually well specified. Before treatment, the therapist conducts a careful evaluation to identify what the problem is, how the client and others are affected by it, and the circumstances under which it emerges. Once the problem has been carefully identified and assessed, the procedures and the goals toward which they will be directed can be specified. Explicit formulation of the procedures and goals is an important characteristic of behavior modification.

> Third, the effects of treatment are assessed to determine whether the desired outcomes have been obtained. In research, behavior modification places major emphasis on measuring outcome and evaluating treatment. . . . Evaluation is also very important in clinical work with individual clients. In this context, evaluation refers to measuring the specific behaviors of interest and thus to monitoring the progress that the client makes during the course of treatment. Such evaluation may be accomplished by having the patient complete various questionnaires about the severity of specific symptoms or by having the patient keep a record or diary of activities.

In addition to the obvious emphasis on careful baseline assessments and monitoring of progress, a second major feature of behavior modification programs is their reliance on direct action and participation of the learner. Little time is spent talking about what one should do whereas the bulk of the sessions often consist of actually practicing the desired behavior or the alternative behavior to undesirable behavior. Moreover, the learner is not only an active participant in the target behavior but, in most cases, in the decisions involved in the development of the program itself. The chances for program success are greatly enhanced when the learner has a role in setting goals, deadlines, rewards, penalties, and so forth.

Specific Techniques

Depending on the demands of the particular situation, the best behavior modification program for implementing favorable change in a particular behavior may require attention to the discriminating stimulus, the behavior itself, the reinforcing stimulus, or perhaps to some combination of these basic three elements. Depending on the particular mix, emphasis, and form of these elements, a wide variety of behavior change patterns can be devised. Many of these techniques have been highly refined in clinical situations wherein the focus was on various types of behavior pathology, rather than on health behavior per se. However, many of these provide implications for health education/promotion. The broad range of operant conditioning techniques as described by Karoly and Harris (1986) are summarized in table 10.1.

This broad array of techniques tends to emphasis tangible rewards and sanctions somewhat to the neglect of less dramatic devices such as verbal feedback, record keeping, and social support that are often very useful to the health educator. Moreover, health educators seldom have the luxury of dealing with single individuals in tightly controlled situations. More often they will be targeting groups in more loosely structured situations. Here, operant principles have been more effective with behavioral situations that occur frequently in everyday life, such as seat belt use, eating habits, and various types of substance abuse. This general approach has shown less success with behavior that occurs less frequently as, for example, drinking and driving, adolescent sexual behavior, or the use of preventive health care services.

Applications in Health Education/Promotion

As noted, the technology of behavior modification has many useful applications in health education/promotion; however, health educators generally find it best to combine this technology with one or more additional educational approaches. Many smoking-cessation programs, for example, begin with a conventional presentation of the factual information related to the health risks smokers incur,

Table 10.1 Behavior Change Techniques Based on Operant Principles

Technique	Definition	Application
Positive Reinforcement	Reinforcing desirable behavior with favorable consequences	Used most often to add behavior to one's repertoire
Negative Reinforcement	Reinforcing behavior by removing aversive stimuli	Few applications in health education
Extinction	Removing rewards or favorable consequences linked with poor behavior	Often used to discourage attention-getting behavior
Prompting and Fading	Providing cues or reminders for desirable behavior	Useful when there is little resistance to change
Shaping	Rewarding successive approximations until target behavior is achieved	Useful when target behavior is complex
Chaining	Rewarding first steps and successive steps of a behavior chain	Used when target behavior is a series of distinct actions
Differential Reinforcement	"Crowds-out" poor behavior by rewarding alternative behaviors	Useful when poor behavior is inherently satisfying
Satiation and Restraint	Poor behavior repeated until it becomes unpleasant	Difficult method; best left to specialists
Time Out	Removing subject from situation that is rewarding poor behavior	Often used to control behavior of young children
Overcorrection, Positive Practice, and Habit Reversal	Desirable behavior is "overlearned" to effect permanent change	Often used to correct postural defects
Response Cost	Establishing graduated system of penalties for poor behavior	Similar to punishment but protects client autonomy
Response-Contingent	Discourages poor behavior with aversive consequences	Pure punishment with all its hazards; used infrequently

Source: Karoly, Paul, and Anne Harris. "Operant Methods." In *Helping People Change: A Textbook of Methods*, eds., F. H. Kanfer and A. P. Goldstein. New York: Pergamon, 1986:111–144.

followed by instruction in self-applied behavior modification techniques for handling the addictive aspects; these two modalities are then supported by a third strategy in the form of regular meetings based on the group process in which social support and social pressure help firm up the client's resolve to stick with the program.

These very common "mixed modality" programs actually represent a "natural marriage" for the health educator. The use of reinforcement and stimulus control, i.e., the management of environmental cues for desirable or undesirable behavior, are standard aspects of health education/promotion programs. Indeed, one of the most important features of all educational/behavior change programs is the exercise of control over environmental factors that shape behavior. Creating unique ways of controlling the environment is a particularly challenging task, as is the equally important role of teaching learners to control their own environments. These points are illustrated in more concrete form in the two examples that follow, one involving safety belt use and the other, weight control.

Safety Belt Use

In research conducted at a medical center in Galveston, Texas, four groups of hospital personnel were used as subjects in a study designed to investigate methods of encouraging safety belt use (Simons-Morton BG, Brink, and Bates, 1987). The groups were organized on the basis of each subject's parking lot assignment. All four groups received persuasive messages concerning safety belt use by mail during each of the four weeks of the investigation; this was the only method used with the first group. Prominent signs encouraging seat belt use were posted at the entrance of the second group's parking lot and their use or nonuse was also periodically monitored by a very visible parking lot attendant observer. The third group was also monitored in addition to receiving the mailed fliers; however, the observers in this case gave out free food coupons and similar prizes to those wearing belts and printed reminders to those who did not. The investigators used an ''all-out'' approach on the fourth group which included all the previous measures plus the addition of a ''Buckle-Up'' message displayed on an eight-foot balloon floating over the parking lot along with a six-foot high barometer showing the current rate of use. Messages were placed on car windshields; moreover, monitors periodically provided verbal encouragement, prizes, and reminders as cars entered the lot and offered the chance to win additional prizes in a later drawing.

As might be expected, this fourth group showed the greatest gains with use improving from 17 percent to 45 percent during the four-week period of the study. The third group also improved substantially—moving from 18 percent to 38 percent. The first two groups, who were presented with less intense programs, also improved but their gains were not significantly better than the 7 percent gain posted by a community comparison group. This latter group was included in the study to monitor any normal ''secular'' change that might be occurring in the community as a whole in response to general media programs, recent news events, or similar factors. Although the fourth group improved the most, the costs for their more elaborate program was quite high—an average expenditure of $97 for each person who was apparently influenced to adopt safety belt use. The gains in the third group were achieved at a lower cost of $37 per new adoptee.

In their report the researchers noted certain limitations in their methodology and cautioned against assumptions that the same results could be achieved within other work groups; however, their results were generally consistent with similar studies conducted in other locations. Generally, more elaborate intervention programs achieve better results and the behavior modification components—which in this study included the various prompts, the incentives, and the verbal encouragement—typically hold their own when compared with purely persuasive techniques.

Weight Control

A highly successful weight loss program was conducted in three business/industrial sites in central Pennsylvania with competition for cash rewards used as the primary incentive (Brownell, 1984). The clients who volunteered at each site were organized into three teams. Although five dollars was allotted for each participant, all the money at each site was pooled and subsequently awarded to the team that recorded the best weight loss record during the program. In another standard behavior modification technique, a four-by-five-foot bulletin board was placed at each workplace to show each team's progress as determined by weekly weigh-ins. Also, a treatment manual (Brownell, 1979) was distributed to participants in weekly installments. It provided basic information on nutrition and exercise along with specific instruction on self-management devices such as stimulus control, slowing eating, reinforcement, and social support.

The three programs in this study ranged from 12 to 15 weeks in length and involved a total 213 subjects who were an average 34 percent overweight at the beginning of the study. The subjects lost an average of approximately 12 pounds and reduced their overweight status by an average of 9 percent. A six-month follow-up study of 94 of the participants revealed that they had retained 80 percent of their weight loss. Of particular importance was the fact that a majority of the participants reported improvement in their morale and energy level on the job and substantial percentages, ranging from 17 percent to 43 percent, reported improvement in work performance, relations with supervisors, and absenteeism; none of the 213 subjects reported any deterioration in these factors. Only one person dropped out of the study; 75 percent of the managers reported improvement in worker morale and none reported any decline. When all the expenses were analyzed, it was found that it cost $2.93 per 1 percent reduction in a worker's overweight status; at the time of the study, this was the lowest figure yet reported.

The most common criticism of behavior modification is that it is dehumanizing and achieves its results at the expense of adverse side-effects. However, this study represents an example of an intervention which relied heavily on such methods as goal setting, positive reinforcement, and feedback yet yielded uniformly positive outcomes on morale, interpersonal relations, and other broader concerns. Among the probable reasons for the absence of any negative effects was the attention given to both the ethical treatment of the workers and the provisions for keeping them informed about all aspects of the program. Their participation was voluntary; they could drop out at any time if they so chose; they were never encouraged to lose weight at an unhealthy rate. The use of the manual provided information on both dietary aspects of weight loss and tips on behavior management which, no doubt, tended to empower them and enable them to take charge of their own program.

The Self-Management of Health Behavior

Throughout the literature of health education/promotion there are constant reminders of the philosophical imperative that the favorable changes in behavior that result from our various programs be voluntarily adopted by clients rather than externally imposed. This issue, which is seldom if ever resolved under the best of circumstances, can be particularly troublesome in programs whose main inducements to behavior change involve reinforcement, aversive barriers, stimulus control, and other techniques based on the theory of behaviorism. However, a close look at this issue soon reveals that (1) whatever problems may exist are not specific to behavior modification programs and (2) the practice of shifting more control of the program to the client actually improves the prospects of effecting desirable behavior change.

Better results are possible when clients are put in charge of their own programs. When this general strategy is adopted practitioners find that (1) a wider range of behaviors can be addressed, such as eating and smoking in everyday situations beyond the program setting, (2) the reinforcements can often be more consistently administered because, in contrast to the program leader who may miss instances of critical behavior, the subject usually is aware of them, and (3) any favorable change is more likely to become "internalized" and thus endure beyond the time frame of the formal program (Kazdin, 1989).

Spontaneous Self-Management

As with many other aspects of psychology, operant conditioning is based on everyday observations of human behavior; consequently, it should not be surprising to find that people regularly use rather well structured self-management techniques in many instances without any outside assistance. Throughout history writer and authors, who tend to record their own personal behavior in journals and autobiographies, have provided us with many examples. A particularly clear description is found in the autobiography of the very prolific Anthony Trollope, a nineteenth century English author.

> When I have commenced a new book, I have always prepared a diary, divided into weeks, and carried on for the period which I have allowed myself for the completion of the work. In this I have entered, day by day, the number of pages I have written, so that if I have slipped into idleness for a day or two, the record of that idleness has been there, staring me in the face. . . . Nothing surely is so potent as a law that cannot be disobeyed. It has the force of water that hollows the stone. (Trollope, 1980:118–120).

Trollope had thus developed a well structured and apparently effective program of self-management which took the form of the modern technique of self-monitoring. It took another 150 years or so for psychologists to develop the technical vocabulary to define self-monitoring which, according to Kazdin:

> ... consists of systematically observing one's own behavior. ... The information conveys whether the behavior departs from a culturally or self-imposed standard of performance. If the behavior departs from an acceptable level, corrective action may be initiated until the level has been met. (Kazdin, 1989:219)

Client-Centered Programs

Natural wisdom notwithstanding, the successful application of behavior modification requires more than simply leaving clients to their own devices. In most cases the individual should be the dominant figure in the process; however, the process requires the optimal mix of individual autonomy and professional guidance. The individual, for example, may walk in off the street into the educator's office and announce, "I'm tired of being fat—please help me lose weight." If they are to succeed they may need to receive information on the caloric value of foods, caloric cost of specific exercise, and advice on specific self-management techniques; however, it is their responsibility to decide when the program begins, what goals are to be achieved, and the specific incentives and/or disincentives that are to be imposed.

The success of client-centered programs also depends to a large degree on the aforementioned factor of motivation and the skill and innovation of both client and helper. Fortunately, there are a number of well established techniques available. Kazdin (1989) describes five basic categories, namely, (1) self-monitoring, (2) stimulus control, (3) self-reinforcement and self-punishment, (4) alternate response training, and (5) biofeedback.

As previously described, **self-monitoring** simply takes a normal everyday behavior, formalizes it, and makes it more precise. It may be used as a free-standing strategy or combined with self-reinforcement and/or self-punishment to enhance the prospects of long-term change. **Stimulus control** techniques most often involve changing or avoiding the situation that "triggers" or elicits the undesirable behavior. Someone on a weight reduction diet, for example, may choose to put tempting snack foods out of sight or, perhaps, in the garbage can. Placing one's required medications alongside the never forgotten morning coffee pot can serve as a cue or stimulus to a desirable behavior.

Regardless of whether the program be externally directed or self-administered, **self-reinforcement** techniques tend to be more effective and less troubled by undesirable side-effects than **self-punishment**. The professional literature contains many reports of successful programs of this type. For example, Hailey and associates (1992) compared the effectiveness of self-reinforcement, peer reinforcement, and simple encouragement with no subsequent reinforcement on the frequency of breast self-examination among college women. They found both types of reinforcements to be effective and approximately equal in their effects. The form of reward selected most often was frozen yogurt/ice cream; the researchers also found that, consistent with self-management theory, the self-reinforcement group tended to retain the desirable behavior longer after the formal reinforcement period than did those reinforced by their peers.

Both **alternate response training** and **biofeedback** generally require more professional guidance than other self-management techniques; however, their implementation is heavily dependent upon the client. The practice of whistling a pleasant tune to crowd out the anxiety one might suffer while walking by a cemetery on a dark night is a simple example of this technique. In another example a therapist advised a deeply religious but depressed patient to translate biblical passages whenever she felt deeply depressed; she found that this activity, which she perhaps should have discovered by herself, greatly improved her mood (Stuart, 1967). Biofeedback is a bit more complex in that it involves training one's involuntary (autonomic) system to respond differently to certain situations or stimuli. The process often begins in a clinical setting wherein some undesirable physiological response, such as extreme muscle tension, is monitored and displayed to the patient, who subsequently learns to practice relaxation techniques as a means of relief. Once the patient learns to recognize the onset of this condition, then the relaxation procedures can be self-administered in real-life situations. Although health educators are not frequently involved with biofeedback procedures, familiarity with its general principles provides a more complete understanding of human behavior in all its forms.

Behavior Modification and Health Promotion

During its relatively brief span of existence, health education's technology has evolved from a simple practice of providing information to people based on the naive assumption that if they know what is right they will do it, to a modern process of health promotion based on a "combination of educational, organizational, economic, and environmental supports for behavior conducive to health" (Green and Johnson, 1983). After many years of indifferent success we now know that people have a multitude of competing motives and frequently do not respond to simple appeals in behalf of their health.

One response to this problem has been the incorporation of behavior modification technology into the general mix of health education/promotion methodology. Elder and associates (1985), for example, completed a review of the major community health intervention programs directed at the single area of heart disease prevention which have been conducted since 1976. They counted seven instances of procedures based on positive reinforcement and eleven instances of procedures based on negative reinforcement and the increase of restrictions. They also emphasized one additional advantage of behavior modification, namely, it has been studied and used by professionals from such a wide variety of health and related fields that it serves as a universal language of sorts. As they state:

> Perhaps the single greatest advantage of behavior modification is that it is readily conceptualized into a parsimonious and yet complete system, thereby facilitating communication between researchers and practitioners from a variety of disciplines pertinent to health education. (Elder et al., 1985:167)

This widespread use attests to the general effectiveness of behavior modification. Granted, this very effectiveness in implementing predictable behavior change on occasion raises ethical concerns; however, any such problems are quite manageable.

Public concern about the ethical questions surrounding behavior modification has persisted for half a century since it was raised to unrealistic levels by such popular books as *Brave New World* (Huxley, 1946) and *1984* (Orwell, 1949) and later revived by B. F. Skinner's controversial *Beyond Freedom and Dignity* (1971). Consequently, those professionals who choose to use this technology have found it prudent to give extra care to ethical matters. It is possible to draw a clear distinction between *education*, in which there is an emphasis on the empowerment of the individual or an enhancement of their ability to achieve self selected goals, and *persuasion*, in which there is an effort to impose external values consistent with preselected behavior patterns (McAlister et al., 1989). However, as one examines these processes closely, it becomes apparent that they seldom exist in any pure form. The most straightforward effort to educate tends to exert a persuasive effect along with the intended enlightenment; the most blatant effort at persuasion generally provides some degree of enlightenment as a beneficial by-product. Our political system protects the rights of a variety of commercial and public interest groups to present their messages in our open ideological marketplace. In other words, "In participatory political systems, publicly directed efforts to influence personal and collective behaviors are justifiable if methods are used without exploiting human nature in ways that reduce dignity and individual responsibility" (McAlister et al., 1989). Generally, health educators have been able to devise effective procedures that meet this standard.

In clinical and quasi-clinical situations the practice of fully informing the clients of the procedures and their rationale is routinely practiced. In other instances criticism is minimized by selecting behavior change goals that are supported by a strong community consensus. The health educator who finds ways to discourage drinking and driving or violence against children is seldom accused of being too manipulative. Also, in a recommendation presented both to improve the effectiveness and maintain the ethical standards of these programs, Elder (et al., 1985) counsels that behavioral technologies must be compatible with existing community norms. It would not be wise to dispense lipstick or other cosmetics as rewards for seat belt use, for example, in a Quaker community that did not condone the use of such items. In general, following such common sense guidelines will serve to enhance rather than detract from the effectiveness of behavior modification.

Summary

The salient feature of behaviorism as a theoretical approach is its rigorous concentration on the external, observable conditions associated with the target behavior. This feature places it in sharp contrast with cognitive theories which emphasize such internal factors as attitudes, values, and beliefs. The behavioral concept of operant conditioning, which is based on the simple premise that behavior that is rewarded tends to be repeated, is used to change voluntary behavior. Although simple in principle, operant conditioning becomes complex in its application. Depending on the demands of specific situations, behavior may be shaped into more complex forms, reinforced to effect a more frequent or regular pattern, reduced in frequency, or extinguished completely. These changes in voluntary behavior are brought about by carefully orchestrated presentations of rewarding or aversive stimuli. The use of a broad array of behavior change techniques based on the principles of operant conditioning is generally termed "behavior modification."

Behavior modification technology has found wide application in health education/promotion programs in its pure form, particularly in the management of eating disorders and substance abuse; however, it is more often used in combination with informational and persuasive strategies. An important feature of most applications of behavior modification has been the active involvement of the learner/client in program formulation and management. This practice both enhances the chances of internalization and long-term behavior change and deflects any potential criticism based on charges of excessive manipulation. Such concerns also have been held to a minimum by such practices as informed consent, careful selection of rewards or contingencies, and attention to the norms and sensitivities of the surrounding community.

Social Cognitive Theory

In the social cognitive view people are neither driven by inner forces nor automatically shaped and controlled by external stimuli. Rather, human functioning is explained in terms of a model of triadic reciprocality in which behavior, cognitive and other personal factors, and environmental events all operate as interacting determinants of each other.

—Albert Bandura

Introduction

Health educators dealing with all the usual obstacles and frustrations that come with actively planning and implementing programs in very real situations may tend to regard theories of behavior change as mere classroom exercises that have little to do with the real world. Those developing theory-based programs, however, tend to find that each theory has some degree of validity yet is not entirely satisfactory in providing useful explanations of behavior change and effective guidance in the development of health promotion programs. Thus, they tend to adopt an eclectic position as they piece together program components suggested by several different theories. In years past this eclecticism was no doubt a logical response to limitations in the state of art; however, these previously disenchanted and eclectic practitioners now have an attractive alternative. Social learning theory (Rotter, Chance, and Phares, 1972; Bandura, 1977), particularly Bandura's social cognitive theory (Bandura, 1986), has become an extremely useful approach for programs directed at general personality development, behavior pathology, and health promotion.

Reciprocal Determinism

One of the more appealing qualities of social cognitive theory (SCT) is its broad scope. Unlike the many intrapersonal theories of chapter 9 with their emphasis on hypothetical "inside the head" constructs such as knowledge, beliefs, and attitudes, social cognitive theory gives due attention to the external environment with its capacity to reward and punish. Unlike the operant conditioning theory of chapter 10, it gives due attention to such human qualities as expectations, values, confidence, and self-control. It incorporates these widely diverse elements into an integrated whole and, in the process, provides clear implications for virtually all field situations.

The historic search for the root causes of behavior has centered around the possible alternatives of (1) genetically based instincts or propensities, (2) environmental influences, and (3) the application of "free will" by the individual. Belief in the existence of free will as a behavioral determinant is attractive to many health educators who place value in the concept of charging individuals with the responsibility for their own health (which is, incidentally, a good strategy regardless of one's views on free will); however, scientific explanations of human behavior generally reject free will entirely, reduce genetic influences to a few generalized drives such as sex and hunger, and seek environmental explanations for almost all complex human behavior that requires decision making. SCT theorists restore a semblance of integrity to human behavior while staying within the bounds of science; this accommodation of human qualities and scientific rigor is based mainly on the concept of **reciprocal determinism**.

Bandura (1986), the leading SCT theorist, recognizes the potency of the behavioral consequences experienced by individuals as determinants of future actions; however, such consequences or "feedback" arising from the **environment** do not hold the dominant position accorded them by behaviorists. They are only one of three factors that interact dynamically to determine behavior. The remaining two are intrapersonal factors within the individual that Bandura categorizes as **personal** factors, which are mainly related to prior history in the form of knowledge and attitudes pertinent to the issue at hand; and **behavioral** factors, which are mainly related to individuals' ability to exert self-control as they determine their response to the situation. Behavioral factors are a learned set of processes based on habits of self-observation, self-judgment, and self-reaction. Also behavior has a reciprocal impact on the environment and thus may exert an effect on subsequent actions.

Environmental Influences

Although proponents of SCT recognize the importance of environmental factors on behavior, they tend to reject any mechanical view of the process by which these factors exert their influence; their explanation is consistent with their strong cognitive theme. "Behavior is regulated by its consequences (reinforcements), but only as those consequences are interpreted and understood by the individual" (Rosenstock et al., 1988:176). Simply stated, it is not only events that influence behavior, but also our perception of events.

According to SCT, there are at least three major processes by which the environment exerts its influence, namely, (1) the reinforcement or inhibition of behavior provided by its consequences for particular actions, (2) the opportunity it provides for observational learning or the modeling of behavior after that of other persons, and (3) the vicarious reinforcement it provides as individuals experience gratification when they see others rewarded for particular actions.

Reinforcement

Proponents of SCT accord reinforcement a central role in the determination of behavior but provide a complex explanation of its mechanisms. SCT adopts the standard operant dogma that the consequences of our actions affect the likelihood and frequency of future such actions. But in SCT three other aspects of reinforcement are also emphasized. First, the individual's interpretation of the consequences (**perceived consequences**) of a particular action are paramount, more important than the actual consequences. For example, two middle-aged adults embarking on an exercise program might experience noticeable muscular soreness and stiffness. One, however, might view such symptoms as signs of damage and pathology and become discouraged, whereas the other might regard this mild discomfort as an indication of an effective workout and thus become even more committed to the program. Second, SCT includes the concept of **vicarious reinforcement**, whereby reinforcement occurs for behaviors that the individual has observed but not yet expressed. As we see attractive people in TV commercials reaping vast benefits from their actions, we are encouraged to try the same strategies if similar situations arise. Third, individuals engage in **self-reinforcement**, a process that is under the control of the individual and independent of the environment. Self-reinforcement is an integral part of the self-regulation system that is a part of the human personality structure.

Observational Learning

In addition to its natural capacity to reward and punish behavior, the environment constitutes an obvious source of information to the individual; the daily flow of events provides a virtual training film for the average individual. If people are asked how they learned to prepare a meal, comb their hair, throw a ball, or do any of a multitude of similar behaviors, it is not surprising to hear them say that they simply watched someone who seemed to know what they were doing. In other words, they learned by observation from a model. And while the most obvious examples involve behavior with a skill component, for example, "how-to" comb one's hair, the process may be easily extended into the realm of the attitudinal or motivational aspects of behavior, for example, "why" the hair should be combed or "why" the seat belts should be worn. Although other theorists made passing references to the concept of modeling or observational learning, it remained for the social learning theorists, particularly Bandura and Walters, to deal with it in a serious manner (Bandura and Walters, 1963).

One of the reasons for this apparent lack of interest in observational learning on the part of the behaviorists provides a further insight into the distinctive features of SCT. The behaviorists investigated observational learning in experiments using lower animals, such as rats and pigeons, as subjects and found that their behavior was little affected by exposure to the examples of trained models. Rats didn't seem to learn from other rats; they all seemed to blunder along by trial and error until they found a pattern that worked. The SCT theorists, however, did considerable work with human subjects, as was their natural inclination, and obtained much more positive results. Bandura felt that the ability of human subjects to use symbols to aid their retention was responsible for their greater effectiveness. He viewed retention processes as the second of the four-stage sequence of observational learning (described below). He hypothesized that animals must rely on imagery alone in retention, while humans can use both imagery and verbal descriptions in this process (see figure 11.1)

Attentional processes.   Bandura observed that "people cannot learn much from observing unless they attend to, and perceive accurately, the significant features of the modeled behavior" (Bandura, 1986:51). A number of factors, including the attractiveness of the model, the nature and complexity of the behavior being demonstrated, and the needs of the observer, have been found to affect the degree of attention observers accord to specific events.

Retentional processes.   If the behavior is to be replicated by the observer it must be retained in memory for future use when appropriate. Of course, retentional capabilities vary among individuals, but retention is better when stimuli are salient, the words and images are relevant to the observer, there are few distractions and an immediate opportunity to recall and apply this information.

Motor reproductive processes.   The third component of observational learning, **motor reproductive processes**, consists of the physical task of actually duplicating the observed behavior. This process can be quite simple as in lighting a cigarette,

Figure 11.1

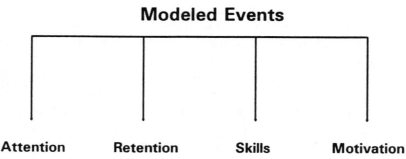

Modeled Events

Attention   Retention   Skills   Motivation

Observational learning. A modeled event may capture the learner's attention, facilitate retention of information, foster skills acquisition, and provide vicarious reinforcement.

Source: Bandura, Albert. *Social Foundations of Thought and Action: A Social Cognitive Theory.* © 1986, Fig. 3, pp. 52. Reprinted by permission of Prentice-Hall, Inc.

or quite complex as in administering CPR. In this latter case, the modeling process itself may lead the observer into a rough approximation of the behavior; it must then be smoothed out with self-corrections assisted by the verbal instruction of others wherein language and symbols again become obvious tools.

Acquisitional processes.   After one gains a basic understanding of how the process of observational learning works, the next step is to determine what types of behaviors can be acquired through its application. Given its central role within this comprehensive approach to learning, it is not surprising to find that SCT advocates maintain that a wide variety of learned outcomes may be explained by use of observational learning. As noted, such specific behaviors as face washing and teeth brushing can be acquired by observation. The scope of such acquisitions can be enlarged by the action of **abstract modeling** wherein the learner derives a concept out of a group of related learning experiences and begins to make applications that were not specifically observed. For example, those persons who develop the generalization that "many factors affect personal appearance" may then go beyond washing and brushing and begin reading about nutritional factors and skin care, the selection and care of clothing, and other actions not specifically modeled.

This process may be extended to ethical behavior; children who observe their parents treat many different people with dignity and respect regardless of their age, race, educational level, or occupation may naturally display similar behavior. In a closely related process, unique behaviors may be elicited by a process termed **creative modeling**. As learners observe different examples of behaviors they often combine bits and pieces from different models into unique types of behavior. As Bandura describes it:

> Beethoven adopted the classic forms of Haydn and Mozart, though with greater emotional expressiveness . . . . Wagner fused Beethoven's symphonic mode with Weber's naturalistic enchantment and Meyerbeer's dramatic virtuosity to evolve a new operatic form (1986:105).

Observational learning may also be used to explain a wide variety of motivational and emotional responses as opposed to the primarily cognitive effects which have been discussed. Often the learner is not shown "how" to do something as much as encouraged to do it or not do it under certain circumstances. When the driver of a car buckles up his or her seat belt, for instance, the passengers are often influenced to do the same; in SCT terminology, the driver elicited the response of a preexisting behavior since the passengers presumably already knew how to use their seat belts. This example is most valid in those cases where the driver's behavior serves to remind the riders that the belts are available and that it is prudent to use them. A somewhat different set of mental dynamics comes into play in those instances when the passengers are initially aware of the belts but somewhat reluctant to use them for fear of appearing to be "safety nuts" or perhaps feeling that their action would display a lack of confidence in the ability of the driver. Here the driver's behavior served to modify the inhibitions of the passengers. According to SCT, models can strengthen or weaken inhibitions, well documented in the clinical treatment of phobias.

Personal Factors

As people approach a situation that calls for some action or response, they seldom proceed purely on the basis of trial and error. Each individual brings grist to the decision-making mill in the form of myriad facts, concepts, skills, beliefs, attitudes, and vague impressions. Although these entities exist in the present as they exert their affects on behavior, they are the product of past experiences that the decision maker brings to the current scene. Once the person makes a decision and acts, there will always be some immediate consequences which then impact on this historical self-structure and change it to a greater or lesser degree. But even this feedback will be filtered through the complex maze of the self-structure for its assessment as positive or negative, important or trivial. This experiential baggage is retained cognitively as expectations and expectancies about the action that the individual is considering.

Outcome Expectations

Perry and others (1990) describe outcome expectations as the result the individual anticipates from taking a given course of action. For example, positive expectations about drinking alcohol increase the likelihood that an adolescent will drink, while concerns about consequences of getting caught drinking as a minor increase the likelihood of abstinence (Augustyn and Simons-Morton, 1995). Similarly, a young woman considering initiating a fitness program might anticipate better control of her weight and increased strength, making her less dependent on others for assistance. However, she may also anticipate that exercising will take away from her other leisure pursuits. These various expectations result from a combination of her past experience in similar situations, her observations of others, and the available information on the prospective program.

Outcome Expectancies

Expectancies are the values that one attaches to a particular outcome. In the example just provided, the young woman expected to become stronger and more independent by initiating a fitness program. Although most women would have positive expectancies related to such an outcome, some might view strength and independence as negative outcomes that might disturb valued relationships with those on whom they routinely depend for help. Thus the prospects of becoming stronger would carry a negative expectancy. The analysis of expectations and expectancies is based on the common sense observation that an individual's decision on a given behavior is based on (1) beliefs of what the outcomes will be and (2) beliefs concerning how desirable these outcomes would be.

Efficacy Expectations

Some of the most promising research related to health behavior in recent years has focused on the concept of self-efficacy. As defined by Bandura (1986:391), **self-efficacy** is "people's judgments of their capabilities to organize and execute courses of action required to attain designated types of performances." Related to one's **behavioral capability**—the knowledge and skills necessary to perform the task—it is the individual's subjective perception of his or her ability to perform the behavior in question. As such it is, in effect, a specialized set of expectations that apply to the performance, not to the outcome, of a given behavior.

Self-efficacy is a surprisingly good predictor of behavior (Kok et al., 1991). Both everyday observations and structured research support the common belief that people tend to do things that they believe will lead to valued outcomes. However, the recent evidence that people are affected by their relative confidence in their ability to carry out behaviors, although not surprising in itself, suggests that self-efficacy is more important than anticipated. Apparently people have a strong aversion to trying things that might make them appear awkward, inept, or that might lead to outright failure, regardless of the desirability of the possible outcomes. Strecher and associates (1986), provide a review of research supporting the usefulness of self-efficacy in health education, noting Bandura's distinction between an individual's expectations of possible outcomes and expectations about his or her self-efficacy.

In addition to the considerable research showing the potency of self-efficacy as a behavioral determinant, several studies have focused on the factors that enhance and strengthen self-efficacy itself. Thus far it appears that four main factors are involved.

Performance accomplishments. One of the better and more obvious ways to develop self-efficacy is by experiencing success in performing the target behavior. Whether one is learning to ski or trying to lose weight, early success builds confidence and leads to more persistent effort. Successful leaders in a wide variety of fields have discovered by practical experience, if not by studying theory, that success breeds success and that it is important to structure the program to provide this experience.

Vicarious experience. One of the authors noted that his 17-year-old son did quite a good job riding a horse on his first attempt. When questioned the young rider explained that he "already knew how to ride" before this first attempt because of his opportunity to watch others both in real life and on film. He not only had learned some skills vicariously but, more to our point, acquired considerable confidence in his ability to perform. His self-efficacy could have been drastically reduced, however, if someone had selected the wrong horse for this first ride. This process of developing self-efficacy vicariously is, of course, simply a specific application of observational learning.

Verbal persuasion. One's confidence in his or her ability to perform a specific task can be markedly increased or reduced by the encouraging or discouraging remarks of other persons whose opinions are respected. Many factors affect the impact of a given instance of persuasion, including the subject's prior experience, the plausibility of the message, and other personal qualities of the subject, such as the extent to which he or she is inner- or outer-directed.

Physiological state.   Pain, fatigue, and illness all affect a person's confidence in his or her ability to perform a demanding task. As with most other psychological variables, the perception of one's physiological state, as well as the actual state, has a direct effect on self-efficacy. The success of efforts to persuade older clients or patients to engage in specific forms of exercise for purposes of fitness or rehabilitation, for example, may depend not only on their actual physical condition, but also on their perceptions of the general capabilities of older people and their own potential as well.

Self-Regulated Behavior

Perhaps the most challenging task of psychologists who take a rigorously scientific view of human behavior is to provide an explanation of behavior that appears to be self-directed and thus to have its very origins within the psyche of the individual. Frequently we see people who seem simply to "reach down inside themselves" and decide to do something that appears inconsistent with either their past history or the external factors in the situation. Indeed, **resilience**, the ability of people to overcome overwhelmingly negative experience, is the topic of considerable current research. SCT does not shy away from the challenge and, in fact, embraces this phenomena and accords it an important place in its overall framework under the heading of self-regulation. Bandura (1986), for example, argues that self-regulatory behavior is not only real but also explainable by the laws of cause and effect. This human quality of self-regulation takes on a mystical appearance because human beings are capable of developing mental mechanisms so complex that their functioning appears to be autonomous; this important component of our self-structure merits a closer look.

Much worthwhile human activity involves doing chores and meeting responsibilities in the absence of any visible reward or reinforcement. Bandura offers an explanation of this human quality that recognizes the uniqueness and complexity of human behavior, while recognizing the importance of reinforcement. He suggests that humans have the capability of rewarding themselves internally through a process of self-reinforcement. As he explains in a widely quoted statement:

> If actions were determined solely by external rewards and punishments, people would behave like weathervanes, constantly shifting in different directions to conform to the momentary influences impinging upon them. They would act corruptly with unprincipled individuals and honorably with righteous ones, and liberally with libertarians and dogmatically with authoritarians (Bandura, 1986:335).

The tendency for human behavior to be consistent, rather than constantly shifting in accordance with the environment, Bandura maintains, is the result of individual, internalized sets of performance standards, and moral codes. These components are supported by the very human abilities of self-observation, self-judgment, and self-reinforcement. These in turn rely to a large extent on the ability of humans to use symbols in their thought processes of memory, cognition, and the like. People think in words and use words both in the analytical task of evaluating their behavior and in their subsequent act of praising or chastising themselves. Humans, more so than any other species, are aware of their own existence; they are self-conscious in a positive sense. They are able to develop the capability of observing their own actions with a considerable degree of detachment, then use their power of language to reinforce or inhibit their behavior. This capability depends on three important sub-processes.

Self-Observation

Clearly, people have an inherent tendency to be attentive to their environment and the events that take place around them. But, in addition, there is evidence that this natural attentiveness to external factors is also turned inward as individuals observe and evaluate their own actions. Much of this tendency to monitor our own behavior is no doubt acquired through the normal give and take of everyday life. As specific actions lead to either desirable or unpleasant results, people find that it is in their interest to keep tabs on their actions so as to maximize the favorable outcomes.

Although all people practice self-observation, there are great variations in the accuracy, objectivity, and intensity different individuals bring to the task. Because self-observation is such a powerful learning experience, teachers, parents, and behavior change specialists may encourage it and even make it a formal assignment. For example, a mother of a teenage son might become concerned about his many and long phone conversations, which diminish the time available for school work, and require him to keep a phone log as a first step toward exerting some control over the practice. Gaining knowledge also can sharpen self-observation. As individuals learn more about the various aspects of human behavior through formal or informal learning experiences, they become more attentive to many of their own actions that they may have previously viewed as unimportant. People also vary greatly in their ability to view their own behavior objectively. The proponents of SCT believe that emotions can distort individuals' views of their actions. The interference of emotions is even more potent in the subsequent process of self-judgment; however, it also applies to the simple perception of what one actually did.

Self-Judgment

As people observe their own behavior they are constantly judging individual actions in terms of both their effectiveness in getting something done and in terms of their relative "goodness or badness" in an ethical or socially useful sense. These judgments are based on an internalized set of standards that the individual believes to be valid and applicable to his or her situation. As Bandura explains, such standards "can be established by direct tuition, by evaluative social reactions to one's behavior, and by the self-evaluative standards modeled by others" (Bandura, 1986:340). Examples of **direct tuition** occur when children are explicitly taught what behaviors are right and wrong, and what achievements are laudatory or below standard. Evaluative social reactions refer to the way people generally respond to what one does in terms of praise, disdain, or indifference; it is simply the pressure of the prevailing social norms. The self-evaluative standards modeled by others refer to the influence of particular people in the social environment who the individual may admire and with whom the individual identifies. These models stand out from the general social milieu and exert an especially potent influence.

These standards must be believed and accepted by the individual if they are to be used for self-evaluation but, unfortunately, such internalized criteria need not be valid and appropriate in an objective sense in order to be fully functional. Therein lies the basis for many human problems. Most of us have known friends and acquaintances who had unrealistically high standards and made themselves chronically discontent or even ill by their subsequent reaction to their level of achievement. Some criminal sub-cultures teach their members that the only sin is "getting caught" and then set standards for the number of assaults or killings needed for full acceptance into the "gang." Fortunately, most of our self-judgment activities fall between these extremes and serve as a favorable influence on our behavior.

Self-Reaction

People see themselves do a particular thing, judge it on a scale that may extend from laudatory to despicable, then reward or punish themselves accordingly. This latter process, termed **self-reaction** by the SCT theorists, may take the form of a pleasant raising or unpleasant lowering of self-esteem, both of which take place covertly or internally with nonetheless significant long-term effects. Self-reaction may also take the form of direct overt action to reward or punish one's self. There are numerous examples of authors rewarding themselves with a period of relaxation or a special treat after the completion of a self-prescribed number of words or pages. Persons on weight-loss diets often reward themselves with new clothes, or even a self-indulgent dinner in a fine restaurant when they reach a specific goal. Self-reactions can also be punitive ranging from mild self-chastisement to suicide. In the extreme these negative forms are the focus of much research into the dynamics of mental illness; however, within the more normal range of everyday activities, self-reactions can be orchestrated both by the individual or by parents and educators, for example, in the individual's behalf.

Practical Applications

A review of the basic tenets of SCT can equip health educators with a valid general orientation to their overall task of facilitating behavior change. It provides a constant reminder that much of what an individual learns about anything takes place in a social context with interpersonal relationships playing a key role. This emphasis on social influences, however, is tempered to some degree by the recognition that human beings are quite rational in their behavior; they remember things and rework previous experiences in their minds as they make decisions. The influence of this inner dynamic process will sometimes result in behavior that seems inconsistent with the realities of the external situation.

General Implications

Social influences play prominently in many learning situations. The powerful influence on behavior of best friends and significant others, group membership, and even perceptions of social norms is well documented. Also, learning is facilitated by words and symbols that capture the essence of a behavior, as a century of tobacco advertising attests.

Social Influences

The principles of SCT can very quickly lead the beginning health educator to a conclusion that most experienced teachers make after some years on the job; namely, their students are more readily persuaded to adopt new behavior patterns by other people's actions than by what the teacher says. The old saw, "Your actions speak so loudly I can't hear what you say," applies. Ideas are also important, but at a later stage and for a different purpose.

The most obvious application of this concept pertains to the life-style of the health educator. Although most students who select health education as a field of study are oriented toward good personal health habits, they often find either during their professional preparation or in the first year or two of their working careers, that situational stress, resulting from heavy work loads and conflicting responsibilities, can start moving them toward a sedentary life-style, poor eating habits, excessive use of pills or alcohol, and other less than ideal behavior. It's easy to say, "You of all people ought to know how to take care of yourself"; however, health educators who don't work hard in pressure situations may lose their jobs or programs or both and find themselves with no clients to admire their slim waistlines and clear, well-rested eyes. The answer to such frequent conflicts is not easy but, at least, health educators have dual motivations for resolving them: their good health is not only a personal asset but a professional tool. There are many other applications of the modeling process, as will be discussed in a following section.

Symbols Help

Although SCT seems focused on concrete demonstrations of favorable behavior, we should not forget the contention by Bandura and others that the human capacity to describe actions with words helps them retain and replicate the observed behavior. A group of overweight clients might be impressed by a film showing a model (actor) demonstrating the use of good weight-control strategies, but fail to retain the details without a thorough follow-up discussion. Such a discussion allows them to collectively recall, verbalize, and list the things they saw, such as putting all snack food out of sight, eating while seated at the table, using a small plate, chewing food slowly and thoroughly, and so forth. In addition to increasing the precision or thoroughness of the retention process, the use of discussion and printed information can serve to broaden the scope and hence the applications of the general type of behavior observed. Post-coronary patients, for instance, might be skeptical in regard to their ability to rehabilitate themselves prior to observing others in similar circumstances participating successfully in their own rehabilitation by use of appropriate exercise, stress management techniques, and so forth. However, once they have "bought" the general concept through observational learning, they often will be ready to learn about other aspects of a healthy life-style by means of reading, listening, and other less direct means of instruction. SCT thus supports the concept of person-to-person experiences for both their persuasive and informational value, but also recognizes the value of printed materials, lectures, and so forth to extend the scope of behavior change. This makes for a well-balanced, somewhat confluent, i.e., cognitive and affective, approach.

Specific Methods

The health educator who embraces SCT will typically find that its principles can provide guidance for the refinement of virtually all standard techniques for improving knowledge, development, attitudes, or behavior. Moreover, a number of specific techniques either have arisen directly from the theoretical work or have become closely associated with SCT. Examples include modeling, skill training, contracting, and self-monitoring. These techniques can be used alone or in combination with one another depending upon the demands of the instructional situation.

Modeling

The theory underlying modeling has been discussed previously under the heading of observational learning; the points in this section generally follow those provided by Blomquist (1986) for use in school settings; however, they also seem appropriate for a variety of other situations:

1. The attention that the learner gives both to the model and the target behavior is crucial. It is best to select models who are similar to the learners in age, gender, race, and competence. Such qualities as likability, prestige, and status also enhance appeal as do models who already occupy the learners' aspired station in life. The use of multiple models helps increase the odds of including qualities that will impress individual learners. Also, the behavior modeled should not seriously conflict with the values of the learners. Modeling has been shown to

be effective when presented with live models as in dramatizations, role playing, or, when practical, in real-life situations; film and videotape presentations are also effective as are puppets and clearly illustrated stories for children.

2. Once learners have taken a positive view of the target behavior, the next step is to encourage its acquisition and retention. It is often helpful if the model describes the target behavior as it is demonstrated. Also, discussions following the modeling event that can clarify and put the behavior into words are helpful. When it is not feasible to practice the desired behavior in the learning situation it may be useful to provide for its mental rehearsal.

3. The direct practice of the behavior following the modeling event can be very important even for simple actions that require no appreciable skill development. The motor reproductive process provides an additional way of remembering the behavior. When some degree of skill is required, e.g., as in breast self-examination, then instruction and practice will increase both the odds that the practice will be used and the effectiveness with which it is applied.

4. The consequences of behavior learned through modeling provide the same reinforcing or inhibiting effect as behavior resulting from other sources; thus both artificial incentives and efforts to provide positive interpretations to natural consequences are recommended. Also, according to SCT vicarious rewards or negative outcomes produce potent effects; thus, observations of models experiencing positive results can encourage the learner to make the initial effort. However, there is considerable evidence that overly dramatic scenes of models experiencing unhappy or tragic consequences for unfavorable behavior, as with drugs or unprotected sex, tend to be blocked out and ignored.

The task of the health educator is to be creative in identifying role models and learning activities that model targeted health behaviors. While qualitative needs assessments are useful in identifying appropriate models of the target behavior for a specific population, modeling is a particularly adaptable method. It can be accomplished in a variety of ways—through story telling, in photographs, and by videotape. Consequently, it is possible to expose the learner to appropriate role models within the context of the classroom or other setting.

For example, in the "Great Sensations" school-based program to promote low-fat, low-salt eating among high school students, groups of students in focus groups identified themes that would be likely to resonate with the students and a variety of models (Simons-Morton BG et al., 1984). Subsequently, posters were developed around specific themes—such as selecting low-salt snacks—and contained photographs of student role models with appropriate snacks and a direct quote from the student about how terrific that low-salt snack was. The posters were placed prominently in the cafeteria and other point-of-purchase locations. Each week a different student role model was portrayed on the poster with a photograph and quote (see figure 11.2).

In the "Safety Belt Connection" (Simons-Morton BG et al., 1987), a worksite project to increase safety belt and shoulder harness use, a variety of models were selected from among workers by parking lot observers. These models properly buckled up and were asked to provide a testimonial about safety belt use, which was printed on a poster along with the person's photograph. The

Figure 11.2

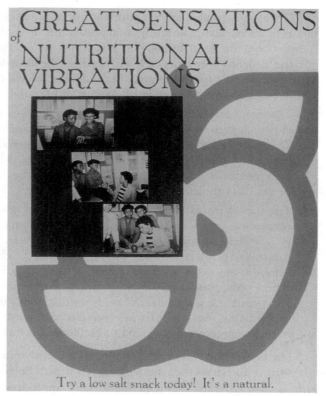

Poster used in "Great Sensations" study modeling low-salt snacking.

posters were displayed at various parking lot entrances and at strategic points about the worksite. By selecting workers in different parking lots who left the lot at different times, a variety of representative models were displayed (see figure 11.3).

Skill Training

Skill training includes psychomotor and social skills, such as refusing an offer to use illegal drugs or asking someone of the opposite sex for a date. Skilled behavior, regardless of whether or not psychomotor skill is involved, generally involves a precise sequence of behavioral sub-components and presents a challenge to the inexperienced performer. As noted, skill development both enhances the effectiveness of the target behavior and the probability that the learner will try it at all. As Bandura (1986:391) states, "Competent functioning requires both skills and self-beliefs of efficacy to use them effectively."

Figure 11.3

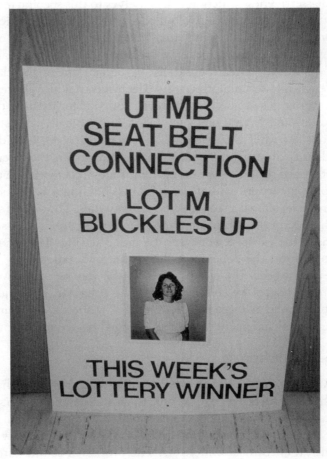

Poster used in "Safety Belt Connection" study modeling the use of safety belts.

Bartlett and others (1986) provide a concise description of the typical steps involved in skill development:

1. Describe and demonstrate the skill to the learner.
2. Ask the learner to demonstrate the skill back to you.
3. Provide any needed correction and ask the learner to repeat the skill again.

Complex skills should be broken down into component parts and learned separately. Social skills, such as assertiveness training, can often be presented effectively through role playing when learners have developed sufficient trust in the learning situation. Here the learner is not told exactly what to say but must learn to respond to a variety of possible situations. The ability to refuse gracefully a cigarette, an alcoholic beverage, or a calorie-laden dessert are forms of assertiveness which lend themselves to this specific technique. For example, students can first observe a model refusing, then practice refusing predictable preplanned overtures, and finally, they can be given the opportunity to practice against a variety of clever approaches designed to break down their resolve.

In the "Great Sensations" program, one of the classroom activities was designed to teach ninth-grade students refusal skills. The teacher told the students how to refuse something that was not good for them or that they did not want to do, and gave them some examples. Basically, the students were asked to consider what they were being requested to do, consider the consequences, identify an acceptable alternative, and act on the alternative. The students practiced several of the component skills and engaged in a **behavioral rehearsal** role play where one of the students, holding a bag of salty potato chips and an apple, offered a second student some chips. The second student was to consider the offer, reject the chips, and then request the apple as an alternative. What made the exercise work was the group setting. The second student was asked to perform the behavior in his or her own unique way, refusing the chips in a manner that the group judged to the way he or she would really do it. The group judged the style as well as the behavior. If the judgment was that the student did not get into it, then he or she did it again (see figure 11.4). A successful judgment was acknowledged by group approval and the apple.

Self-Monitoring

A basic tenet of health education is the admonition that people should take charge of their lives or "become their own parents" so to speak. Self-monitoring translates this general recommendation into operational terms; it is essentially a contract with oneself. People, of course, generally try to act in accordance with their own best interests. The process of self-monitoring simply serves as a method of thinking through the intended change and setting specific goals. It tends to remove ambiguities and reduce the chances of vacillation and excuses. For example, some years ago one of the authors decided that the quality of his skiing was hampered by a waistline too large and equipment too old. He self-contracted for a 15-pound weight reduction in return for a pair of high performance skis and discovered the only serious flaw in the technique: the "self" also must pay for the reward.

The "Go For Health" school health promotion project (Simons-Morton BG et al., 1991) was designed to facilitate a heart-healthy diet and physical activity among elementary school students. Self-monitoring was one of the curriculum methods. At various times, students were asked to monitor the heart-healthy foods they ate and the vigorous activities in which they engaged. They recorded all such foods and activities until they reached a pre-specified number, at which time they added their name to a poster that served as a visual monitor for the entire class. The healthful foods and activities were considered to be

Figure 11.4

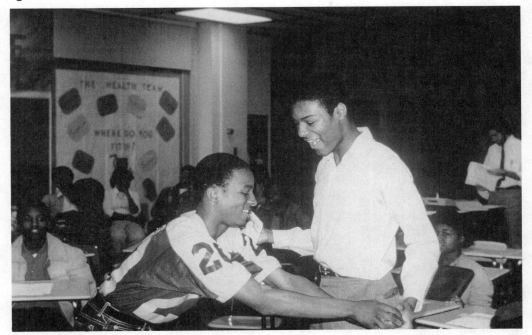

Example of behavioral rehearsal role play conducted as part of "Great Sensations" healthy snacking study.

part of the students' behavioral repertoire, and they were encouraged to increase the frequency with which they ate these foods and engaged in these activities. Although this was not a time limited assignment, the students wanted to reach their specified number of foods and activities and be recognized for it. Hence, not only was the behavior of each student and of the class monitored, but also the act of adding to the group record was visually monitored and reinforced.

In the "Safety Belt Connection" the authors used a group monitoring method popular with fund raisers. Giant thermometers were created to register the percentage of drivers entering and leaving the parking lot who were properly buckled. The percentage of correct use at baseline, the most recent observation, and the target percent were prominently marked. These thermometers were placed at the entrance and exits of the parking lot for the workers to see (figure 11.5).

Contracting

The close affiliation of SCT with behaviorism is demonstrated in the highly useful behavior change skill known as **contracting**. It is in one sense a program

Figure 11.5

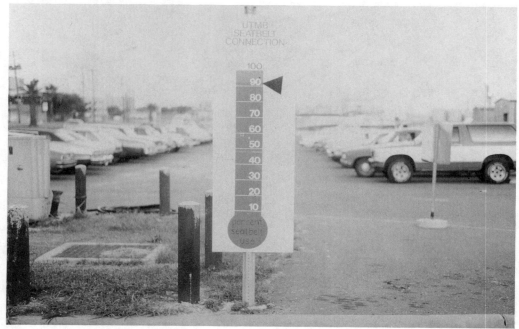

Visual reference for group monitoring of safety belt use in the "Safety Belt Connection" study.

of behavior modification with social influence involved as a principal environmental contingency. Although a token or other reward may be involved, the desire to impress or please another person represents the added SCT feature. As described by Parcel and Baranowski (1981:17), contracting involves some combination of the following information:

- which two or more parties are involved in the agreement
- what specific behaviors each will perform
- some measure and criterion (goal) for successful performance
- some self-identified contingency, or reward, for successful performance
- the signatures of the participants

The contracting method was successfully employed in the "Great Sensations" project. Students contracted to substitute one more healthful snack from a list provided for one less healthful snack. The contract was co-signed by the student and a student partner. Shown in figure 11.6, the contract specified what healthful snack the student would add to his or her diet within a two-day period.

Figure 11.6

```
┌─────────────────────────────────────────────────────────────┐
│                                                             │
│        Goal for the Day                                     │
│        ───────────────                                      │
│                                                             │
│        Today is   _____    _____      │
│                   DAY OF WEEK          DATE                  │
│                                                             │
│        Yesterday I ate the following salty snack:           │
│                                                             │
│                   _____  │
│                                                             │
│        Today I am going to try a low-salt snack             │
│                                                             │
│                   _____  │
│                   WRITE HERE THE SNACK YOU WILL TRY         │
│                                                             │
│        Signature  _____  │
│                                                             │
└─────────────────────────────────────────────────────────────┘
```

Example of a personal contract employed in the "Great Sensations" study.

The contract stipulated that success would be judged by the student partner and rewarded by a coupon for a healthful snack available in the cafeteria.

Summary

Social cognitive theory provides a broad but well integrated explanation of human behavior. It recognizes the strong influence that positive and negative consequences—arising from both the social and the physical environment—have on our behavior, but it places perhaps more emphasis on such internal factors as knowledge, attitudes, skills, and values as behavioral determinants. However, its most useful contribution lies in the very plausible explanation it provides for the way these internal factors are formed and the way they interact in the decision-making process.

The importance of person-to-person influences on behavior is a continuing theme throughout all components of SCT as is the human ability to think and remember by use of language based on symbols. Although an individual can learn much from observing the world of nature, the specific actions of other people, especially those important to us, have particularly strong effects on our subsequent behavior. We watch others and find out how to do things; through this observation we may also gain confidence in our ability to do something similar; when we see them succeed, we receive vicarious satisfaction from their accomplishments and the behavior thus becomes reinforced even before we make our initial effort.

Both these observations and direct experiences provided by the environment lead internally to the placing of value, the development of knowledge, the early beginning of skills, and the formation of self-confidence (self-efficacy) with respect to a particular behavior. Together these products of perception and cognition form an important set of personal factors which become a second force, in addition the environment, in the determination of behavior. A third force is provided by a close-knit set of processes that acts as a self-regulatory mechanism. Its functioning is based on the fact that behavior does not typically occur in single, discrete units but in chains or sequences of actions that produce feedback. In what may be a uniquely human capability wherein behavior helps determine behavior, the individual monitors, evaluates, and reacts to his or her own behavioral components and makes changes, adjustments, or perhaps abandons the entire effort. These three major components, (1) the environment, (2) the personal qualities of the individual, (3) the response of the self-regulatory mechanism to aspects of the behavior, all interact in a process of reciprocal determinism.

All of these various components are fraught with the complexities characteristic of any realistic effort to explain human behavior. However, the comprehensiveness of SCT, the precise definition of its processes, and its internal consistency enable it to both present useful implications for program design and provide for its own elaboration and improvement through research.

Organizational Change

Organizations exist to enable ordinary people to do
extraordinary things.
            —Ted Levitt (former editor of the *Harvard*
                        Business Review)

Introduction

Organizations are "goal-directed, boundary-maintaining, activity systems" (Aldrich, 1979:4). They are purposive, coordinating resources toward accomplishing a goal, such as making a profit, providing a specific service, or producing a product. Policies and procedures govern activities within organizations. Each organization has its own norms and culture. To work effectively with organizations, health educators need a framework for understanding organizational systems and how to change organizational behavior.
    Consider the following:

- Students at a university want to establish a Designated Driver Program (i.e., taxicab services for students who need assistance with rides home) following the tragic death of one of their friends who had an accident while driving home from a party at which he had been drinking heavily.
- A health educator at a community health center thinks that single parents would be more likely to bring their children for immunizations if patient services could be extended for one evening a week.
- Employees in a small manufacturing plant want their environment to be smoke-free.

In the examples above, organizations were targeted to provide programs and policies that would be supportive of individual behavior change. Outcomes specific to organizations, such as a health-promoting culture and a safe environment, are important in their own right. The Multilevel Approach to Community Health (MATCH) planning model discussed in chapter 6 provides the framework we will use to consider health promotion at the organizational level.

Health Education and Organizational Change

MATCH and Organizational Health Promotion Objectives

MATCH takes an ecological approach to health promotion, with intervention objectives and targets of intervention at the individual, interpersonal, organizational, community, and governmental levels. Figure 6.1, which provided an overview of the model, indicated that intervention approaches at the level of the organization included organizational change, consulting, training, and networking. Organizational decision makers listed as targets of intervention were administrators, managers, internal change agents, workers/employees, and union members and leaders. Intervention objectives for healthful organizations included policies, practices, programs, facilities, and resources. Organizational culture and norms are also important intervention objectives.

Figure 6.8 contained intervention objectives at each level of change across the settings of schools, worksites, health care institutions, and community for preventing alcohol misuse. In this chapter we will discuss how to facilitate changes within organizations to accomplish these objectives. How do we influence organizations in these different settings to adopt curricula, policies, and programs? How do we influence the cultural norms of these organizations so they are more promoting of health for their workers, students, patients, and clients? To accomplish these goals, health educators need a working knowledge of the process of organizational change.

Health Educators as Internal and External Change Agents

Health educators find themselves working with organizations in several ways. For example, many health educators are employed by such organizations as health departments, community health centers, schools, and corporations, and must work within their own organizations to accomplish their goals. Other health educators may work in a consulting capacity, in which case they are brought in by an organization to provide specific health education services, such as conducting a needs assessment or evaluation or planning a health promotion program. Alternatively, they may be in the position of trying to get community organizations to adopt new programs or collaborate with other organizations.

The health educator, in the role of an internal change agent, may work within his or her own organization to implement programs and policies to improve employee health. For example, directors of worksite health promotion programs must understand the dynamics of organizational change if they are to get their programs fully implemented within the organization and achieve high levels of participation among employees. This requires such skills as obtaining management support to provide resources for the program and to allow employees time off for participation; using communication systems effectively to market the program; changing the norms and culture of the organization to be more supportive of health promotion; and ensuring that the health promotion program is continued.

Almost all health educators work within an organizational setting. To be effective managers, they must learn the skills of administration and understand organizational structure and processes. Program planning and coordination, staff management, budget and financial control, marketing management and (for worksite health/fitness programs) facility and equipment management will be discussed in chapter 15, Practice Settings.

As an external change agent, the health educator may work to get organizations to adopt new programs and policies that affect the health of employees or students. For example, a key performance objective of program staff in voluntary health agencies—such as the American Cancer Society and American Heart Association—is that school districts within their region adopt and implement comprehensive school health programs. In such a situation, the health educator would try to influence a school district decision maker, such as a curriculum coordinator, to review and decide to use the agency's health curriculum in the school district. Once the decision to use the curriculum was made, the agency staff and volunteers would coordinate with the district to set up training sessions for the teachers so they can implement the curriculum effectively. Agency personnel also work with school management to change the school environment, including the food services, physical activity program, and health service.

In addition, many public health programs are carried out through coalitions of organizations. As representatives of their organizations on coalitions, health educators need to know how interorganizational networks function and how to carry out the role of boundary spanner between their home organization and the coalition. A health educator from a voluntary agency serving on an interagency council for smoking or health must assess how the goals and activities of the coalition match those of his or her organization, have an understanding of how much discretion he or she has in committing the agency to provide staff and other resources to coalition activities, and be able to work collaboratively with other coalition members.

In these examples, health educators have worked as either internal or external change agents to get a program adopted by an organization, to add new services and staff to their organization, to change the way existing staff relate to each other, or to coordinate activities among organizations. Health educators with knowledge and skills in planned organizational change will be more effective in achieving such objectives than those who have not developed these competencies.

Planned organizational change may be directed to people, technology, or organizational structure. People-focused change involves training to enable staff to carry out their roles more effectively. Technological change refers to changes in programs or policies that the organization uses to accomplish its goals. Structural change includes changes in how the members of an organization relate to each other, their job descriptions, and how rewards are distributed. Typically it is easiest to change people and hardest to change structure. However, the impact and maintenance of the change is strongest with structural change and weakest with people-focused change (Brager and Holloway, 1978).

Concepts for Understanding Organizations

In this chapter, we introduce concepts important to structural change in organizations and then discuss a multi-faceted approach to planned organizational change. The concepts, which may at first appear dry and useless, provide both a blueprint and the nuts and bolts to assist the practitioner in approaching change of the organization as a system, which is more effective than targeting individual change.

To plan and carry out organizational change, it is important to understand the structure of organizations, organization culture, and human processes within organizations. For example, in beginning a worksite health promotion program, the health promotion manager must know who within the organization has decision-making power regarding the program's budget, how to obtain support for the program from management and from employees, what the existing norms related to health promotion are within the organization, and how to influence the norms to become more supportive of physical, mental, and social health.

Organizational Structure

Organizational structure includes the locus of authority (where decisions are made) and the degree of participativeness in decision making, the division of labor (how specialized each job is), and formalization (the extent to which rules and procedures are written). One can think of organizational structure as the blueprint for a house showing its frame as well as its plumbing, electric, and heating systems.

All organizations have an authority structure, which is reflected in the organizational chart. Authority, which is the power one person has over another person's action, may be centralized, decentralized, or dispersed (Mayer, 1979). Figure 12.1 shows these three types of organizational authority structures.

Centralized Authority Structure

A centralized authority structure is typified by a bureaucracy with a pyramid or hierarchical structure. Decision-making power is vested in the organization's executive officer. There is a clear chain of command; decisions are made at the top and carried out by organization members at lower levels. Military organizations and government agencies exemplify this authority structure.

Decentralized Authority Structure

In a decentralized authority structure, power to make some decisions is delegated to units within the organization. For example, in a school system, some decisions are made at the level of central administration and others at the level of the school or classroom. In large companies, authority for some decisions is located at headquarters and authority for other decisions at branch offices.

Figure 12.1 Types of Organizational/Authority Structures

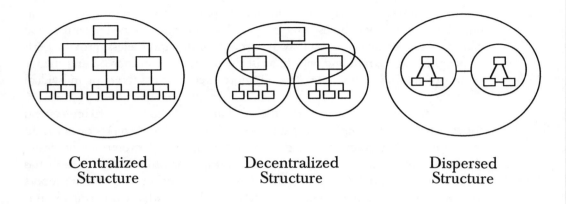

Centralized	Decentralized	Dispersed
Structure	Structure	Structure

Dispersed Authority Structure

In an organization with a dispersed authority structure, all actors are co-equal with each other. Examples of this are a university faculty or research organization. In organizations of this type, it is not possible to have a high level manager make decisions that affect what activities organizational members carry out. In these organizations, strong cultures and values hold the group together and make joint activity possible.

Participation in Decision Making

The degree of participativeness in decision making varies with organizational type, with centralized authority structures typically having the least and dispersed authority structures having the most participation. However, this varies within organization type. In all types of organizations, there has been a movement toward participatory management and employee involvement in decision making. Productivity growth rates in American industry have declined and international competition increased since the mid-1960s. Innovations designed to address these concerns have included self-managed work teams, employee involvement teams, labor-management committees, and decreasing the number of levels of authority within an organization. Increasing participation in decision making by employees leads to their increased ownership of the decisions and commitment to the organization (Mayer, 1979; Rosow and Zager, 1982).

Formalization

Formalization, the extent to which rules and procedures are written, determines how much discretion the individual actor has in his or her job activities. In organizations with high formalization, changing policies and job descriptions will initiate change in activities carried out within the organization. However, when rules and regulations are highly specified, it is difficult for new ideas to be tried and there is little room for creativity. Thus, formal procedures inhibit the initiation of change but are important for the implementation of a specific change and the institutionalization of a change.

Mission

The mission and core technology of the organization are also important. In some organizations, such as a company developing health promotion products to sell, health education is central to accomplishing the mission of the organization. However, in most settings where health educators work, health education is supportive to accomplishing the organization's mission. In schools, health education is an instructional element (though it is given less emphasis than major subjects) and thus is congruent with the mission. Comprehensive school health, however, is based on the school's mission and supports the core technology: good health and nutrition enable children to learn. For worksite health promotion, the focus is on increasing the health and productivity of workers so that they can better perform their jobs. At public health departments, health education supports infectious and chronic disease control efforts to decrease morbidity and mortality in the population.

Organizational Culture

Culture has been defined as "(a) a pattern of basic assumptions, (b) invented, discovered, or developed by a given group, (c) as it learns to cope with its problems of external adaptation and internal integration, (d) that has worked well enough to be considered valid and, therefore, (e) is to be taught to new members as the (f) correct way to perceive, think, and feel in relation to those problems" (Schein, 1990). External adaptation involves the organization's relationship to its environment. The organization must develop a consensus on its core mission, goals, and means for accomplishing those goals. Internal integration involves coordination of human and physical resources for accomplishing the mission and goals. Organizational cultures develop over time, and there is disagreement among theorists on the extent to which organizational cultures can be managed and intentionally changed (Ouichi and Wilkins, 1985). There is general agreement, however, that culture forms the context for the adoption and implementation of organizational innovations and must be considered in any organizational change effort. The organizational culture and subcultures can be supportive or resistant to a particular change. Not surprisingly, change attempts will be more successful if they are compatible with the organizational culture.

    Your text authors agree that culture is powerful and stable and must be taken into account in planned organizational change. However, they also believe that interventions to change culture are possible, and, although cultural shifts may require patience and long-term intervention, they will be effective and long lasting. An example of effective cultural change for health promotion at the societal level has been the dramatic shift in cultural norms for smoking, which was fueled by numerous public health interventions.

Typologies

Trice and Beyer (1993) summarize typologies of general organizational culture described by different researchers. For example, Ouichi (1981) contrasts Type A organizations, characterized by hierarchical control, high specialization, short-term employment, individual responsibility and individual decision making, with Type Z organizations that have clan control, long-term employment, individual responsibility and consensual decision making. Depending on whether the culture displayed high or low concern for employees and high or low concern for performance, Sethia and von Glinow (1985) characterized organizations as apathetic, caring, exacting, or integrative (see table 12.1). Depending on the level of risk, structure, and pace of feedback, Deal and Kennedy (1982) named four organizational types: process, tough-guy/macho, work-hard/play-hard, and bet-your-company. These different cultural types have different orientations toward health promotion and require different types of health promotion programs. Also, different strategies are needed to influence the adoption and implementation of new policies and programs.

Table 12.1 Corporate Culture Characterized by Level of Concern for Employees and Performance

Concern for Performance

		High	*Low*
Concern for Employees	*High*	Integrating	Caring
	Low	Exacting	Apathetic

Source: Adapted from Sethia and von Glinow, 1985.

Shared Beliefs

The substance of a culture is a shared belief system. Values, beliefs, and norms enable people to make sense of their world and to bind people together. Values are preferences for certain outcomes, such as personal achievement, humanitarianism, self-reliance, freedom, and equality. Beliefs relate to the cause and effect relationships, e.g., "If I work hard, I will get ahead." Norms are expectations of others for a person's behavior. For example, "My coworkers expect me to work through lunch."

Expressions of Culture

The expression of a culture is through observable forms, including symbols, language, stories, and practices. Organizations differ in their logos, style of dress, whether or not they use uniforms, and office arrangement and furnishings. Key information is also conveyed through characteristic jargon and slang, humor, gossip, and slogans. Stories are another way to convey cultural meanings, such as how much a company cares for its employees or whether/how a person can rise to the top of the organization. Rites or public performances—such as orientations, annual meetings, company parties, farewell parties, and awards ceremonies—reaffirm values, move persons from one status to another, strengthen the ties between organizational members, and link members more closely to the organization (Trice and Beyer, 1993).

Health Promoting Cultures

Allen and colleagues have written extensively on fostering health-promoting cultures within organizations (Allen and Bellingham, 1994; Allen et al., 1987; Allen and Allen, 1986, 1987). Values they see as implicit in the wellness movement are (1) living fully, beyond freedom from disease; (2) self-responsibility; (3) life-style integration emphasizing balance and harmony; and (4) caring for others and the environment.

A first step is to identify whether or not these values are congruent with current cultural norms within the organization. A norm is the expectations others have for your behavior, or, in this case, what is expected and accepted in the organization. In a survey, employees could be asked the extent to which they agree or disagree with a variety of statements that reflect the wellness values. An example of an item would be "In our organization, people tend to work so hard that they lose contact with other important parts of their lives (Allen and Allen, 1986:47). Table 12.2 contains additional items drawn from the work of Allen and his colleagues.

Besides measuring norms, the health educator should examine the systems and structures of the organization to see whether they are supportive of health. Are the rewards and recognition system and the allocation of resources reinforcing of the wellness values? Is an appreciation of wellness shown in the organization's rites and rituals? Do top managers model a wellness life-style?

Table 12.2 Indicators of Organizational Norms Related to Wellness

In our organization, it is accepted and expected:

1. for people to see desserts, such as cake, pie, pudding, and ice cream, as an expected part of lunch.
2. for people to associate overindulging in food with work celebrations and social events.
3. for people to go out for a drink after work.
4. for people to exercise as much as would be healthy for them.
5. for people to look upon work stress as something they can do something about.
6. for people to take on more responsibility than they can handle.
7. for people to ask for help if their work load becomes too heavy.
8. for people to handle conflict situations with other people constructively.

Source: Allen and Allen, 1986.

Using information from this assessment, the health promotion change agent would work with managers and employees to create more healthful norms, structures, and systems. This is done through a process involving employee task forces, training, and programming for behavioral and environmental change.

Planned Organizational Change

Brager and Holloway (1978) have included five stages in the process of planned change: initial assessment, preinitiation, initiation, implementation, and institutionalization. As seen in table 12.3, initial assessment begins with an analysis of the problem, the gap between how things are and how the change agent(s) would like for them to be and what strategies can be used to move the organization to close the gap. During the preinitiation stage, the change agent prepares the organization for the change and works to increase its readiness and receptivity for the change. This is followed by initiation of the change, in which the change idea is formally introduced and the change agent works for the adoption of the innovation. Adoption is followed by implementation in which the innovation is translated into action. All changes, however, are not maintained by the organization. Institutionalization ensures that the change is anchored in the organization through budgets, job descriptions, and other structural changes. To be effective, organizational change must proceed through all five stages.

Table 12.3 Stages and Strategies for Planned Organizational Change

Stage	Tasks
Initial assessment	1. Problem assessment and selection of change goals 2. Force field analysis of driving and restraining forces 3. Choice of tactics for change
Preinitiation	1. Choice of a change agent with credibility and legitimacy 2. Increase awareness within the organization of the need for change through evaluations and formal and informal discussion
Initiation	1. Selection of "top down" or "bottom up" change strategies 2. Specification of any policies or procedures in the change
Implementation	1. Choice of formal and informal communication channels for the change 2. Development of administrative procedures for the change 3. Analysis of driving and restraining forces for implementation 4. Monitoring of change process
Institutionalization	1. Inclusion of change in strategic plans and organizational goals and objectives 2. Written job descriptions 3. Hiring permanent staff 4. Stable source of funding

Source: Adapted from Brager and Holloway, 1978.

Initial Assessment

The first task the change agent carries out is a **force field analysis,** an assessment of organizational forces that promote the change or restrain it. Lewin's field theory has provided the framework for this activity. This model holds that an organization is a system that is dynamic, with the current situation representing the equilibrium between driving and restraining forces for change. Thus, shifts in either the driving or restraining forces will disrupt the equilibrium, resulting in a movement that either supports the change or the status quo. In a planned change intervention, the change agents act to either reduce the forces restraining change or to increase the forces for change. Reducing the forces that restrain change is often less threatening to the organization and thus meets with less resistance than increasing the forces for change. Thus, decreasing the forces that uphold the status quo is usually a more effective strategy for initiating change within an organization.

Figure 12.2 is a worksheet for conducting a force field analysis for a specific change. First the driving and restraining forces are identified and then rated in terms of their importance and changeability. These forces may be related to the beliefs of organizational members and leaders, organizational structure, the technology, or the environment. Organizational members with the power to adopt the change are identified. Based on this assessment, a strategy for change is selected that addresses changeable forces that act to resist change. As the organization becomes more receptive to change, introducing strategies that drive change is appropriate.

Preinitiation

At this point, the change agent has analyzed those forces that act to drive or restrain the organizational change desired. It is now time to prepare the organization for the change. In order to surface the need for change effectively, it is important that the change agent have credibility and legitimacy. The health educator acting as an *internal* change agent has had the opportunity to develop trusting relationships with coworkers and supervisors, to be part of the political give and take within the organization, and to demonstrate his or her expertise

Figure 12.2 Force Field of Driving and Restraining Forces for Organizational Change

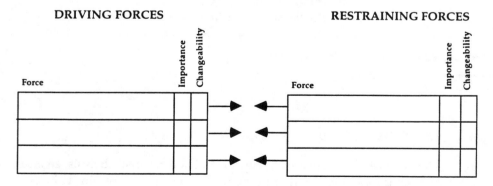

Use 2 "+" signs to indicate most important or most changeable, 1 "+" for somewhat important or changeable, 1 "−" for somewhat unimportant or unchangeable and 2 "−" signs for very unimportant or very unchangeable.

in practice. This is built up over time, through countless encounters with other organization members over many different situations and issues. Also, the position of the change agent within the organization, and thus his or her power and access to top decision makers, will influence his or her ability to introduce change. An external change agent, on the other hand, has usually been invited into the organization by top management to initiate a change and is typically hired on the basis of his or her expertise and credibility.

Next the change agent must increase organizational awareness of the situation requiring change. This can be done through informal discussions with coworkers and supervisors and routine formal meetings in which the situation can be linked to issues of organizational concern. Frequently, evaluation results focus attention on a problem. Thus an important change strategy is to conduct an evaluation, demonstrate the need for change, and have the evaluation stakeholders propose change strategies. (See chapter 8 for more information on evaluation.) The goal of this step is to increase organizational awareness of the change idea and to foster positive attitudes toward the proposed change.

Initiation

At this point, the goal of the change agent is adoption of the change by the organization. The strategy chosen to achieve this goal may be "top down" or "bottom up" or a combination of the two, depending on the situation. If key decision makers are change-oriented and supportive of the change, the change agent may simply present the need for change and suggested strategies to the decision maker and the change may be adopted outright. On the other hand, if the key decision makers resist change and are strong supporters of the status-quo, a "bottom-up" strategy in which organizational members with less authority build the momentum for change is necessary. This process may be confrontational and involve shifts in power.

A combination of the two approaches is usually most effective. Rarely are the need for change and its costs to the organization so clear-cut that one manager can make the decision. Also, having a unilateral management decision for change will make implementation among those who carry out the program more time consuming and difficult. Change is typically a negotiated process both up and down the organization. Goals and strategies may be modified when both top and bottom organizational members are included in the discussions regarding the proposed change and come to a consensus about what should be done. In this case, there is more ownership of the change and implementation will proceed more smoothly.

Implementation

Implementation has been defined as "an interactive process in which ideas, expressed as policy, are transformed into behavior, expressed as social action" (Ottoson and Green, 1987). Ottoson and Green offer a metaphor for understanding implementation. They view implementation as a drama, with policy as the plot, context as the stage, and the CEO, managers, employees, and policy beneficiaries as actors.

Figure 12.3 provides a visual model of implementation—showing the relationships of concept and context, process, and outcomes—that was used in a study of the implementation of smoking policy by Gottlieb and colleagues (1992). The concept, or the innovation to be adopted, is characterized by its goals and assumptions, its developers and their relationship to the organization, its specifications (including its scope and procedures, any incentives or penalties, and how flexible it is), and how much change of the organization's activities and employees' behavior is required.

The concept has to be implemented within the context of the organization. The context includes the organizational structure—including the degree of centralization of the authority structure, the level of formalization, and the number and types of employees. These have been discussed earlier in this chapter. Also important are the characteristics of the core technology; for example, whether work involves production of materials, people processing, or information processing. The physical and social/cultural environment of the organization must be considered, as well as the supportiveness of the organization's external environment.

The implementation process includes formal and informal communication regarding the innovation, the administrative policy and procedures related to the innovation, and the level and visibility of top and mid-level management support. Change agents must be alert to both intended and unintended outcomes of the innovations they are implementing. Often, there are unexpected outcomes

Figure 12.3 Innovation Implementation Model

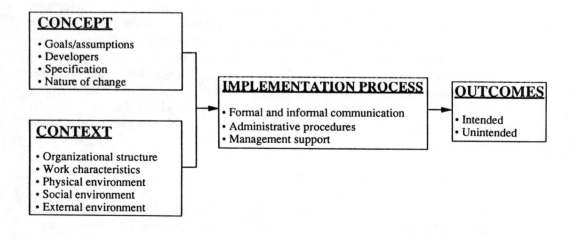

that may be negative and require fine-tuning of the innovation or its implementation. For example, implementation of a smoking policy in a large agency was found to have both the intended outcomes of improved air quality, decreased smoking frequency at work, and increased employee satisfaction and some unintended consequences, including disruption of work, diminished air quality around smoking areas, and decreased interaction between smokers and nonsmokers.

If the change is highly specific and the organizational structure is hierarchical, one administrator can designate what changes are to be made by whom in the authority structure. Usually, however, translation of the new policy into practice may not be clearly specified. The change may be complex, requiring a number of steps by different actors over a long period of time.

A number of barriers can present themselves during the implementation period, and management of the implementation process must overcome these problems if the change is to be realized. Lack of staff commitment; conflict with other organizational goals and objectives; poor communication of new policy and procedures; lack of familiarity with the program; too rapid or radical a change; insufficient budget, staff, and space resources; and difficulty in coordinating efforts across organizational units have all been identified as barriers to implementation (Green and Kreuter, 1991; Ottoson and Green, 1987; Brager and Holloway, 1978).

Implementation offers a somewhat different set of restraining and driving forces for the change, as organizational members confront what the new program or policy actually means to them as they carry it out. Some of the same forces that were identified in the initial assessment phase will continue to be felt; others will emerge. Conducting another force field analysis will point to specific issues that must be addressed if the program is to be implemented and identify strategies for reinforcing the change process.

Management strategies that are key to smooth implementation include: staff participation in decisions regarding implementation, providing training and coaching for new staff roles; being empathetic to problems of change; rewarding and recognizing performance; communicating openly and clearly with all affected through memos and newsletters; committing sufficient resources; continuing demonstration of top management support for the innovation; and using cross-disciplinary teams. The manager needs to monitor the implementation process, getting feedback from staff as to what is working well and what is not, whether the outcomes are those that were intended, and what technical assistance for staff and modifications in the program are needed for successful implementation.

Institutionalization

Institutionalization can be considered as "freezing" the change within the organization. It assures that the new program or policy will become part of routine organizational operations and will survive beyond the initial program implementation, across budget cycles and turnover of staff. Steckler and colleagues (1992) have identified a number of indicators of institutionalization, including written goals and objectives, written plans, formal program evaluations, presence of permanent staff, permanent space, a stable source of funding, written job descriptions and formal supervision.

Case Study: Change in a Voluntary Health Agency

One of the authors, as leader of a multi-organizational team had the opportunity to work with the state office of a voluntary health agency—the American Cancer Society Texas Division—as an external change agent promoting the development of a worksite health promotion program to be offered by the agency across the state. When the relationship was initiated, the author's research group at the University of Texas in collaboration with the health fitness program at Tenneco, Inc., had already developed some model worksite cancer control materials with funding by the Texas Cancer Council. However, funding for the production and dissemination of the materials had not been obtained.

Initial Assessment

The assessment process in this case study was directed first to understanding the needs of worksites in Texas for cancer prevention and control and second to the problem of disseminating the educational materials. It was later in the process that the analysis of the need for organizational change in the delivery organization was carried out.

Preinitiation of Organizational Change

The university/Tenneco team introduced the idea of providing the educational materials to the ACS for dissemination. The ACS was interested. However, at that point in time, the public education director of the ACS believed the critical need was to establish a process for building the capacity of Texas worksites to offer health promotion programs, including those in cancer prevention and control, rather than simply providing worksites with new cancer risk reduction materials. After some negotiation between the two groups, the concept of "Top Priority," a team approach to worksite health promotion, was born. It required a completely different set of supporting materials and processes built around *The Team Leaders' Guide to Health Promotion*, and only used a small portion of the curricular materials developed by the university. It was to be conducted as a collaborative effort between the University of Texas, the ACS, and Tenneco, Inc., with external funding from the Texas Cancer Council.

Initiation

It was now time for the public education director to "sell" the concept within the organization, to the volunteer worksite committee, and to top management. There were several important policy concepts that had to be sold. This would mark the first time that the Texas ACS as an organization had engaged in collaborative program development. The program was a process, not a risk-factor reduction educational product; it was comprehensive and not specific to cancer control. The program required that worksite representatives from companies and agencies all across Texas be trained by the ACS to establish worksite health promotion teams. This involved a major redirection of ACS program staff and internal resources to worksite health promotion.

The program director had strong legitimacy and credibility within and outside the organization. He had been with the organization for over three decades, had established the strong, grassroots community-organization philosophy of programming within the division, and had many ties with both state and national health agencies. He promoted the idea across the ACS organization, linking it to fund-raising opportunities and community leadership development. During the preinitiation period, there was a turnover in the organization's CEO; and the new CEO, who was promoted from within, was supportive of the concept. At a formal meeting of the agency's Employee Education Subcommittee of the Public Education Committee, the university team was invited to present the findings of a statewide survey they had conducted that showed that only 6 percent of worksites were providing cancer education or screening. The plan for the university, Tenneco, and ACS collaboration was brought forward. The volunteers were enthusiastic, especially as one of their committee members, a nurse from Tenneco, had been involved in the development of the initial educational materials by the university. The decision to do the program and to collaborate was approved by the Employee Education Subcommittee and moved up through the official channels of the ACS structure and was approved by the Board of Directors. At this point the program had been adopted.

The ACS conducted a roundtable conference with staff and key industries from their area to explore the experience with, need for, and benefits of worksite health promotion programs. New materials were developed, including the *Team Leaders' Guide* and a series of training manuals, agendas, and presentation materials for staff and volunteers to conduct training across the state. Program staff for the six metropolitan offices in the state were brought into the process early on, as they would be responsible for identifying participants, organizing Team Leader Forums—four-hour seminars on developing worksite health promotion teams—and for organizing community resource exchange network meetings quarterly thereafter in each of their cities. Figure 12.4 shows the overview of the project activities. To initiate the program, a statewide training session on "Top Priority" for 24 lead companies, area education staff, and volunteers was sponsored by the division. Following the metropolitan Team

Figure 12.4 Overview of the Organizational Units for "Top Priority" Programming

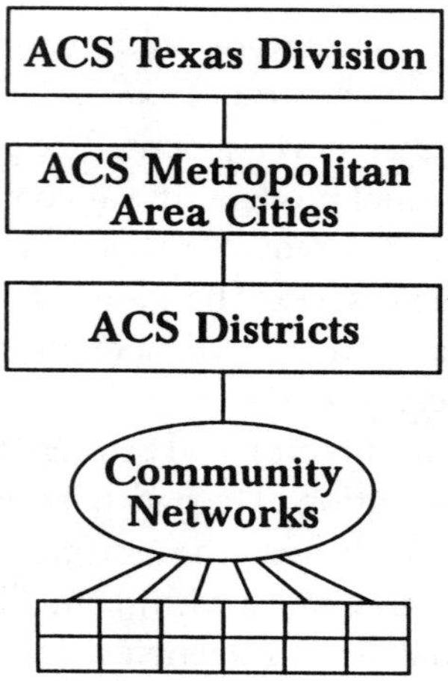

Leader Forums during the first year, trainings were to be held through field offices that served smaller cities and towns in the state, under the responsibility of the metropolitan program staff and the field staff responsible for the ACS organization in the districts where the towns were located.

Implementation

Issues of implementation then came to the fore. Figure 12.5 is a force field analysis for implementing "Top Priority" within the ACS. Driving forces included the commitment and enthusiasm of the public education director, of key volunteers at both the state level and in several of the regions, and several of the metropolitan area program staff. The *Team Leaders' Guide* was viewed as an excellent resource, and participants were highly satisfied with the materials and the training forums. The university was responsive to feedback, and the materials were improved and revised during the early phase of the project.

A significant restraining force grew from the authority structure of the organization (see figure 12.6 for the organizational chart). Note that the division's director of public education does not directly supervise the area public education directors. Information about the program was communicated through public education staff meetings, memoranda, and telephone calls. Resources had not been adequately allocated for formal staff training; each area education director visited a team leader forum in another region prior to organizing the one in his or her city. Informal communication, thus, became very important.

Figure 12.5

Driving Forces	Restraining Forces
• Division program director's leadership	• Lines of authority in program area
• Close informal relationships	• Need for fund raising
• Enthusiasm of staff	• Lack of training resources
• Key volunteer enthusiasm	• Continuous revision of materials
• University consultant input	• Not local staff's idea
• Excellent materials	• Lack of volunteers
• External funding for materials development and evaluation	• Staff already had full roles
	• Downsizing in target companies

Force field analysis for implementation of the "Top Priority" program within the ACS.

Fund-raising needs occupied staff attention and became a strong restraining force during this period, as the poor economy had diminished contributions. This diverted the energies of the field staff, as they were responsible for all aspects of the ACS cancer-control efforts in their district. Each staff had about 8–10 counties to cover. While we have noted the enthusiasm of many staff and volunteers, others did not see the benefits of the program, were new staff, had competing priorities, and/or had poor volunteer leadership in some of the units for which they were responsible. In these cases, staff did not provide as much support to the program effort. Many companies were downsizing the number of employees during this period and were perceived by staff as unready to begin a new initiative such as "Top Priority." The university's evaluation activities and program revisions were also viewed by some as a barrier that interfered with effective implementation.

As implementation progressed, the university and ACS partners tried to decrease the strength of the restraining forces. The revisions on the materials were completed. The evaluation was streamlined, requiring less time for program participants, and integrated more fully into training activities. Field staff were asked to do as little as provide the room for the training session and a list of companies to be invited. They were encouraged to do more, if they wished and were able. The area education directors assumed the administrative responsibility for organizing the forums. To support the activities in the second year, a core group of ACS volunteers were recruited and trained to present the programs and facilitate the community resource exchange networks. At the same time, the driving forces were strengthened. As the "Top Priority" training sessions and network meetings proved to be successful in most sites, staff and volunteers

Figure 12.6 ACS, Texas Division Staff Organization

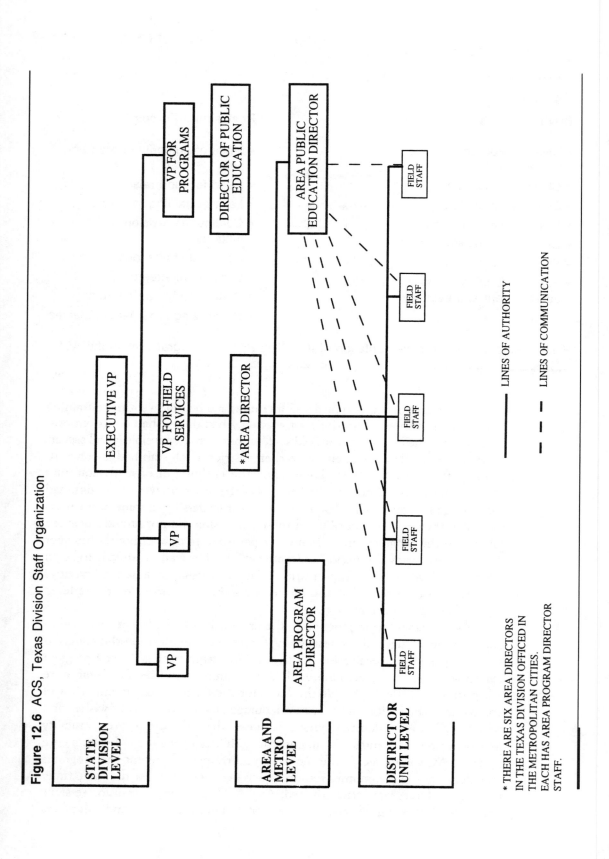

STATE
DIVISION
LEVEL

AREA AND
METRO
LEVEL

DISTRICT OR
UNIT LEVEL

EXECUTIVE VP

VP FOR PROGRAMS

DIRECTOR OF PUBLIC EDUCATION

VP FOR FIELD SERVICES

*AREA DIRECTOR

AREA PUBLIC EDUCATION DIRECTOR

VP

VP

AREA PROGRAM DIRECTOR

FIELD STAFF

FIELD STAFF

FIELD STAFF

FIELD STAFF

FIELD STAFF

——— LINES OF AUTHORITY

– – – LINES OF COMMUNICATION

* THERE ARE SIX AREA DIRECTORS
IN THE TEXAS DIVISION OFFICED IN
THE METROPOLITAN CITIES.
EACH HAS AREA PROGRAM DIRECTOR
STAFF.

became more committed and enthusiastic. During the first two years, 517 worksites were trained in six metropolitan areas and 18 towns.

Institutionalization

"Top Priority" has continued to flourish and appears to have been successfully institutionalized. The division public education director was promoted. His replacement has expanded the program to include Team Leader Forums at the statewide comprehensive school health conference and in jointly sponsored "Top Priority" training programs with the occupational nurses association. Area education staffs have had turnover, and, in each case, the new staff has carried out the program activities. Worksite health promotion through the "Top Priority" program was included in the division's strategic plan, which was written following a reorganization around key cancer control priorities. Funding for the program has been included as part of the program budget, and a grant to extend the program to high risk populations has been received from the national ACS. Process evaluation of the program tracks the number and types of worksites represented at training as well as the resource exchange networks and participant satisfaction with program activities.

This case study has provided a real-life example of a health educator working as an external change agent and the initiation, implementation, and institutionalization of a new program within the American Cancer Society Texas Division to establish worksite cancer control education in Texas. There was mutual adaptation between the university and the voluntary agency during the initial stages of change, molding the program to be adopted. Then, the ACS program director became the champion for the "Top Priority" program and the internal change agent for its adoption and implementation. A force field analysis of implementation showed restraining forces that the university and state ACS staff worked to reduce and driving forces that promoted the full implementation of the program. Institutionalization of the program occurred, as the program continued across changes in staff, strategic plans, and budgets, indicating that the change process was complete.

Summary

Health educators act as organizational change agents to change policies and procedures and to get organizations to adopt and implement health promotion programs. They may be internal change agents within their organization, or external change agents acting on other organizations. Organizational structure and culture provide both the context and target for organizational change. The change process occurs in five stages: initial assessment, preinitiation, initiation, implementation, and institutionalization. Strategies to be used at each stage were discussed in the chapter, and a case study illustrating the change process was presented.

Community and Social Change

To get the bad customs of a country changed and new ones, though better, introduced, it is necessary first to remove the prejudices of the people, enlighten their ignorance, and convince them that their interests will be promoted by the proposed changes; and this is not the work of a day.

—Benjamin Franklin, 1781

Introduction

Social change is the process by which alteration occurs in the structure and function of social systems (Rogers, 1983). Political decisions, technological and organizational innovations, and new ways of thinking about things all bring about social changes that can have profound effects on health. Social Security, Medicare, and current health care reforms are examples of political actions important to health. The advent of automobiles and the development of antibiotics and anesthesia are examples of technological changes with great health impacts. Recent changes in thinking about the rights and status of women, homosexuals, and racial minority groups are other examples of social change. Not all social change, however, occurs at such highly visible levels. Some social change is the product of small groups of people meeting to increase their understanding of important issues, organizing to make better use of existing resources, or acting to alter a policy or practice or redirect public resources.

In health education commonly we are more concerned with changes in particular health behaviors than with the widespread changes in society. Sometimes we are interested in diffusing an important health-related attitude (the use of condoms makes sex safe and enjoyable), behavior (always using a condom during sexual intercourse), practice (making condoms available through school health services), or policy (confidentiality of adolescent users of family planning services). Often social conditions cause the health problems and unhealthful behaviors of concern, and consequently, the social forces themselves become the targets of change. Logically, if the social and political environments contribute to illness, then they can also be made to contribute to health. The process by which this can be accomplished is social change.

Consider the following examples of social change activities:

- The National High Blood Pressure Education Program and National Cholesterol Education Program include continuing education to health professionals and national media campaigns directed at the public to increase awareness and improve detection of heart disease risk factors and treatment of heart disease in the population.

- In a Colorado school district concerned parents and teachers worked for years to get health education fully integrated into the kindergarten through twelfth-grade curriculum.
- Peace Corps volunteers are trained as change agents to develop community resources and provide health services and health education to villagers in developing countries.
- In San Francisco health educators organized impoverished elderly residents into support groups to work together for healthful changes in their housing and community.
- Policy advocates have been working at local, state, and federal levels for the adoption of policies and legislation restricting tobacco and alcohol sales and use.
- Media advocates have gradually been altering the way the press understands, interprets, and reports violent crime, HIV infection, drunk driving, and other health-related topics.
- In eastern Finland residents of a community are working with government officials to organize community resources to reduce the risk of cardiovascular disease in the population.

Each of these vignettes provides a different example of a social change strategy in action. In the following pages the authors describe the general characteristics of planned social change and the targets for social change activities. Some of the various strategies employed by health educators acting as change agents to facilitate social change are then examined.

The Process of Social Change

Social change is hardly a new concept. Indeed, the process of social change is at the very heart of democracy. It is one of the ways the citizens of a political entity force change. Some of the social change concepts most relevant to health education and health promotion grew out of the heightened political consciousness of social activities during the 1960s and 1970s among social workers, political scientists, and social activists. Social change is partly about changing the social environment, the social institutions, policies, and practices such that they are health promoting rather than health damaging. But social change also is about personal awareness, attitudes, and behavior. According to Zaltman and Duncan (1977), "a person changes his or her behavior when they define the situation as being different and now requiring different behavior."

In this chapter we are concerned with how health educators facilitate this process of individuals and groups redefining their situations and acting on the resulting new ways of thinking. The unique feature of social change processes is the emphasis on altering social norms and social conditions. In social change approaches to altering health behavior, individuals and groups can be either the vehicles of social change, as when they organize into self-help groups, or the targets of social change, as when national programs seek to influence general health knowledge, perceptions, attitudes, or behavior.

Before proceeding to describe the approaches to social change, the following characteristics of social change programs deserve mention: (1) planned versus unplanned change; (2) level of change; (3) top-down versus bottom-up change; and (4) change agent functions.

Planned Versus Unplanned Change

Change can be planned or unplanned. Planned change is the product of deliberate efforts to bring about well-defined changes. The intended impact of planning on change is to hasten its initiation, increase the speed of its diffusion, and broaden the number of people involved. Social change occurs on a continuum from unplanned to planned, and the change process can move along this continuum. For example, the civil rights and anti-Vietnam war movements initially were spontaneous social protest movements which later became highly organized and planned. In contrast to the shift in consumer preferences for processed versus fresh foods, which was a highly planned social change orchestrated by food conglomerates, the countermovement toward organic foods has been largely an unplanned social movement. In general, changes in society like the ones just mentioned become more organized once they become sufficiently popular or successful enough to gain the attention of change agents or institutions that begin to provide support for them.

Many social changes have come about inadvertently. Technological advances in transportation and communications have caused dramatic social changes in recent decades. It is now possible to commute to work from home as far as 50 miles each way. At the same time, computers have enabled many individuals to work efficiently from their home offices or at remote sites close to home (a process called **telecommuting**). Computers have created new forms of communication and have increased the speed with which people can be connected to new ideas and events. But computers have also contributed to some negative trends. Computer games have become increasingly graphic and realistic in their portrayal of violence, reinforcing trends in movies and the daily reality of communities infested with weapons and drugs. The unprecedented level of violence in our communities and schools was an unplanned social change. It is not something that any sane person wants, but has resulted from an unfortunate coming together of social and technological events. Current efforts on the part of politicians, police, social workers, and public health activists to restrict weapons and reduce crime and violence is an example of planned social change.

Level of Change

Change occurs at individual, group, organizational, and societal levels. The forces of change at these various levels interact and reinforce each other so that most change occurs simultaneously at all levels.

Change in health knowledge, attitudes, and behavior of individuals have been discussed extensively in this text and need no further explanation here, except to note that individual change occurs within a social context. Indeed, from a social change perspective, the individual is never divorced from his or her social environment and individual-level change is considered largely to be a function of changes in social norms and social conditions.

Group-level change is primarily concerned with normative beliefs, values, and behaviors. The basic units at this level are families, organizations, and naturally occurring community groups. Families have a tremendous influence on their members. Many health behaviors are highly resistant to change without the active participation of key family members. Families and family members belong to groups such as the PTA, organizations such as churches and businesses, and institutions such as schools. Sometimes it is the group rather than its individual members that is the target for social change. Organizational change focuses on work policies, practices, and programs.

Interrelated families, groups, organizations, and institutions make up communities. Communities can be identified by the residents' values, traditions, socioeconomic class, race, ethnicity, geography, and interests. Individuals may belong to several communities simultaneously. For example, health educators see themselves as members of the professional communities of education and health professionals, as well as members of their neighborhoods.

Changes at the societal level cut across and include the many communities that make up a region, a state, or a nation. This level of change is brought about only by major and pervasive influences. Federal health legislation and programs, profound technological innovations (such as immunizations), educational innovations (such as comprehensive K-12 health education), and massive grassroots movements (such as the civil rights, women's liberation, and nuclear freeze movements) are examples.

Top-down Versus Bottom-up Change

Social change can be stimulated or organized from the top-down (imposed by those in power) or the bottom-up (stimulated within social groups). In terms of health, grassroots movements to gain control over resources, power, or decision making are typically bottom-up efforts; for example, self-help groups and health care advocacy groups. Organizational or governmental efforts to get people to adopt certain actions or habits are typically top-down. One example of a planned, top-down approach is the decades-old effort by the tobacco industry to make smoking acceptable and normative. Until recently, most efforts to protect the rights of nonsmokers were bottom-up. Now, tobacco control policies are being advocated and institutionalized by government and worksite policy and practice changes. Attempts to encourage screening for high blood pressure has been both top-down governmental or institutional imposition, pharmaceutical company self-interest, and bottom-up community involvement to combat the silent killer.

The Health Educator As Change Agent

The role of the health educator in social change programs is best described as a change agent. A change agent is an individual "operating to change the status quo in a system such that the individual or individuals involved must relearn how to perform their roles" (Zaltman and Duncan, 1977). A change agent is "an individual who influences clients' innovation decision in a direction deemed desirable by a change agency" (Rogers, 1983). According to Freudenberg (1984), to be effective change agents, health educators need to focus on the environmental causes of health problems, on social change methods, and on populations most in need of help.

Change agents can be internal to the system, organization, or social group that is being targeted, or external to that group, serving in a capacity similar to a consultant. Internal change agents have the advantage of being part of the system and knowing how things work. They have the disadvantage of being a part of a system on which they are dependent. External change agents, although lacking insight about the particular system in question, may have experience from working with many other systems. External change agents also have the advantage of being more or less independent of the system and therefore, more objective.

The task of a change agent is to create, stimulate, and/or facilitate change. Rogers (1983) describes seven functions of change agents in the process of planned change:

1. Develops a need for change
2. Establishes an information-exchange relationship
3. Diagnoses problems
4. Creates the client's intent to change
5. Translates intent into action
6. Stabilizes adoption and prevents discontinuance
7. Achieves a terminal relationship

These functions are familiar to health educators who serve as consultants because the role of the change agent is very similar to that of a consultant. However, while consultants are generally impartial, somewhat passive experts, change agents tend to be highly committed and involved. In practice, change agents tend to be idealistic and activist.

Health educators serving as change agents function actively in institutional and informal settings, facilitating change that is system dependent. This could mean working to introduce a drop-in center on a high school campus, removing barriers to health services access in an inner city area, setting up a self-care organization in a rural community, developing smoking control or gun control policies, or promoting AIDS awareness.

Based on a practical understanding of the process, Rogers (1983) suggests that certain actions may influence the extent to which a change agent's actions may be successful.

Client Orientation

Essentially, a change agent is more effective when oriented more toward the target population than the change agency. The change agent can be effective only if the target population deems her or him credible and trustworthy. Therefore, the change agent must adapt to the needs of the target population, sometimes even to the disadvantage of the change agency. Success may depend on the extent to which the health educator can disregard the expectations of the change bureaucracy in favor of those held by the clients. In organizational settings and in top-down community situations, the agent works for the change agency which may be the funding source (for example, the federal government) or a third party (for example, a local university). Because change agents are intermediaries, or communication links between clients and change agencies, they often suffer from role conflict.

Number and Variety of Contacts

Success is encouraged when a change agent has a large number and variety of contacts with clients. Because people who are alike (homophilic) tend to communicate more often with each other than do those who are not alike (heterophilic), most change agents tend to have greater contact with the small percentage of clients who are more innovative, of higher social class, and are more educated than the rest—in short, more like the change agent. Therefore, change agents are often guilty of elitist bias. Communication is not only less frequent but also less effective when a low degree of homophily is present, unless the source has a high degree of empathy with the receiver. Still, the greatest asset of the change agent is his or her ability to communicate with clients. Consequently, one important focus of education for change agents is empathy training, which is designed to help them understand the perspectives and values of the client. Empathy training includes values clarification exercises, role playing, and directed contact with diverse groups of people in fieldwork activities.

Because the change agent is often heterophilic with the clients, paraprofessional aids or peer leaders are often recruited and trained to provide the needed client contact. Peer leaders have the advantage of being drawn from the target population and therefore may be more credible than professional health educators. Numerous programs have demonstrated that it is possible to train peer leaders, even uneducated community workers, so that they can successfully conduct many of the functions of the change agent.

Client Involvement

Change agent success may depend on the extent to which the clients are involved in planning the change process. Involving clients both (1) encourages a sense of commitment to the project; and (2) provides valuable insight into how the project should be developed.

Client Education

One of the important tasks of the change agent is to educate the client in how to evaluate the success of the innovation. Unrealistic expectations on the part of the client can lead to frustration and discontinuance. Clients, however, can be taught to make accurate assessments of interim progress and to identify markers of success, thus allowing sufficient period of trial.

Marketing

The change agent looks for ways to present the innovation such that it fits the clients' cultural beliefs and values and markets it accordingly.

There are numerous examples of health educators serving as change agents in the United States. The effort of Minkler and Cox (1980) in training health educators to work with destitute elderly in the Tenderloin area of San Francisco is notable. In developing nations, change agents are ubiquitous because foreign aid tends to include money for programs for social change, especially in health care and health education. Foreign service professionals and Peace Corps volunteers usually are the designated agents to carry out these programs.

The Diffusion of Innovations

An innovation is a new or novel idea, attitude, behavior, policy, practice, or program. At the outset these novel, or novel-appearing, practices are not always recognized or perceived as being necessary, important, or even useful. As the innovation is introduced people learn about it, many try it, and some adopt it. Examples of recent innovations in health behavior include exercising, low-fat diets, automobile safety belt use, and responsible drinking. None of these behaviors is truly new but they at least represent a reconsidered or reorganized response to health and social problems.

As noted, innovation also occurs at other societal levels. Recent examples include the adoption by worksites of no-smoking policies, statewide restrictions on handguns, and federal requirements mandating the installation of air bags and anti-lock brakes on new automobiles.

Since a great deal of social change can be conceived of in terms of the adoption of innovations, the literature on the diffusion of such innovations is important to our discussion of social change. Theoretically the progressive adoption of an innovation by members of a community or society can be understood in terms of the cumulative diffusion curve shown in figure 13.1. According to this conceptualization, the adoption of an innovation begins very slowly as a few people or groups try it. Gradually the number of adopters grows until the number of people left who are likely or available to adopt the innovation has diminished. The diffusion curve, reflecting the number of new adopters, then begins to decline and gradually flattens.

Figure 13.1

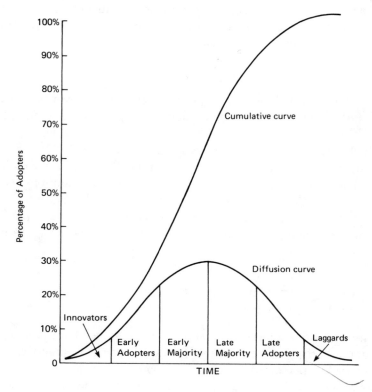

The cumulative adoption curve represents the rate of eventual adoption, while the bell-shaped curve indicates the categories of adopters.

Hypothetically, all of the eventual adopters of an innovation can be classified according to certain characteristics and earliness or lateness in adopting the innovation. The completed pattern forms a normal curve, and if you plotted the diffusion of many innovations on a graph, the resulting curve probably would approximate this curve, although the pattern of adoption of any one innovation may be irregular.

Taking a specific example, suppose you were interested in organizing self-help groups for parents of children with terminal illnesses. This can be perceived of as a novel or innovative response to an acknowledged health and social problem. At a local level, for example at a hospital, the total population available to adopt this innovation would consist of the parents of terminally ill children treated at the hospital over a period of time. Not all of the eligible people would be likely to join or help form a self-help group. The cumulative curve for the adoption of this innovation would indicate the rate at which adoption occurred. For any group of people, some would adopt this innovation soon after learning about it, while others would delay. Still others might never adopt the innovation and would not be reflected in the diffusion curves, which include only adopters. The number of people who eventually participate in such a group, and the rate of adoption among this eligible population, could be recorded to create a diffusion curve. The same process holds if your concerns were national in scope, although the pool of eligible people would be much larger. Another difference is that you might deal mainly with the adoption by hospitals of the innovation, rather than with individual parents.

The health educator working as a change agent seeks to decrease the length of time it takes for an innovation to be diffused and increase the proportion of people or groups who adopt the innovation. In general, the literature on the diffusion of innovations suggests that the extent and distribution of adoption of an innovation depends upon (1) the characteristics of the target population, (2) the characteristics of the innovation or change itself, and (3) the stages of adoption. Each of these three areas must be taken into account by the change agent in developing a plan for facilitating adoption.

Characteristics of the Target Population

The diffusion of an innovation is the progressive adoption by members of a community or society of an idea or practice over time (Zaltman and Duncan, 1977). Accordingly, a successful innovation is likely to be adopted first by innovators and early adopters, then by the majority, and finally by the late adopters and the laggards (see figure 13.1).

Innovators tend to be rather independent, change-oriented, risk-taking individuals. Innovators tend to be venturesome, eager to try new ideas. They are not necessarily the most respected people in a community and they tend to communicate mainly with other innovators and not with a broad cross-section of people. They are important to the diffusion process because they seek information on their own, rely on their own judgement in making decisions about adoption, and are risk oriented. They try out new ideas and provide the first tests of the utility of the innovation.

Early adopters tend to be respected members of the community and opinion leaders, exerting powerful influences on other potential adopters of the innovation. Generally, early adopters have relatively high socioeconomic status within their local organizations or communities, tend to have complex communication networks, and like to be up on what is new and good, but do not like to be too far out in their behavior. They are trendy, but not innovators. These opinion leaders are often sought out by change agents eager to learn how an innovation might be received and how it could be presented to others in ways that would make it acceptable.

Early majority are influenced greatly by opinion leaders and mass media, and over time begin to adopt the innovation. By virtue of their numbers they begin to form a new norm with respect to the innovation. These individuals tend to have frequent contact with their peers but do not hold leadership positions. They are deliberate but willing. By virtue of their social contacts they are the connection between early and late adopters. Many people will adopt a successful innovation only after the early adopters have done so, indicating that it is an acceptable and worthwhile practice.

Late majority are skeptical of change and tend to wait until the innovation is established as the norm before eventually adopting it, by which time it has become a social or economic necessity. They can be persuaded that a new idea is a good one, but their motivation is influenced greatly by their peers. Given their modest resources, they are adverse to risk and tend to prefer that uncertainty about the relative advantages of an innovation be reduced.

Laggards tend to be traditional and conservative, be of relatively lower socioeconomic status, have less education, be socially or geographically mobile, and have narrow and restricted communication networks. They are suspicious of innovations and adverse to risk. They may not adopt an innovation until very late, even when it is obvious to most people that adoption would be advantageous.

This is a general description of any population in diffusion terms. Innovators tend to be ahead of their time, but are not that influential with other people. Early adopters are among the first to adopt the innovation and because of their extensive communication networks and high status, they are highly influential with other people. **Opinion leaders**, whether early adopters or early majority, are highly influential within their spheres of influence, which may be as small as a family or a much larger social unit, for example a neighborhood, a worksite, or a trade union. Opinion leaders set the trends by their adoption of innovations because their attitudes and behaviors are seen by many other people as appropriate, acceptable, and desirable. Thus they serve as role models and norm setters. Consequently, the rest of the early majority and then the late majority begin to adopt. These groups are characteristically influenced by their perceptions of the normative patterns. Finally, the late adopters begin to get in on the action. These classifications tend to be remarkably consistent when one considers a large number of innovations. Therefore, they provide a useful framework for understanding the characteristics of the target population of all kinds of innovations.

In order to illustrate how an innovation might be diffused in society, consider a hypothetical example concerning responsible drinking behavior. Innovators would figure out on their own that driving after drinking is unacceptably risky and would be among the first to identify and adopt responsible drinking practices. They may decide not to drink at all or at least not in situations where driving might be involved. As college students they may have experimented with designated drivers and other responsible drinking behavior. As adults they may continue to innovate in this area and generate new ideas about responsible drinking, but their efforts are not generally influential and they do not necessarily become part of organized efforts to promote responsible drinking.

As information about drinking and driving becomes generally available in the popular press, increasing numbers of people become aware of the findings. Ideas pioneered by innovators become more generally known and some of them are adopted by the early adopters. These individuals assume the new behaviors, limiting themselves to not more than two drinks at a time, establishing a designated driver, switching to nonalcoholic beverages as easily as they change clothing styles. As opinion leaders these early adopters have frequent contacts with a variety of people and during these contacts they model and discuss their responsible drinking behavior. Their adoption of responsible drinking behaviors is noticed and gradually becomes established as or perceived as the acceptable or preferred behavior. The early majority are impressed with the behavior of the opinion leaders and begin to adopt similar behavior.

The adoption of responsible drinking practices by the early adopters indicates that the potential for change is substantial and parallels new information about the extent of the problem and innovations to prevent these problems. Government and private institutions begin to support planned informational and programmatic efforts to diffuse the concepts of designated drivers, responsible hosts, and roadside screening, leading to social pressures favoring responsible drinking behavior, particularly among the early majority. At this point in the diffusion curve, organizations such as Mothers Against Drunk Drivers (MADD) become viable and accelerate the rate of adoption.

The late majority, ever vigilant of what their friends and others are doing but slow to change, begin now to adopt some responsible drinking practices. At this point many forces begin to amass. A social change has been set in motion. Policies restricting alcohol sales and legal penalties for drinking and driving are put in place making responsible drinking a mandatory innovation rather than an elective one. Several health education demonstration programs to discourage drinking and driving show substantial success. Education about responsible drinking becomes part of health education programs in schools, communities, and hospitals. On the defensive, alcohol manufacturers take the high road and begin to market nonalcoholic beverages and create advertisements supporting responsible drinking practices.

Gradually the late adopters begin to adopt the practice. As the beneficial effects of the innovation become apparent, special community-based programs are established. The message is everywhere—posters in health clinics, advertisements on television, and articles in newspapers and popular magazines. Eventually, the laggards find themselves out of step with the new widespread practice so they too adopt responsible drinking practices.

This example illustrates the interdependence of multiple levels of change. Responsible drinking is not really one innovation, but many innovations, some of which are appropriate for individuals and groups (attitudes about appropriate drinking behavior), others for organizations and institutions (responsible drinking programs). As new information about responsible drinking becomes more available, social norms are shaped, which in turn influence public policy. Of course this illustration is simplistic. Complex behaviors do not change readily or consistently. Also, it is unclear how many years or decades it takes for an important innovation or set of innovations, like responsible drinking, to become a generally accepted practice. However, the general illustration provides a useful description of an idealized diffusion process.

The Stages of Adoption

The adoption of an innovation is thought to occur in stages similar to the stages of change discussed in chapter 10. Eventual adopters pass through the stages of (1) awareness, (2) interest, (3) trial, (4) decision, and (5) adoption. Theoretically, the process of adoption of any innovation is the same for all adopters, early or late. Early adopters may be reached via different channels, messages, or processes than late adopters, but they probably go through the same decision-making steps.

Awareness

Awareness of the existence of an innovation and its relative advantages is the first stage in the adoption process. The extent to which a target population is aware of an innovation can be increased through simple communications that effectively penetrate the market. A pregnant woman may become aware of breast-feeding from being around mothers with infants, from informational campaigns, or from medical providers. When this awareness has positive associations it is likely to stimulate interest in the innovation.

Interest

Interest does not necessarily result from awareness. A pregnant woman can be aware that breast-feeding is an option, but not have any personal interest in it. It is personal interest in the innovation that is important here—not abstract, academic interest. Personal interest is stimulated by information about the relative advantages from credible sources and observation of the innovation by relevant role models. Interest in breast-feeding must occur before birth or it is unlikely to be adopted.

Trial

The next stage of adoption is trial. The characteristics of the innovation are important determinants of trial because the cost of trying some innovations is greater than for others. Trial is very important because the adopter will learn from the experience. How-to knowledge that increases efficacy and leads to a positive trial is important to the next stage of adoption. For the mother of a newborn, there is a narrow window of opportunity to try breast-feeding before it becomes impossible. Hence, it is important for interventions to encourage trial immediately after birth.

Decision

Based on experience from the trial, including how other people react to the adoption of the innovation, the adopter decides to continue, quit, or re-create the innovation. Breast-feeding is not natural and easy for all women. Many women have difficulty at first or find it uncomfortable or inconvenient. Such experiences in the absence of supportive intervention are likely to lead to a decision to quit.

Adoption

Adoption here refers to continuation or integration of the innovation into one's life-style. In the case of breast-feeding, such a decision has many implications not only for the health of the baby but also for the life-style of the mother and her family. Problem-solving skills and environmental support may be important for continuation.

Understanding the stages of adoption may enable health educators to develop effective methods and to fine-tune the timing of the implementation. The more the health educator knows about the characteristics of the target population and its stage of adoption, the better he or she is able to intervene.

Characteristics of the Innovation or Change

The rate and extent of adoption of any innovation is a product not only of characteristics of the adopters but also of characteristics of the change itself. Obviously, some innovations are very simple, while others are very complex.

Relative Advantage

Any change must compete in the marketplace of ideas and behaviors. Innovations that have important advantages over current practice or competing innovations will be adopted by more people. Of course, the relative advantages of an innovation are not always apparent immediately. Indeed, the advantages of some innovations become apparent only after a period of use, as in the case of diet or exercise. Therefore, it is not just a matter of the relative advantages of the innovation, but also a question of the perceived relative advantages of the innovation. Perceived advantages of an innovation that has not yet been tried may be different from the perceived advantages after it has been tried. Therefore, separate intervention strategies often are developed to encourage trial and to foster continuance. Some innovations appear advantageous at the outset, but less so in practice, while other innovations do not appear to be so advantageous until they are tried.

Returning to our earlier example, responsible drinking behavior must compete with social and market forces favoring the current standards of drinking behavior, which generally are not responsible. Let's take the case of a single responsible behavior, that of the designated driver. A potential adopter of this innovation may have a variety of opportunities to evaluate its relative advantages. At the awareness stage some information about the innovation may be shared. For example, a waiter at area drinking establishments frequented by young adults may introduce the availability of free soft drinks for the designated driver when he takes the drink orders. Other information about the program in the form of signs or leaflets may also be available in the establishment to increase awareness of the program and emphasize its relative advantages.

Impact on Social Relations

Many attitudes and behaviors are socially mediated, meaning that the perceptions and actions of other people are critical to their adoption. The designated driver program may provide additional status for a group member who does not really care about drinking that much, but likes to be with the group. It also may appear advantageous to members of the group who like to drink but do not like driving home afterward. Of course, this same program may be perceived by some groups as disadvantageous for a number of reasons. Needs assessments of the perceived impact of adopting the innovation on social relations among the variety of targeted groups would be useful for developing interventions to increase the rate of adoption of the innovation.

Divisibility and Reversibility

Divisibility is the extent to which a change can be tried on a limited scale. Highly divisible actions are easier to try. In our example, the designated driver concept can be tried one time and then discontinued. However, it is not infinitely divisible because it only works if the designated driver abstains totally from drinking and remains available to drive the members of the party home. Similarly, being a designated driver is reversible in that one person would not always have to be the designated driver. However, it may not be entirely reversible in that a person could quickly become labeled or known as the designated driver, making it difficult to escape from this role and responsibility.

Complexity

The more complex to understand and use, the less likely the change will be adopted or even tried. Ideas that are difficult to understand are adopted very slowly. Complex ideas and behaviors are very difficult to introduce without great resistance. Simplifying the innovation becomes an important educational challenge. The more simply and clearly the designated driver program can be developed and described, the more likely it will be adopted.

Compatibility

There are psychological, social, and cultural factors to consider in analyzing the likelihood of change. Lifelong and culturally endemic habits do not change easily. The change agent must seek to link the innovation to existing cultural patterns or present it in a way compatible with how the learner would like to see himself or herself and with the values and beliefs of the social group. Hence, the success of a designated driver program may depend on the extent to which it can be made compatible with current attitudes and practices and the extent to which the target population perceives that the concept is compatible with its values.

Communicability

Frequently discussed practices, such as drinking, are likely to be given a quicker and fuller test by more people than practices that are difficult to communicate or less likely to be communicated.

Time

An idea that is introduced prematurely may not achieve great adoption because there is no supporting structure for it. In other words, it must be "an idea whose time has come." As H.G. Wells stated about his country in 1931: "In England we have come to rely on a comfortable time lag of fifty years or a century intervening between the perception that something ought to be done and a serious attempt to do it." In addition to needing fertile ground for a planted idea to grow, once that idea sprouts it takes some time for it to spread throughout the population. The spread of any change is uneven over time. In general the rate of future adoption can be predicted from the rate of adoption up to that point in time. The faster its adoption and more widespread a change becomes, the greater will be the number who finally adopt it. As adoption increases, the social, environmental, and political structures to support the innovation tend to increase. For example, media attention to the problem of drinking and driving, increased law enforcement efforts, plus evidence from successful designated driver programs, combine to encourage adoption.

Approaches to Social Change

Our discussion of diffusion provides a general perspective of how change occurs naturally and provides some ideas about how the extent and pace of diffusion might be increased by a change agent. In the following pages we address approaches to social change that can be employed to diffuse a health promotion innovation, whether it is a new social norm, health behavior, policy, or process.

In this chapter we have been discussing education for change primarily at the group and societal levels. The strategies useful for this kind of education differ from strategies commonly employed strictly for personal behavior change primarily in their focus on the structure and influence of social forces. Many theories and strategies discussed in previous chapters have applications within the broader context of strategies for social change. For example, principles of operant conditioning, knowledge and attitude change, and social learning are relevant (Parcel et al., 1989). Many of these principles and methods are integral to the broad educational approaches for social change described in the following pages: (1) empirical-rational education; (2) normative re-education; (3) community organizing; (4) media advocacy; (5) policy advocacy; and (6) social marketing. Principles of organizational change, described in chapter 12, also are relevant.

All approaches to planned change are primarily educational, but the target of education, the variables of interest, and the methods are unique. Education may be directed at increasing knowledge about the function of things, people, or systems. When attempting to introduce new information into a human system, we need to know how people come to adopt this innovation and how human systems might enable or discourage it. The task necessarily shifts from how to do this thing to how to overcome resistance to change by individuals and systems.

The educational approaches for social change are not completely discrete in that they overlap somewhat in terms of the role of the change agent, extent of external (top-down) pressure, educational methods, and in other ways.

Empirical-Rational Education

The goal of empirical-rational education is to introduce rationally justifiable proposals for change to people who will benefit from their adoption. Theoretically, a body of knowledge or set of skills exists that the learners, who theoretically are rational, want to know or be able to do because it serves their self-interest. The role of the change agent is to disseminate the information and teach the skills. Empirical-rational education is a universally accepted method

Figure 13.2

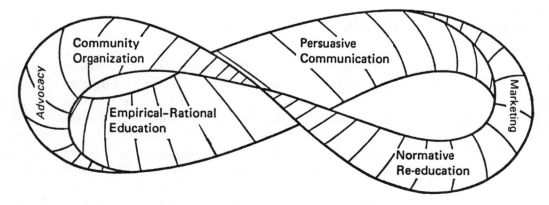

Six theoretical approaches to social change on a circular continuum (Mobius strip).

of implementing planned social change. Public school education is the greatest example of such an approach, and it is difficult to deny the importance of compulsory education as a normative influence. Indeed, formal education of all sorts, including training in public health and medicine, are based on this approach.

Theoretically, in the empirical-rational approach to education new information derived from research is synthesized and disseminated to the population by means of schools and other agencies. Students are exposed to this body of knowledge and develop the relevant skills. Self-interested individuals see the utility and value of the new information and put it to use in their lives.

Empirical-rational education is the process by which students are trained and professionals become prepared. Curricula, conferences, continuing education, and public information campaigns are all based on the principle that information and skills lead to informed decision making. In a democratic society it is the responsibility of the state to make new knowledge available to the public so that people can make knowledgeable choices. The empirical-rational approach is extremely important for introducing new knowledge and technology into society. One can hardly imagine a modern society not investing heavily in such education because of the tremendous flow of new information that is vital to the advancement of contemporary societies. For example, in the United States the federal government has the ability and the obligation to mobilize the nation's resources for health research in order to expand the knowledge base for prevention (USDHEW, 1990).

The traditional classroom teacher is a good example of an empirical-rational change agent. Lecture, Socratic dialogue, guided discovery, and demonstration are typical methods of imparting information from those who know (the teachers) to those who want or need to know (the learners). The learner is best conceptualized as a self-interested consumer of information. Empirical-rational education of this sort is common in many teaching, training, and counseling situations.

The development of a curriculum is the best evidence of empirical-rational education in practice. In such diverse areas as public school education, military training, higher education for health professionals, or on-the-job training, curricula are created to assure that the important information is identified for transmission to all the learners. In modern practice, curricula tend to be organized by goals, objectives, content, learning activities, and measurable outcomes.

In public schools the very existence of health education in the curriculum is a powerful legitimatizing force. Where health education content is subsumed under other subjects (such as physical education, science, humanities, and home economics), health education cannot be addressed in a comprehensive and consistent manner and the teachers are not necessarily trained to teach this material comfortably and capably. Even when a health education curriculum exists, the content that is included is very often controversial or the product of political or social pressures. For example, not too long ago it was difficult to introduce drug education into the school curriculum, but today it is a national priority and nearly every school district includes it in the curriculum.

While the empirical-rational system of education is the foundation of a modern society, there are limits to its effectiveness. One of the problems is there is a lot more information than there is time to teach it and the competition for curriculum time is fierce. In medical school, public health content must compete with anatomy, physiology, and clinical courses. In public education, health education must compete with science, math, physical education, and other courses. Relatedly, even when health education is included in the curriculum, it is effective only when it is taught well—and it is a difficult subject to teach because it is necessarily interactive. The content simply does not lend itself to straightforward lectures; the most effective approaches are interactive, involving the students in discussions, role plays, and practical learning activities.

Another problem is content changes, with new information being added and old information being replaced. For example, it has only been in the last twenty-five years that empirical studies have demonstrated the relationship between cigarette smoking and a host of health problems including cancer and cardiovascular disease. During this time schools and public health education programs have been instrumental in disseminating the information to the public in forms that are understandable and convincing. This process has been influential in encouraging many people to quit smoking, to not start, or to smoke less than they might otherwise. It has been a powerful influence on the knowledge and attitudes of the public about smoking. New studies about the dangers of smoking are constantly being published, while the tobacco industry produces a constant stream of information in an attempt to cast doubt about the dangers of smoking. Thus, it can be difficult for educators to remain current.

Empirical-rational approaches to education must also compete with other influences on health knowledge, particularly advertising, which often relies on counter-intuitive associations (e.g., smoking is glamorous, a new car will increase the owner's esteem, cleaner collars will make a spouse happy), rather than on the dissemination of logical information. The tobacco industry, for example, spends millions of dollars annually to promote smoking, mainly through appeals to non-rational motives. This type of advertising tends to dilute, distort, and overwhelm the influence of the empirical-rational education provided by schools and public health agencies.

Nevertheless, curricula are powerful socializing and professionalizing forces. Curricula standardize the content that is taught to the learners. The content selected (or omitted or deleted), the target population, and the teachers are aspects of empirical-rational education that are influenced by social and political pressures. The development of formal accreditation of academic departments of health education and the development of standards for the certification of health education practitioners are examples of rational empirical education. Of course, even with these accreditation and certification standards, within the profession of health education there is competition among those who would prefer to see the professional training of health educators emphasize programmatic skills, individual change methods, or social change (Freudenberg, 1984; McLeroy et al., 1993). By developing and implementing effective curriculum, professional training, continuing education, and standards of practice it is possible to affect substantial numbers of people, and therefore to diffuse this new learning.

Normative Re-Education

The goal of normative re-education (NR) is to raise consciousness, develop understanding about underlying causes, and identify strategies for action. Normative re-education is highly learner centered. The health educator or change agent may serve as advisor, counselor, critic, or facilitator. The learner identifies what he or she needs to know and, given the proper support, acts on this knowledge.

Normative re-education is so named because it is based on assumptions that learning is social (normative) and that learning new knowledge, attitudes, and behaviors requires unlearning old ones (re-education). The critical emphasis in these strategies is on the social character of learning. Theoretically, learning is influenced by social norms and values.

Normative re-education approaches to change invariably focus on engaging participants in a process of critical analysis of the causes of problems such that they can identify actions that can alter the situation. The role of the change agent is to facilitate the clients' efforts to understand the situation in which they find themselves and the dispositions required to alter it. The clients are active and critical participants in the process. They must identify the problem and develop plans for action. The focus is not on changing the behavior of the target population, but on increasing their understanding of the underlying causes of health and social problems, and facilitating the change process. The process of education is a dynamic exchange between educator and learner.

Because of the social nature of learning, groups are the logical units for normative re-education strategies. Naturally occurring social groups provide the best opportunities for these strategies. Groups can be influenced in a number of ways: (1) the composition of the group can be varied, (2) the content of the sessions can be altered, and (3) the process of the group can be modified.

Paulo Freire's education for critical consciousness (conscientizacion) provides an example of normative re-education. Freire advocates a very decentralized and learner-oriented approach to education. **Conscientizacion** involves the participants in a process which includes (1) reflection upon problems, (2) identification of root causes, (3) examination of the implications and consequences of the issues, and (4) development of a plan. This is accomplished primarily through a process of dialogue in small groups. The change agent has several unique roles in this process:

1. Tuning into the "vocabular universe" of the people through a process of participant observation. Minkler and Cox (1980) recommend living with the target population over an extended time period.

2. Working with small groups and key informants to identify key words and "generative themes" that suggest the hopes and concerns of the target population.

3. Synthesizing the ideas of the target population and codifying them in visual images and symbols.

4. Giving these symbols and images back to the people for decoding through "cultural circles," which are small groups of people who suggest solutions and the generative themes for programmatic use. (Minkler and Cox, 1980; Wallerstein and Bernstein, 1988)

A variety of health promotion programs have employed normative re-education theory and methods (Minkler and Cox, 1980; Wallerstein and Bernstein, 1988; Freudenberg and Golub, 1987). A general example of normative re-education comes out of the personal growth and human liberation movements. Consciousness-raising groups of all kinds are formed to enable people to cast off the restraints of their socializations. Successful consciousness-raising groups have been formed for ethnic minority groups, feminists, homosexuals, environmentalists, and peace activists, to name a few. Typically, groups meet on a regular basis to discuss the problems of being an oppressed minority in modern society. The sessions develop the members' confidence that the prejudice or persecution that they experience is not their fault. Further, the process emphasizes positive thinking, studying the history of oppressed minorities, developing coping strategies, and sometimes organizing to counteract wrongs. The groups provide a safe forum for the members to discuss their frustrations and their hopes for the future. Whether such sessions are organized and facilitated by professionals or trained laypersons, they provide a supporting atmosphere within which problems can be specified, underlying causes identified, and plans of action developed.

Community Organizing

Community organizing is the process by which community groups seek to achieve common goals. The goals of community organizing are to promote better use, organization, and availability of resources and to change the standards of acceptable behavior in a community by changing community norms about health behavior (Abrams et al., 1986). Hence, community organization approaches are useful in situations where material and human resources are poorly organized, inefficiently employed, or unevenly distributed among the population and where social norms fail to support health promoting behavior, practices, and policies. Community organization can be highly centralized as in many health planning efforts, or it can be decentralized as in the development of grassroots organizations and self-help groups. Social action and locality development approaches to community organization provide the context for health promotion programming (Rothman, 1970).

Social/Political Action

The goal of social action is to change the distribution of resources, power, and decision making. The basic strategies involve organizing the population around salient issues. Conflict methods are appropriate, including demonstrations, boycotts, protests, and rallies. The change agent serves as an activist, an agitator, negotiator, and a partisan. The women's movement, the gay rights movement, and the environmental health movement of the last several decades are examples of broad programs of social action. These actions are generally directed at existing institutions that represent traditional, entrenched forces and biased policies.

Locality Development

The goal of locality development is to create economic or social progress. This approach applies especially to disorganized and disenfranchised groups. Themes emphasized in this process are self-help, cooperation, and democratic decision making. The change agent may teach problem-solving skills and facilitate the organization of the group, but self-help is the rule.

Many communities employ social action and locality development principles to rid their neighborhoods of crime and drugs, prevent dumping of environmental toxins in their neighborhoods, or to prevent development that may pollute or undermine the integrity of the local community (Freudenberg, 1984). Minkler (1990) described several important locality development concepts for contemporary community organization practice:

Empowerment. Empowerment is ". . . the process by which communities are enabled to act effectively in transforming their lives and their environments" (Rappaport, 1984). Empowerment is the ability to influence the conditions of life that results from increased awareness, social support, and problem-solving skills.

Community competence. Community competence is the ability of the community to function such that it can solve its problems. This requires that various segments of society be able to collaborate and work together, often through coalitions, but also in informal ways.

Participation. This term highlights the principles of inclusion and "starting where the people are" in terms of their perceived needs, rather than with the needs and goals of the change agency. Genuine participation in the social change process is important because participants become empowered by their ownership of the project.

An Example of Normative Re-Education and Community Organizing

Minkler and Cox (1980) describe a health education program based on community organizing principles and Freire's ideas of normative re-education. In an impoverished area of downtown San Francisco called the Tenderloin District, a concentration of poor, elderly people live in cheap hotels among drug addicts, prostitutes, and criminals. The goal of the project was to help develop groups of elderly in each hotel to provide support, raise consciousness, and become empowered to improve their situation through social action. Also, the program sought to unite the support groups in the different hotels into a coalition that could make demands on local agencies and government. Health fairs were conducted at the various hotels to stimulate interest and facilitators organized interaction/support groups. Peer leaders among the elderly were identified to facilitate discussion and help guide the program. Through dialogue they developed a list of twelve generative themes for the interaction/support group meetings. Social change activities of various sorts continue in the Tenderloin District to this day. This project is noted for its creative application of normative re-education and community organizing principles to facilitate social change and promote health among a disadvantaged target population.

Advocacy

Advocacy refers to a set of skills that can be employed to alter public opinion and mobilize resources in favor of a policy or issue. Advocacy is an important aspect of social justice, which concerns the extent to which societal conditions are fair and resource distribution is equal. Public health is a social good of which democratic governments are responsible for assuring the equitable distribution. We are referring here, of course, not only to the distribution of health services, but also the distribution of economic opportunity and social justice. Real participation and representation in the political process is central to social justice. Advocacy, however, is not necessarily a national issue—it is just as important at local levels.

There is a wide range of advocacy approaches and methods. Here we discuss two approaches to advocacy that are of particular importance in health promotion—media advocacy and policy advocacy.

Media Advocacy

Media advocacy is the use of media to apply pressure for changes in public health policy (Wallack et al., 1993). Media advocacy seeks to change the way media reports and presents certain issues. It seeks to alter the vocabulary, the content, and the selection of news such that it favors public health rather than entrenched interests and the status quo. Media advocacy is an approach to changing the normative behavior of the media. It attempts to raise the consciousness of media professionals and alter the practices of policymakers and corporate leaders who are influential in structuring the environment within which individual health behavior occurs.

The electronic and print media are major American businesses. The selection of stories and their presentation is a product of professional decisions and commercial considerations about what stories and what story angles are likely to gain the largest number of viewers or readers, and therefore, to generate the most advertisement revenues. Media attention is precious, since there are many more possible stories than time and space permit. Therefore, there is fierce competition for news coverage. News coverage of a particular health issue, for example, AIDS or breast cancer, not only increases the awareness of the viewers about that issue, it also confers status and legitimacy. Critics of the mass media, the ownership of which has become increasingly centralized, argue that they favor the interests of the most powerful groups in society in terms of the selection and content of stories (Wallack et al., 1993). Much of this criticism applies equally to national and local media.

Media advocacy uses and influences media in some unique ways. It is more interested in healthful public policies and environmental change than in the delivery of messages about personal health behavior. It seeks to develop coalitions and encourage community organization as a base of support for agenda setting and framing issues. Such groups are more powerful than individuals acting alone. The goals and work of these groups—identifying problems, creating programs, and making policy statements—can be fostered greatly through media advocacy. Understanding how the media work can enable media advocates to improve the quantity and quality of coverage of health issues. Two critical processes are agenda setting and issue framing.

Agenda setting.   Media advocacy is concerned with gaining and increasing the attention of media on a particular topic to increase its visibility, salience, and legitimacy. Remarkably, health issues, such as the proliferation of weapons and violent crime, or unintended pregnancies among teenagers, can languish without policy direction and without public action until they receive concentrated and sustained media attention. Such attention alters the perception of their importance relative to other health-related issues. Wallack and associates (1993) describe successful efforts to alter the media agenda such that greater attention was devoted to AIDS, the environment, and other important issues.

Issue framing.   The media first identifies a story and then frames it by selecting certain people and events to relate the story, thereby telling the public what is important about that topic. The content that is included tells people what aspects of the topic are noteworthy, while the content that is excluded is not legitimized. In contemporary society news is presented in small digestible bites; hence, not very much can be presented about any particular topic. The words and pictures that are selected slant the story greatly. For example, the coverage of a local protest against the siting of a waste disposal dump in a neighborhood can be framed in pictures and words that either present the protest leaders as radical troublemakers or as committed citizens acting in the best interests of their neighbors.

Policy Advocacy

Policy advocacy is another important social change approach for health promotion. Policy advocacy is one of several policy-related activities of health educators, focusing on organizing citizen participation and influencing policy adoption. Other policy functions include policy analysis, development, and administration.

Briefly, health educators frequently have an opportunity to analyze and develop policies. Policy analysis involves evaluating alternative courses of action and making recommendations to policymakers. Policy analysis can focus on the relative advantages of alternative policies regarding costs, efficacy, effectiveness, outcomes, possible side effects, and other issues. Policy analysis can also be evaluative, focusing on the extent to which a certain policy has been implemented and enforced and the degree to which its objectives and outcomes have been met. For example, worksites increasingly have adopted smoke-free policies. Policy analysis would focus on the options to accommodate nonsmokers, policy administration, resource allocation, penalties for policy violations, education for policy administrators and workers, and the like.

Health educators often are well positioned to serve as policy developers. In this capacity they may provide relevant sources of information, provide policy briefings, and prepare drafts of policies and procedures. Policy development requires careful problem identification, objective setting, consideration of alternative actions, estimation of consequences, allocation of resources, and consideration of other implementation issues. For example, worksite health educators are frequently asked to develop policies on smoking and to develop procedures and programs to facilitate the acceptance and administration of the policies.

Health educators also have policy advocacy responsibilities, as described by Steckler and associates (1987). From a social change and social justice perspective, health educators should serve not merely as content and process experts, but also as advocates for those who would be affected by the policies.

Target population participation.   Too often policies are established without input from the populations that are affected by them. Again, worksite smoking-control policies are relevant. Clearly, smoking-control policies are in the public interest and worksite smoking-control policies are the products of years of effort on the part of social change advocates. However, in developing a specific worksite policy one of the health educator's responsibilities is to assure that there is sufficient worker input into the policy. The participation by smoking and nonsmoking workers in policy analysis and development should lead to a result that is appropriate and acceptable.

Coalitions.   Health educators frequently are involved in developing coalitions that have policy objectives. Coalitions can serve to provide information and support among the leaders and members of groups with common interests. Coalitions can also be more influential in policy advocacy than single groups. It is common, for example, for coalitions to form around topics such as AIDS, child health, tobacco control, and substance abuse prevention, where many public agencies and citizen groups are concerned but not administratively connected. Successful coalitions can have important influences on policy development and implementation. For example, in many states coalitions of groups concerned about drunk driving have managed, through concerted effort, to influence the statewide adoption of prevention policies and strategies.

Influencing policymakers.   Health educators are well trained in influencing knowledge, attitudes, and behavior in ways that are relevant and effective with policymakers. These efforts may include persuasive communications, direct lobbying, development of influence networks, training, and the use of mass media. Restrictions on smoking in public places are just now becoming the rule rather than the exception. In county by county and state by state, the efforts of health educators and others over many years have helped influence policymakers to adopt such restrictions.

Example.   Freudenberg and colleagues (1987) used principles of normative re-education in efforts to increase awareness and promote activism on the part of citizens and advocacy groups to reduce lead poisoning in New York City. The program was initiated by the formation of small groups that studied the problem of lead poisoning and redefined it as a political and resource problem rather than a personal health problem. Mass media coverage of the problem was elicited, increasing public support for policy changes. The critical press coverage seemed to predispose officials of the City of New York to give more attention and resources to the problem. A coalition of concerned groups from housing, public health, children's rights, and public interest law formed to advocate for changes in laws to prevent lead poisoning and increases in resources for screening and education.

Social Change and Conventional Health Promotion Programming

The social change methods described so far have their roots in the era of political activism and radical social change popularized in the United States in the 1960s. This approach to social change remains relevant today in the United States and other countries where many subgroups are disenfranchised, impoverished, and disorganized. Not surprisingly, many of these methods of social change have been modified for use in mainstream health promotion programs. Generally, these modifications lean toward conservative adaptations that are probably more acceptable to funding agencies and perhaps more consistent with conventional programmatic perspectives on the change process. Indeed, some social change principles have become part of conventional health promotion practice.

Bracht and Kingsbury (1990) present an example of a programmatic adaption of a social change process in their five-stage model for community organizing for health promotion.

Stage 1: Community Analysis. Base interventions on accurate analysis of the community's needs, values, resources, and social structure. Assessment should include (a) the capacity of the community; (b) limitations of and barriers to change; and (c) readiness for change. The analysis should lead to a set of priorities established with the participation of community leaders.

Stage 2: Design and Initiation. Develop an organizational structure, usually involving a core planning group and local coordinator (Green and McAlister, 1984). The mission, goals, and roles and responsibilities of the leaders and members of the organization should be clarified, preferably in writing.

Stage 3: Implementation. Develop a plan of action with the benefit of substantial and meaningful citizen participation. The plan of action should involve multiple approaches and strategies that can largely be integrated into existing programs.

Stage 4: Program Maintenance-Consolidation. As the staff and participants gain experience with the program activities, the inevitable problems of design and implementation must be addressed. Hence, in a good program there is a balance between implementation fidelity to the original activities and appropriate modification or recreation. This process is enhanced when the activities are integrated into existing structures and there is good communication between the implementers and the developers of the program.

Stage 5: Dissemination-Reassessment. Reassessment is a continuous process and programs naturally change over time, given appropriate feedback mechanisms. Most programs start small and expand if they are successful. Successful programs must develop plans for the future and marshall resources to reach future goals. Descriptions of the program activities and evidence of success can be produced as a way of documenting the importance of the program and disseminating its principles to other communities.

Social Marketing

Social marketing is an amalgam of social change approaches and product marketing. Social marketing seeks to increase the acceptability of a social idea or practice among a target population (Kotler, 1982). Social marketing uses media to promote a product, idea, or attitude, applying marketing techniques to social issues. Social marketing, like marketing in general, is based on the assumptions that consumers in different socioeconomic groups and geographic regions have unique attitudes and behaviors that are the product of their experiences; in other words, learned. Hence, the task in social marketing is to offer an attractive product, which might be a tangible good (e.g., a condom), a service (e.g., contraceptive counseling), or an idea (e.g., using condoms is protective against STDs), in exchange for the consumer's resources, which might be money, time, or effort. Consumers who perceive that the product is worth the cost are likely to purchase or adopt it.

Social marketing employs research (market analyses) of the target population's needs, wants, and expectations regarding products to segment the population into target audiences (Lefebvre and Flora, 1988; Novelli, 1990). Based on market analysis the product is positioned with respect to advantages, nature of the product, price, distribution, and promotion (communication). Products are promoted by advertising, public relations, direct marketing (e.g., direct mail or telephone solicitations), special promotions (e.g., coupons or incentives), and interpersonal, face-to-face communication. Great attention is given to market integration, where product demand and availability are coordinated with advertising and promotions to maximize the effectiveness of the effort.

The process of social marketing is consistent with conventional health promotion programming. Based on a survey or market analysis, a marketing plan is developed and the products and services of the plan are developed, tested, and refined. The market plan is then implemented, followed by market assessment and feedback. Hence, the plan can be modified constantly in keeping with the changing nature of the marketplace.

It is easy to see the appeal of social marketing for health education and promotion. Social marketing is a highly dynamic process that seeks to respond to the needs of the target population by changing the nature of the product, its distribution and availability, and promotional activities to maximize the number of adopters. Too many health promotion programs have failed to analyze the market and develop and promote products accordingly. Additionally, too many health promotion programs fail to adapt to changes in consumer needs and wants, thereby becoming ineffective. Marketing is an aggressive activity, based as it is on the view that there is a limited market for each product and competition from similar products. Successful products not only have to be better, they have to be competitive in terms of relative advantages, cost, and the like.

Examples from Community Studies

Community studies that have been developed to address major chronic diseases provide examples of conventional social change methods in practice. The unique features of several important community studies are described in the following paragraphs. In particular it is interesting to note differences in emphasis, the use of volunteers and peer leaders, and the integration of community organization and social marketing principles.

North Karelia

Two decades ago in eastern Finland residents of the rural county of North Karelia became concerned about the high rates of cardiovascular disease in their community, caused by the prevalence of cigarette smoking, obesity, high blood pressure, and high-fat diets. Aware that their health problems were nourished by the prevailing norms, concerned citizens participated in the development of a concerted community effort of planned social change. Ten years later the number of smokers had decreased markedly, the use of low-fat milk had all but replaced whole milk, butter consumption had decreased, and the prevalence of uncontrolled high blood pressure had declined by 25 percent among men and 50 percent among women. Illustrating the potential for planned community action and social change, the highly acclaimed success of the North Karelia project was based on the following planned and coordinated change strategies (McAlister et al., 1982):

1. Public information, persuasion, and social marketing of new attitudes, practices, and products regarding cardiovascular health.
2. Empirical-rational training of medical professionals in risk factor assessment, screening and treatment of cardiovascular disease, and prevention.
3. Reorganization of preventive health services to emphasize prevention.
4. Community organization to create social support and social action.
5. Top-down support for the development and marketing of heart healthy products.
6. Changes in public school curriculum to emphasize health behavior protective against cardiovascular disease.
7. Public health education programs for smokers and other high-risk individuals.

Pawtucket Heart Health Program

The PHHP, located in New England, employed mass media, community organization, and diffusion approaches (Lefebvre et al., 1987). The purpose of the mass media campaign was to increase awareness and interest in participating in the program. The approach to community organization was to mobilize the participation of existing organizations such as worksites and churches. The unique feature of the PHHP was its use of volunteers to deliver the instructional programs. Volunteers were trained to serve as instructional leaders or facilitators for small groups of learners in their organization. Instructional programs for leaders and instructional materials for learners were developed for each major cardiovascular disease risk factor. After a brief training program, the leader was responsible for several instructional programs on that topic. Program staff trained the trainers and facilitated the recruitment of participants into the program. The PHHP provides a unique combined approach to health promotion.

The Stanford Five-Community Study

The Stanford Five-Community Study employed a mass media campaign, health professionals training, along with the implementation of individual education counseling for risk factor modification, implemented through local health clinics (Farquhar et al., 1985). The mass media program focused on increasing knowledge and attitudes about preventive health behaviors such as exercise, low-fat and low-sodium diet, and smoking and was employed to recruit people to screenings and high risk individuals into specific programs established in clinical settings. Specific intervention programs were developed for smokers, those with high blood pressure, and those with elevated cholesterol.

The Minnesota Heart Health Program (MHHP)

In the MHHP, social marketing and community organizing approaches were adapted and employed in each of three communities (Middelmark et al., 1986). The MHHP employed seven specific strategies that were applied to the risk factors of smoking, diet, and physical inactivity: (1) community leaders and organizations were involved in the planning of the program through community advisory boards; (2) mass media informational campaigns were conducted; (3) risk factor screening and education activities were organized in community and clinical settings; (4) point-of-purchase promotions for healthful foods were implemented in local grocery stores and restaurants; (5) adult education classes were organized to educate the population about cardiovascular disease prevention; (6) public school instruction was developed; and (7) professional education was conducted through the medical societies.

A Su Salud (To Your Health)

A Su Salud is a community-based study developed to prevent cancer among Mexican Americans in Texas, mainly by decreasing smoking and encouraging cancer protective behaviors (Ramirez and McAlister, 1988). Unique features of the program, which was based on social learning and social marketing principles, included (1) formative evaluation of the health needs and interests of the target population; (2) collaboration with local print and broadcast media to present news stories about community health-related events, people, and programs and to interview role models who were homophilic with the target population but practiced cancer protective health behaviors; (3) training and support of neighborhood peer leaders who were responsible for informing neighbors about specific media events scheduled on local radio and television by delivering monthly schedules and informing people of upcoming events; (4) presentation of social role models in a variety of media and forums.

Summary

Social change is a process that alters the structure and function of social systems. This may include the adoption of a new social norm or change in policy, practice, or power. Social change is sometimes unplanned, but it can be planned; it occurs at individual, group, and societal levels; and it can be generated from the top-down or from the bottom-up. The health educator working as a change agent is most effective when he or she communicates well, has a great number and variety of contacts with clients, is highly empathetic with the client, and markets the innovation well. The adoption of beneficial innovations tend to occur first among innovators and early adopters and only later among the majority and still later among laggards. Adoption occurs in stages: awareness, interest, trial, decision, adoption, and continuation. Innovations that have relative advantages over current practice or competing innovations are more likely to be adopted, as are those that have little negative impact on social relations, can be tried in increments, are not too complex, and are easily understood.

The change agent may employ a range of social change approaches, including: empirical-rational education, normative re-education, advocacy, community organizing, and social marketing. Some of these approaches are revolutionary in that they seek to alter the environment and the political, economic, and social status and power of the target population. Social change approaches, particularly aspects of community organizing and social marketing, have been incorporated into conventional health promotion programming.

PART IV

PROFESSIONAL PREPARATION AND THE FUTURE

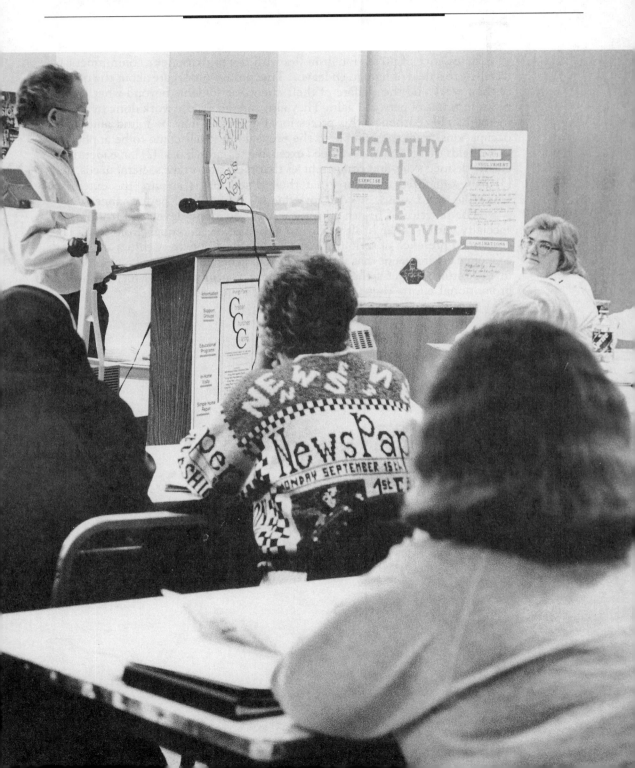

The essence of professionalism lies with the practitioner's commitment to a cause—to a field of human endeavor. True professionals care about the quality of their work and the welfare of their clients or students beyond what it may mean in terms of personal gain. They also care about the work done by others in their field. Although this professional approach may be found among all occupations, from the humble to the prestigious, it has come to be applied to those fields that (1) have developed extensive research bases, (2) have identified clearly defined skills and competencies that meet important societal needs, and (3) have organized to ensure that their practitioners acquire the extensive education and training needed for effective professional performance.

The practice of health education has grown and developed from a sub-specialty within other health fields to a mature, autonomous profession. The continued presence of serious, persistent health problems within a social and economic environment that seems destined to generate even more such problems in the future, suggests that there will be a continuing need for the health promotional efforts that health educators can provide.

Professional Issues in Health Education

On your own, how do you improve your competence and judgment in an area? Read and discuss case studies, talk to practicing health educators about what they do and why they do it, read books, go to professional meetings. When you lead a discussion, plan a meeting, consult or give advice, don't be afraid to ask for feedback. The same is true of decision making—ask why it's good or why it isn't.

—Sigrid Deeds, *The Health Education Specialist*

Introduction

We asked a number of practicing health educators what it meant to them to be a professional and received a variety of answers. Some emphasized the skills and knowledge they had and the quality of services they provided to their clients. "To manage my worksite health promotion program, I stay current by reading journals in my content area and in health promotion. I also attend workshops and research presentations." Others spoke about their involvement in professional associations and the work they did on behalf of the profession of health education. "My first supervisor said that you're really not in health education unless you're in a professional organization doing something. I've been deeply involved in the state and national organizations over the last 20 years. I've gotten to help develop the code of ethics and credentialing from the ground up. My colleagues across the country are a great support to me in my job. I feel good about my work." Service was another theme. "I really feel like I am making a difference. Though I don't do 'hands on' health education, I am committed to helping others and know my community program for drug prevention is literally saving lives."

During the undergraduate and graduate education and internship experiences, students learn more than the skills and knowledge required of health educators. They learn what others—their internship and later job supervisors, coworkers, and clients—expect of them as they practice their profession. This set of skills, knowledge, and role expectations is all part of being a professional.

To understand better what it means to be a professional, we will turn to a sociological view of the professions. This provides a backdrop for examining health education as an emerging profession. We will see that health education displays many of the characteristics of a true profession. However, it does not have licensure as do medicine and the allied health professions and it does not require as prolonged a period of study as medicine, law, or higher education. As we will see, health education has established a voluntary certification process designed to specify education and practice standards for the field.

Following our discussion of professional issues in health education, we turn to the competencies for health education as defined for certification. This will help students understand what they need to know and be able to do as health educators.

What Is a Profession?

The dictionary definition for a profession is "a vocation requiring some knowledge of some department of learning or science" (Random House). The regulation of professionals began with the ancient Babylonian Code of Hammurabi, based on the principle that "the strong shall not injure the weak" (Gross, 1984). Today most professions have a system of credentialing to assure that a minimal level of competence is attained in order to practice. **Accreditation** is a credentialing process for institutions and is defined as "the process by which an agency or organization evaluates and recognizes an institution or program of studies as meeting certain predetermined criteria or standards" (USDHEW, 1971). The processes for credentialing individuals are licensure and certification. **Licensure** is "the process by which an agency of government grants permission to persons to engage in a given profession or occupation by certifying that those licensed have obtained a minimal degree of competency necessary to ensure that the public health, safety and welfare will be reasonably well protected." (USDHEW, 1971). **Certification** is the process by which a "nongovernmental agency or association grants recognition to an individual who has met predetermined qualifications specified by that agency or association" (USDHEW, 1971).

Sociologists have analyzed the professions from two perspectives. The functionalist approach examines the function of the professions for society and, within that framework, a list of criteria for whether an occupation is a profession have been developed. Professions provide society a way to handle a major need, i.e., maintaining health. Professional standards assure quality, and certification and licensure serve to link education and skills to the marketplace. On the other hand, analysts using a power or conflict paradigm focus on who is served by the professions and, within that framework, movements to increase professionalism are seen as stemming from the economic self-interest of the professionals. In this view, certification and licensure are a means to control entry to the market. Our discussion of professionalism in health education in this chapter flows from a functionalist perspective; however, we recognize that valuable insights into the politics of the professions and professional practice have come from a conflict perspective (Gottlieb, 1992; Hall, 1985; Larson, 1977).

Medicine, law, the ministry, and higher education are the ideal type professions, possessing most of the characteristics of a profession. They emerged in the Middle Ages and the term profession comes from "to profess" which means to take vows. Sociologists have examined the characteristics of these professions to determine what criteria define a profession. Occupations can be classified along a continuum from nonprofessional to professional. Movement along the continuum is possible and for the past several decades health education has been working to advance its professional status through its professional associations and academic institutions.

Characteristics of a Profession

The essential characteristics of a profession have been identified as (1) a service mission, (2) a unique body of knowledge, and (3) a period of prolonged training. Related characteristics, which flow from these, are continuing education, a code of ethics, control of standards of education, shaping of legislation related to the profession, and peer review and control of licensure boards. Finally, members of a profession are strongly identified with that profession (Cockerham, 1989).

Essential Characteristics

Within this framework, health education is considered an emerging profession. Health education definitely has a service ideal as seen in the mission statement of the Society for Public Health Education: "The advancement of the health of all people through education." However, health education is an interdisciplinary field and draws knowledge from social and behavioral sciences, epidemiology, and other sources.

Core competencies for health education recently have been identified, and this process has codified the knowledge and skills necessary for academic preparation and certification of practitioners. The bachelor's degree has been designated as the entry level for the profession, which is consistent with other allied health professions yet less restrictive than for the ideal type professions.

Related Characteristics

Continuing education.   Members of a profession must keep up with changing knowledge and practice in their fields after their primary educational preparation is complete. Attending continuing education programs is required for license

---

Table 14.1 Characteristics of a Profession

Essential Characteristics	Related Characteristics
A service mission	Continuing education
A unique body of knowledge	Code of ethics
A prolonged period of training	Standards of education
	Shaping of legislation
	Freedom from lay control
	Strength of identity

retention for physicians, nurses, and other licensed providers and to retain certification for health educators. In the health education field, these programs are provided by professional associations, universities, and other groups, and there is a process for the programs to offer continuing education credits for certification.

Ethics.   Health education has a code of ethics originally developed by the Society for Public Health Education (Taub et al., 1987). This document gives guidance regarding what is right and wrong in professional practice and flows from the service ideal—that the professional's ultimate responsibility is to the client and the public. We will discuss ethical issues in health education later in this chapter. The Hippocratic Oath, with which you may be familiar, is the code of ethics for physicians.

Accreditation of programs.   Besides being accredited through their regional accrediting bodies for higher education, academic programs in health education offering the Master's of Public Health Degree are accredited by the Council of Education in Public Health, on which members of the health education profession serve. Similarly, a voluntary approval process for other bachelor's degree programs is available through two health education professional organizations (the Association for the Advancement of Health Education and the Society for Public Health Education) acting jointly. Also, the competencies for certification are included in the accreditation process for colleges of education offered through the National Council for the Accreditation of Teacher Education. However, professional course work in health education is less tightly controlled by the profession than are medical and nursing curricula by their respective professions.

Legislative advocacy.   Advocacy for legislation related to professional interests is an important part of the agenda of professional organizations. For professions with a state licensure process such as medicine and nursing, the professional practice acts are legislated. Since health educators are not licensed by the state, they are not involved in advocacy related to the scope of their practice.

There are, however, legislative issues that affect the health-related programs funded through the public sector, such as family-planning programs, chronic disease prevention programs, AIDS services, and regulations related to private sector activities in such areas as occupational health and safety, air and water quality, tobacco and alcohol control, and transportation safety. These programs and regulations set the environment in which health educators practice and, more importantly, have a direct effect on the public's health. Health education professional organizations work on behalf of their members to influence legislation and regulations to benefit public health and to advance the causes of health education.

Freedom from lay control and control of licensure boards.   Peer review means that the profession is free from control by members outside the profession. Professions which have licensure are required to have state licensing boards to ensure that providers meet basic standards for practice and exhibit ethical conduct. These are controlled by the profession, although there is consumer membership as well. In general, professional domination of licensure boards has been reduced and public accountability increased since the 1960s. As mentioned earlier, health education is not licensed by the state through a professional practice act. Except for school health educators who must be certified by the state to teach, health education has voluntary certification through the National Commission for Health Education Credentialing.

The establishment of a certification process for health educators in 1988 marked a turning point in the profession of health education. For the purposes of our examination of the professional status of health education, certification represents additional control of entry to the profession based on an academic background linked to a core set of knowledge and skills. Only graduates of accredited programs in health education may sit for the examination to obtain designation as a Certified Health Education Specialist (CHES). However, in contrast to licensure, certification is not required by law for the practice of the profession. As of April 1, 1995, there were more than 4,300 certified health education specialists. The impact of certification is dependent on employers' adoption of certification as a condition of employment in health education. The National Commission for Health Education Credentialing and the health education professional associations are working to increase the recognition of the value of certification and its use by employers.

At this time there is no formal process to censure unethical health education practitioners. Peer review is not tied to the certification process and consists of informal mechanisms, including supervision within organizations and discussions among practitioners.

Strength of identity with the profession.   A professional is strongly identified with his or her profession and the profession is his or her life's work. All of us would probably agree that health educators as a group may not be as strongly identified with their work as are physicians and some other professionals. This is partially due to the lack of a career ladder for advancement in health education. As health educators obtain seniority, they often switch to general administration. There also is not a clear image of a health educator in the public's mind as there is of a physician, a teacher, or a nurse.

A Brief History of Health Education Credentialing

The decade of the 1920s witnessed the formation of the American College Health Association, the Public Health Education Section of the American Public Health Association, the American School Health Association, and the Society of State Directors of Health, Physical Education, and Recreation. Other major professional associations, such as the Association for the Advancement of Health Education and the Society for Public Health Education, were established between

1937 and 1950. In 1971, the Coalition of National Health Education Organizations was formed, with representatives from eight professional associations (Coalition of National Health Education Organizations, 1990).

All of the professional associations maintained a continuing interest in defining the competencies and training needed by health educators. At the same time, curriculum development in health education was proceeding in schools of public health and colleges of education. Table 14.2 outlines key events in the history of curriculum development and credentialing.

In 1978, the process which led to certification was begun with a conference and the resulting formation of a broadly representative National Task Force on the Preparation and Practice of Health Educators. The National Task Force specified the role of health educators through a process of interviewing practitioners and their employers from school, health care, community, and worksite settings. The committee weighted the competencies in terms of their importance and specified levels of supervision for entry level practitioners. The report of this task force, *A Framework for the Development of Competency-based Curricula for Entry Level Health Educators*, was widely disseminated. In 1981, the National Conference for Institutions Preparing Health Educators reviewed and endorsed this report and recommended that voluntary certification be pursued. The core competencies identified through the role delineation process were then used by colleges and universities to modify their curricula to ensure that they were preparing students to carry out these competencies.

The National Commission for Health Education Credentialing was established in 1988, with the National Task Force on the Preparation and

---

Table 14.2 Milestones in Health Education Credentialing

1949 First U.S. Office of Education Conference on Undergraduate Preparation of Health Education Students

1956 College Health Conference on the Professional Preparation of School Health Educators

1966 The Committee on Graduate Curriculum in Health Education offers recommendations for a core curriculum that includes health science, behavioral sciences, and research

1978 National Center for Health Education facilitates the Role Delineation Project

1978 Conference on the Commonalities and Differences in the Preparation and Practice of Health Educators in Bethesda, Maryland

1985 A Competency-based Curriculum Framework for the Professional Preparation of Entry-level Health Educators published

1988 National Commission for Health Education Credentialing, Inc. established

1990 First examination for Certified Health Education Specialist (CHES)

Source: Adapted from Deeds, 1992.

Practice of Health Education serving as the Interim Board of Commissioners. The first task of the National Commission was to develop a test based on the role delineation report using Professional Examination Services, which provides the testing for psychologists and other professions. After the certification process was underway, members of the Board of Commissioners were elected by the certified health educators as their representatives. Following a one-year period during which long-time health education practitioners were grandfathered into certification, testing was begun. Beginning in 1992, only persons graduating from an accredited health education program could sit for the test.

The National Commission for Health Education Credentialing has three divisions that reflect its mission: (1) the Division for Professional Development, (2) the Division for Certification of Health Education Specialists, and (3) the Division for Professional Preparation. Each division has a Board of Directors who are certified health education specialists representing medical care, school, community, business/industry, and professional preparation program settings.

A system for approving continuing education programs to maintain CHES status and reporting individuals' credits earned has been developed by the Division for Professional Development working with the major professional associations. To be approved for continuing education as part of this process, programs must be based on the health education competencies identified for certification and be conducted by qualified professionals.

The Division for Professional Preparation has worked to have the core competencies included as essential to the accreditation of college and university health education programs. As mentioned earlier, the National Council for the Accreditation of Teacher Education, the Council on Education in Public Health, and other accrediting bodies examine whether the curriculum is adequate to provide students with the competencies for certification. Other processes are occurring in the states. For example, the Texas Coordinating Board for Higher Education has used the competencies to define curriculum standards for community health education programs in Texas.

The National Commission and the professional associations are also working to promote certification as a criterion in the hiring process. Obviously, for voluntary certification to have a strong impact, employers must honor the certification and require candidates for health education positions to be certified or, if this is not possible because of the relatively small number of certified professionals nationally, indicate that the credential is preferred. At the present time, many employers cannot know prior to hiring the difference between competent and incompetent health education services, the appropriate professional preparation in health education, and how the skills of health educators fit the employers' needs.

Certification based on core competencies that represent the commonalities of performance among educators working in a variety of settings is leading to the unification of health education. Prior to specializing for work in a specific setting or in a specific content area, health educators must master this common body of knowledge and practice. It has brought the different professional associations together in agreement over what health educators must know and be able to do.

Credentialing: An Alternative Opinion

At the present time, there is not total consensus among health educators on the philosophic underpinnings related to certification. Some health educators believe that increasing professionalism and closing entry to persons not trained in accredited health education programs serves only to raise the salaries and opportunities for certified health education specialists. They believe it can stand between health educators and the clients they serve by increasing the power differential between the two. However, as noted earlier, all the major professional associations have gone on record as supporting certification through the National Commission for Health Education Credentialing, and the majority of health educators endorse the credentialing movement (Gottlieb, 1992).

Health Education Responsibilities and Core Competencies

The role description of a health educator is "an individual prepared to assist individuals, acting separately or collectively, to make informed decisions regarding matters affecting their personal health and that of others" (Bureau of Health Education, 1980).

The health educator may be called upon to carry out any or all of seven basic types of responsibilities:

1. assessing individual and community needs for health education
2. planning effective health education programs
3. implementing health education programs
4. evaluating the effectiveness of health education programs
5. coordinating the provision of health education services
6. acting as a resource person in health education
7. communicating health and health education needs, concerns and resources.

Within each of the seven areas of responsibility, three to four competencies are identified as necessary to the fulfillment of the responsibility. The competencies are broadly defined skills that an entry-level health educator is expected to perform. In turn, each competency is related to specific sub-competencies, upon which measurable general objectives are based. This hierarchy, from the general role to specific objectives, assures that the learning objectives in professional preparation programs and the examination items for certification relate to the responsibilities identified in the role delineation project.

Table 14.3 illustrates the relationships among these components, giving competencies, subcompetencies, and objectives within Responsibility 1. You

Table 14.3 Subcompetencies and Objectives for Responsibility 1: Assessing Individual and Community Needs for Health Education

Core Competency	Subcompetency	Objectives
A. Obtain health related data about social and cultural environments, growth and development factors, needs, and interests.	1. Select valid sources of information about health needs and health knowledge.	a. Differentiate between validity and reliability as indicators of relevance and dependability. b. Evaluate the validity and reliability of sources of health information.
	2. Utilize computerized sources of health-related information.	a. Name easily accessible data banks (e.g., ERIC, Medline, National Clearinghouses, etc.). b. Explain methods of accessing data banks.
	3. Employ or develop appropriate data-gathering information.	a. Describe survey techniques commonly employed by health educators. b. Appraise suitability and validity of various health survey instruments. c. Design valid health behavior inventories of needs assessment procedures.
	4. Apply survey techniques to acquire health data.	a. Develop a plan for effective administration of survey instruments. b. Organize the obtained data in ways facilitative of analysis and interpretation.
B. Distinguish between behaviors that foster and those that hinder well-being.	1. Investigate physical, social, emotional, and intellectual factors influencing health behaviors.	a. Describe behavioral and nonbehavioral causes of health problems. b. List physical, social, emotional, and intellectual factors commonly influencing choices among health behaviors. c. Identify principal determinants of positive or negative health behaviors in specified situations.

Core Competency	Subcompetency	Objectives
	2. Identify behaviors that tend to promote or compromise health.	a. Explain cause and effect relationships between health behavior and well-being. b. Predict immediate and long-range effects of specified health behaviors. c. Advocate potential benefits of a healthful life-style.
	3. Recognize the role of learning and affective experiences in shaping patterns of health behavior.	a. Differentiate between cognitive and affective learning experiences. b. Explain the part played by perceptions and values as health behavior determinants. c. Describe ways health behaviors are learned or changed.
C. Infer needs for health education on the basis of obtained data.	1. Examine needs assessment data.	a. Interpret data gathered through library research or as reported by health agencies. b. Classify health-related data according to specified variables (age, sex, risk factor of interest, etc.).
	2. Determine priority areas of need for health education.	a. Establish criteria for the selection of priority areas of need. b. Apply those criteria to identification of those areas most in need of health education.

Source: National Task Force on the Preparation and Practice of Health Educators, Inc., 1985.

can see from this example that the Competency-Based Curriculum Framework outlines the specific skills and knowledge required by the entry level health educator. Appendix B contains the Self-Assessment for Health Educators of the National Commission for Health Education Credentialing. This document lists all responsibilities, their competencies and subcompetencies. Students will be able to use this tool to assess their own skills so that they may plan their future classroom, volunteer, and internship experiences more effectively.

Assessing Individual and Community Needs

Needs assessment is the first stage of the planning process. It includes the collection of data regarding the health knowledge, beliefs, attitudes, and practices of individuals and the environment in which they live and work. Sources of data include questionnaires, interviews, existing records, observation, and physiological tests. The information obtained can be used to determine whether a health education program is needed and, if so, what its components should be.

The three competencies within Responsibility 1 are:

A. Obtain health related data about social and cultural environments, growth and development factors, needs, and interests.

B. Distinguish between behaviors that foster and those that hinder well-being.

C. Infer needs for health education on the basis of obtained data.

Planning Effective Programs

Once the needs assessment has been completed to determine the scope and direction of the program, a detailed plan is developed for the most effective use of educational resources. The first step is to identify and involve those persons who should participate in the planning process. The health educator then works with this group to facilitate the technical planning process, including (1) the formulation of specific objectives based on the needs assessment and resources available and (2) the selection of interventions consistent with these objectives.

The four competencies for Responsibility 2 are:

A. Recruit community organizations, resource people, and potential participants for support and assistance in program planning.

B. Develop a logical scope and sequence plan for a health education program.

C. Formulate appropriate and measurable program objectives.

D. Design educational programs consistent with specified program objectives.

Implementing Programs

This area of responsibility places the health educator directly in the teaching role and the necessary abilities as counselor, lecturer, group facilitator, and user of audiovisual techniques are stressed. Emphasis is placed on the ability to match the educational methods, activities, and media to the learning objectives and clients and the ability to assess whether the educational program is successful and to revise the program activities if necessary based on this feedback.

The four competencies of Responsibility 3 are:

A. Exhibit competence in carrying out planned educational programs.

B. Infer enabling objectives as needed to implement instructional programs in specified settings.

C. Select methods and media best suited to implement program plans for specific learners.

D. Monitor educational programs, adjusting objectives and activities as necessary.

Evaluating the Effectiveness of Programs

Evaluation begins with the specification of program objectives and a plan for assessing whether or not they have been met. There are three types of evaluation. Process evaluation focuses on whether the program is being implemented as planned; impact evaluation, on whether there have been changes in knowledge, attitudes and behavior; and outcome evaluation, on whether the goals for morbidity and mortality reduction have been reached. Process and impact evaluation are of most concern to the entry level health educator.

Besides the technical aspects of designing the evaluation, selecting the instruments, and analyzing the data, the health educator must also attend to the management of the evaluation process and the interpretation of findings to stakeholders in the evaluation, i.e., to those persons who are interested in the results of the evaluation. The final step is making decisions regarding the future of the program and the utilization of findings for program planning.

The four competencies in Responsibility 4 are:

A. Develop plans to assess achievement of program objectives.

B. Carry out evaluation plans.

C. Interpret results of program evaluation.

D. Infer implications from findings for future program planning.

Coordinating Provision of Services

Health education programs are often sizable enterprises involving many people and considerable resources. They are usually based within larger organizations such as schools, colleges, hospitals, business firms, and public health departments. Community coalitions may be involved in the provision of health education services. To mobilize such resources as money, personnel, space, and time, health educators must have good coordination and management skills.

The four competencies in Responsibility 5 are:

A. Develop a plan for coordinating health education services.

B. Facilitate cooperation between and among levels of program personnel.

C. Formulate practical modes of collaboration among health agencies and organizations.

D. Organize in-service training programs for teachers, volunteers, and other interested personnel.

Acting As a Resource Person

As people go about their personal or work-related activities, they often encounter the need for health information of a limited and specific nature. A homemaker may want to know about the safety of microwave ovens; a prospective resident may want data on the relative purity of the local water supply; a high school teacher may want to find a source of educational materials on alcoholism. Such people are not candidates for educational programs; they simply need answers to their questions. Sometimes as their primary duty and often as an auxiliary one, health educators function as clearinghouses for health or health education information. The community health education section of a public health department often assumes this responsibility. The health educator in such a situation must be able to assemble and organize general information to satisfy a variety of routine requests and, in addition, must become aware of community resources for referral of complex requests.

Sometimes the consumer needs informational services that require consultation on programmatic activities. For example, a producer of industrial chemicals might become concerned over the efficiency of the company's methods of informing its workforce about special hazards and needed precautions that are associated with a new production process. In this case, the health educator must be able to analyze a unique situation in a short time and apply the general principles of information dissemination.

The four competencies for Responsibility 6 are:

A. Utilize computerized health information retrieval systems effectively.
B. Establish effective consultative relationships with those requesting assistance in solving health-related problems.
C. Interpret and respond to requests for health information.
D. Select effective educational resource materials for dissemination.

Communicating Needs, Concerns, and Resources

The work of health educators typically requires communicating many different types of messages using many different types of media. A wide variety of individuals and groups often become involved as the targets of these communications. They may be organized into (1) persons whose support is needed if a program is to be developed or retained and (2) health consumers who need information, education, or counseling. The media or techniques vary with the objectives and task. One-on-one active listening is used in such activities as birth control counseling, group process skills for the leadership of smoking cessation groups, lecture/discussion presentations in lobbying for support from various community councils or corporate boards, and mass media campaigns for encouraging population-wide changes such as drug abuse prevention or immunization. In all communications, the health educator must take into consideration the many value systems and cultures represented in our society today.

The four competencies in Responsibility 7 are:

A. Interpret concepts, purposes, and theories of health education.
B. Predict the impact of societal value systems on health education programs.
C. Select a variety of communication methods and techniques in providing health information.
D. Foster communication between health care providers and consumers.

Overview of the Health Educator's Role

When you ask health educators what they do on the job, the answers you receive are likely to reveal that their job responsibilities are as diverse as their patterns of professional training. As noted throughout this text, health educators work in a variety of settings and interact with a variety of population groups. Following are some examples of tasks performed by health educators. Note the similarities and differences among them in skills required, basic orientation toward health problems, and relationship to health authorities. Each of these tasks, however, falls within the role of the health educator. Performance of each task reflects a unique mix of the health education competencies.

Improve Compliance to Authoritative Recommendations

Through formal classes, one-to-one counseling, media campaigns, and various other means, many clinical and community health educators encourage people to take their medication, improve their diets, wear seat belts, and adopt other such behaviors as prescribed by such sources as physicians, national councils, and state legislatures.

Assist Clients in Behavioral Management

Many people wish to lose weight, improve their physical fitness, stop smoking or drinking, or make some other behavioral change, but find this difficult to accomplish on their own. There is no need to convince the clients of the desirability of the change; the challenge is to assist them to eliminate undesired behaviors and establish more healthful behaviors.

Assist Clients in Decision Making

People often face decisions in which there are a number of acceptable alternatives, such as how to handle an unwanted pregnancy, how to obtain good medical services, or how to select nutritious food on a limited budget. Here the health educator functions as a counselor and makes the client aware of a range of choices and the pros and cons of each.

Help Students Develop Knowledge and Insight

Most school health educators are not pushing for specific behavioral changes, nor do they often focus on the individual problems of students. Their task is to help students develop decision-making skills, knowledge, and insights related to health which will serve as resources throughout life.

Improve the Performance of Health Care Personnel

Some health educators specialize in helping hospital and outpatient clinics provide better services to their patients by providing in-service training to receptionists, nurses, technicians, and physicians on how to improve knowledge, adherence to medical regimens, and satisfaction of patients and their families. Often instructions and information given by clinical specialists are difficult to understand and may not meet the patients' needs. As behavioral specialists, health educators can often assist health care providers to promote patient health.

Help Communities Solve Health Problems

Some problems such as insufficient medical services or excessive exposure to environmental hazards require concerted community action for their amelioration. Health educators are often cast in the role of community organizers who mobilize and resolve conflicts among various groups to achieve the community's aims.

Professional Training

If you asked several health educators where they received their professional training, you would likely receive a variety of answers. The following include the major routes undertaken by individuals to prepare themselves for a career in health education.

Schools of Public Health

There are 26 schools of public health that offer programs of public health education leading to the Master of Public Health (M.P.H.) degree. At the doctoral level many of these schools offer programs in this field leading to either the Doctor of Public Health (Dr. P.H.) or Doctor of Philosophy (Ph.D.) degrees. In addition there are ten accredited M.P.H. programs in community health outside of schools of public health (Association of Schools of Public Health, 1994; Council on Education in Public Health, 1994). Graduates from these programs are generally well grounded in epidemiology and behavioral sciences and tend to specialize for work in public health departments, international health, and community settings.

Departments of Health Education

Approximately 200 colleges and universities other than schools of public health offer professional training programs in health education (Association for the Advancement of Health Education, 1991). Nearly all of these schools offer bachelor's degrees in health education, and many offer master's and doctoral degrees as well. These programs vary greatly along several dimensions. The departments offering such programs may be based in any one of a number of different colleges including education; health sciences; liberal arts; or health, physical education, and recreation. The curriculum and the professional orientation of the faculty also vary, with some departments representing community or public health education, some focused mainly on teacher training for public schools, and still others linked closely to nursing, medical technology, and other allied health programs. Many of the teacher and worksite health promotion training programs are closely associated with the field of physical education.

Related Professional Programs

Many persons whose professional training includes little or no training in health education per se become employed as health educators by virtue of their training in nursing and allied health, social work, biology, psychology, communication, or other related fields. The diversity of background and orientation of this group are obvious. On-the-job training and in-service education in health education is necessary for these persons to carry out their responsibilities. As health education becomes more strongly identified as a profession, this route into health education will be curtailed.

Laypersons

Many people serve as health education volunteers for voluntary health agencies, such as the American Cancer Society or American Heart Association, or for organizations such as family-planning agencies, community clinics, hospitals, or schools. Nonprofessional community liaisons, community health aides, and teacher aides—natural leaders from the community being served—often play a key role in the delivery of health education services. With proper screening, training, and supervision, these persons can function well to carry out specific health education activities. Problems arise when nonprofessionals with a knack for marketing and persuasion "put out their shingle" and offer services that they are not qualified to deliver.

Professional Associations

As discussed earlier in this chapter, professional organizations carry out many of the essential functions that make an occupation a profession. These include conducting continuing education programs, disseminating research findings to broaden the knowledge base for professional practice, legislative advocacy on behalf of the profession, establishing a code of ethics, and establishing standards for education in the profession. Health education associations provide a professional identity and "home" for the health educator, with an informal collegial support network, formal job banks, and other services.

There are seven health education professional associations that make up the Coalition of National Health Education Organizations. These organizations have played key roles in the history and development of health education as a profession. In addition there are other professional organizations to which health educators may belong based on their setting or specialty area, such as the Association for Worksite Health Promotion, the Sex Information and Education Council of the United States (SIECUS), or the American Society for Training and Development.

Descriptions of the major health education professional associations follow. All except the International Union of Health Education are members of the Coalition of National Health Education Organizations. Each membership organization publishes a journal and newsletter and, with exceptions noted, sponsors an annual conference. Students are encouraged to join at reduced rates. Many of the organizations have state affiliates, and the state associations are an excellent entry point to professional life for students and new professionals. Two of the organizations do not have open membership. The Association of State and Territorial Directors of Public Health Education and the Society of State Directors of Health, Physical Education and Recreation have specified members based on their position in state government (Deeds, 1992).

Association for the Advancement of Health Education (AAHE)
AAHE is part of the larger American Alliance for Health, Physical Education, Recreation and Dance. Growing out of an initial focus on school-based health and physical education, it promotes comprehensive health education programming and draws its membership from professionals practicing in schools, universities, and community health settings. It publishes the *Journal of Health Education*. For further information, contact AAHE, 1900 Association Drive, Reston, VA 22091.

American College Health Association (ACHA)
The focus of ACHA is the health of college students, and its membership is predominantly physicians, nurses, and health educators working in college and university health services. Its journal is the *Journal of the American College Health Association*. For further information, contact ACHA, 1300 Picard Drive, Suite 200, Rockville, MD, 20850.

American Public Health Association (APHA)
APHA represents the major disciplines in public health through its sections. The Public Health Education and Health Promotion section and the School Health Education and Services section are the two sections of primary interest to health educators. Its journal is the *American Journal of Public Health*. For further information, contact APHA, 1015 15th Street, NW, Washington, DC, 20015.

American School Health Association (ASHA)
ASHA focuses on issues related to school-age children and draws its membership from school health educators, nurses, and physicians. Research and practice

in comprehensive school health is a major area of concern. Its journal is the *Journal of School Health*. For further information, contact ASHA, P.O. Box 703, Kent, Ohio 44240.

International Union for Health Education (IUHE)

IUHE aims at improving health through education and cooperates closely with the World Health Organization and the United Nation's Educational, Scientific and Cultural Organization. It sponsors a conference every three years and publishes the journal *Hygie*. For further information, contact the North American Regional Office/IUHE, P.O. Box 2305, Station "D", Ottawa, Ontario, Canada, K1P5W5.

Society for Public Health Education (SOPHE)

SOPHE was formed to contribute to the health of all people through education by encouraging research, high standards of professional preparation and practice, and continuing education. It sponsors both an annual meeting, held in conjunction with that of APHA, and a mid-year scientific conference and publishes the journal *Health Education Quarterly*. For further information, contact SOPHE, 2001 Addison Street, Suite 220, Berkeley, CA 94704.

Association of State and Territorial Directors of Health Promotion and Public Health Education (ASTDHPPHE)

As seen from its title, ASTDHPPHE is comprised of the directors of health education from states, territories, and the Indian Health Service. It is an affiliate of the Association of State and Territorial Health Officials. It is concerned with standards of health education practice in state health departments and in liaison activities between federal, state, and local health education programs. For further information, contact your state department of public health.

Society of State Directors of Health, Physical Education, and Recreation (SSDHPER)

Membership in this organization is limited to directors of school health, physical education, and recreation in state agencies. SSDHPER promotes comprehensive statewide programs of school health, physical education, recreation and safety. For further information, contact your state department of education.

Ethics and Health Education

- To whom are professionals in the area of health promotion accountable—their employer(s), the profession, their clients, or themselves?
- For what are professionals accountable—results or how the results are obtained?
- Are there ethical guidelines governing the marketing of health promotion programs and services?

- What impact does marketing and its attendant competition have on professional relationships, collaboration, networking, and social support?
- What are the limits regarding what we are willing and able to do to meet the needs and expectations of employers, clients, and the profession?
- What are the practical and ethical implications of the current emphasis in health promotion on individual behavior change strategies?
- What are the responsibilities of the individual versus the community for promoting and maintaining health behaviors?
- Under what circumstances, if any, are coercive strategies acceptable?

These questions were raised in a discussion on ethical issues by practicing health educators as they struggled to deal with dilemmas they faced in their daily work (Burdine, McLeroy and Gottlieb, 1987). These professionals were concerned with situations in which their employing organizations were more concerned with profits or number of service visits than benefits to clients; in which persons with unhealthful behaviors such as smoking or lack of exercise were being blamed for their poor health or risk status in the face of persuasive advertising for tobacco products and lack of free community facilities for exercise; in which all the strategies for health promotion at a worksite were directed at individuals when the conditions of work were stressful and unsafe; and in which individuals were forced to make behavioral changes because of corporate policies or laws.

Professional health educators look to their code of ethics to guide them in making decisions about what is right and wrong in their professional practice. In 1976, SOPHE published a code of ethics for health education, which was subsequently revised in 1983 (see Appendix C). At the time of this writing, it appears likely that this code will become the basis for a profession-wide code adopted by the major health education organizations. The code is clear as to who should be served: "Health educators' ultimate responsibility is to the general public. When there is a conflict of interest among individuals, groups, agencies, or institutions, health educators must consider all issues and give priority to those whose goals are closest to the principles of self-determination and enhancement of choice."

The code recognizes that coercive strategies may be necessary when an individual's behavior harms others and voluntary approaches to change the individual's behavior have not been effective. However, it advocates the use of voluntary strategies whenever possible and encourages involving the people to be affected in the choice of educational strategies and methods. It requires that all program participants be clearly informed of the benefits and risks to be expected from their involvement in the program. The problem of "blaming the victim" (locating the cause of health problems within the individual, rather than in social and environmental forces) is addressed by stating that health education strategies must not place the exclusive burden of change on the target population and by charging health educators to speak out on issues affecting the public's health.

In addition the code requires that health educators clearly communicate with employers their qualifications, capabilities and aims and holds health educators responsible for maintaining and improving their competence through participating in continuing education, reading the professional literature, and being active in professional associations. Specific responsibilities of faculty to students and of researchers and evaluators to their participants and sponsors also are outlined.

Table 14.4 provides a list of questions generated in a discussion of the "business of health promotion." Health promotion services increasingly have become a marketable commodity, with greater consumer interest in life-style change and corporate and government interest in containing health care costs through primary prevention. The accompanying expansion of the health promotion and fitness industry has created new practice contexts for health educators that require a fresh look at ethical dilemmas. The questions in table 14.4 focus specifically on the practice of health promotion. Think about how you might answer them if you were a health promotion practitioner working in a health and fitness club, in a worksite health promotion program, in a hospital health promotion program, or in a consulting group marketing health promotion services. What are some possible problems that might be encountered in each of these settings? How would you deal with them?

Table 14.4 Questions for an Ethical Health Promotion Practitioner

---

1. On what basis do I or my organization allocate health promotion resources?
2. How do I choose what and to whom to sell?
3. What are the implications of the methods I use in health promotion programs?
4. Am I planning for organizational success or participant success?
5. To whom and what am I accountable?
6. Whose needs am I meeting?
7. Who is being left out of my program?
8. What claims do I use in "selling" health promotion?
9. To what end do I market health promotion?
10. To what extent do I consider how long behavior change will last?
11. Do I fully explain the risk and benefits of my programs to clients?
12. Do I involve the participants in the process?

Source: McLeroy, Gottlieb, and Burdine, 1987.

How to Prepare Yourself: A Guide for Students

Students enroll in health education classes for a variety of reasons. Many specific content classes, such as health concepts, human sexuality, and drug education are of general interest to college students and often are taken for personal development. Others, such as planning and evaluation, epidemiology, and methods of health education, are useful electives for students in a variety of pre-professional programs. The knowledge and skills learned in health education training also provide an excellent preparation for becoming an informed and active citizen, regardless of one's specific profession.

How do you know if you wish to become a health educator? The core competencies of health education provide a clear picture of the day-to-day tasks of the health educator. These are common to the field as a whole, although the exact mix of competencies required for a specific job varies with setting and content area. A school-based health educator, for example, must be highly knowledgeable in the subject matter of health science, highly skilled in teaching methodology, and well-versed in curriculum structure and process; however, he or she may have less need for community organization skills and little need to use the mass media. Conversely, some community-based health educators may have job responsibilities that are almost entirely devoted to the production of press releases and the development of mass media campaigns and have little or no need for group process, discussion leadership, or other teaching skills. Because most students have no direct experience with health education practitioners, other than school health educators, it is helpful to talk with the faculty about what jobs are available in health education and to gain some field experience in health education settings through volunteer work or class projects.

There is no specific personality or set of characteristics that typifies a health educator. Most health educators are greatly interested in health; in health behavior; and in individual, organizational, and community change. Enthusiasm for the content and process of health education may be the most important personal quality required of a health educator. Not surprisingly, this enthusiasm translates into action with respect to personal health habits. While not all health educators are perfect role models, most are working to improve some aspects of their personal health behavior much of the time. In general, health educators are a gregarious and personable group, with a desire to contribute to society and to help others.

What courses to take? The health education student should work closely with his or her academic advisor to plan the program of study. This should begin with a self-assessment of the competencies required for certification found in Appendix B. This, along with the student's interests in settings and content areas, will help define what courses should be taken and what field experiences are important. Course work that fulfills the general undergraduate requirements should be chosen with care, with emphasis on biology and the behavioral sciences. Electives should be selected to provide a minor specialization in such supporting areas as nutrition, psychology, or business, depending on the student's career interests. The undergraduate student should take prerequisite courses for graduate study, usually including statistics, behavioral science, biological sciences, and health education. Competency in a foreign language often is required as well, and many health educators working in community, health care, and international settings find that a Spanish language proficiency is extremely helpful.

Experience, recognized as a great teacher, is the best way for a student to explore various settings and competencies in health education. It is also highly valued by employers. The old adage that you cannot get a job without experience, and you cannot get experience without a job, is only partly true. There are a number of ways of gaining experience in preparation for that coveted first job.

Many courses require a term project in which the student tries out some of the ideas included in the course. This assignment can be used as an opportunity to interview or observe health educators at work, to organize and conduct learning activities, and to evaluate and report results. Projects may serve to broaden the student's experience or provide an early opportunity for specialization.

Serving in a volunteer capacity is another way to gain experience. Good volunteer positions are well-defined, with specific tasks and responsibilities. Short-term training and limited supervision are usually provided. There are a number of advantages to volunteer work. The volunteer obtains valuable training and field experience. He or she usually meets health educators and other professionals and can learn from them. A successful volunteer experience should also lead to a recommendation from the supervisor. Perhaps most important to the educational experience, however, is that the experience of working in the field provides a framework for other learning. The student will understand the applicability of theory and methods to the "real world."

Supervised fieldwork is perhaps the single best form of experience that one can obtain through a college or university professional preparation program. It allows the student to work in the capacity of a health educator in a real situation, supervised by both a faculty member and a qualified field professional. In teacher preparation programs, student teaching provides the student valuable classroom exposure and experience by working with a variety of student groups. In contrast to schools, students in community settings are less familiar with the structure and function of their field placement organizations. Fieldwork provides an opportunity for the student to become acquainted with the workings of the organization and to participate fully in a designated program. An intensive practicum in the core competencies of planning, implementation, coordination, and evaluation is the objective. We suggest that the student repeat the self-assessment in this text prior to the field placement and that the student, faculty advisor, and field supervisor work together to plan an experience that will be maximally useful in the student's development as an entry-level health education professional.

For the student interested in getting the most out of his or her formal professional preparation in health education, the authors have the following suggestions:

1. Put at least as much time and effort, if not more, into your professional preparation courses as your other courses. You will not only learn a great deal this way, but you will also develop an appreciation for what else you need or want to know. At the outset of each course ask yourself what the course is designed to teach in terms of knowledge and skills. Visualize how this knowledge and skill is related to the competencies required of a professional health educator. Seek to master the knowledge and skills.

2. In general, try to excel academically. Better students have an advantage both in learning and in the recognition they gain from their academic performance.

3. Take your course work and course content home with you. Health education is both very personal and highly social. Try out what you learn in the classroom on yourself and on your family and friends. See what works; be analytical and critical.

4. Consider papers and projects in the long-term context of your need to learn about health and health education. Term papers provide an opportunity for the enthusiastic student to begin to develop an area of expertise upon which future learning can build. Projects provide an opportunity to meet people, to try out new concepts and ideas, and to be exposed to the "real world."

5. Get involved in health education activities in your department and at the university. If there is a major's club, a chapter of Eta Sigma Gamma (the national health science honorary), a research project, or community health education program associated with your department, be sure to get involved. If there are health education programs emanating from student health services, the dorms, or elsewhere on campus, try to participate in the planning, the implementation, and the teaching if at all possible. If none of these activities exist where you are studying, take it upon yourself to initiate something.

6. Join a professional organization and attend its regional and/or national conferences. All the professional organizations in health education offer discounted rates for students for both membership and conference fees. Most paid memberships include the cost of the organization's journal. In addition to continuing education through the journal and conference presentations, professional associations offer an opportunity for the student to become part of a network of health educators. Students are able to hear about jobs and to become acquainted with potential employers through participation in local and state professional associations.

7. Become a regular reader of professional journals. Read not only for content, but also to learn what is of interest to health educators and what programs exist, as well as current trends, new methods, and opportunities.

Specialization

Health educators tend to be generalists. The very nature of the profession requires a broad range of interests and skills that are applicable to a variety of settings and content. However, as with any profession, health education is far too vast for anyone to be an expert in all its facets and content. Specialization allows health education students to narrow their interests in the field, to provide a context for learning, and to probe more deeply into issues. Selecting an area of specialization in advance may facilitate the learner's selection of courses, projects, and fieldwork. As mentioned in chapter 4, there are three distinct categories from which areas of specialization may be selected: (1) setting, (2) content, problem, or population group, and (3) function.

Setting

Setting is the most common category of specialization. Setting specialization areas include school, worksite, community, and patient (including hospital, HMO, and student health services) health education. Most professional preparation programs allow a major emphasis for either school or community health education, with all nonschool health education subsumed under the community emphasis. For many students a greater degree of specialization is desirable. For example, employed health professionals who study health education often prefer to focus their learning on their setting of employment. Others prefer to focus on a particular setting they are familiar with or to which they are drawn.

Content, Problem, or Population Group

Some health educators specialize in a particular content area such as sexuality, drugs, or nutrition, or in a particular problem area, such as infectious disease control, accident prevention, cardiovascular disease, or cancer risk reduction. Still others focus on the health problems and health behavior of a particular population group such as women, children, adolescents, older adults, workers, or a minority group such as African Americans or Hispanics. Of course, one health educator who specializes in human sexuality, another who specializes in infectious disease control, and yet another who specializes in women's health issues may all be interested in sexually transmitted disease, for example, or the high risk of cervical cancer among females who have had numerous sexual partners.

Function

A health education function, such as needs assessment, planning, coordination, implementation, teaching, or evaluation, may be selected as an area of specialization. Health educators usually become acknowledged as function specialists only after a great deal of experience in the profession.

Career Planning

Preparing for your initial job search should begin in your undergraduate program. Your field experiences and networking through professional associations will acquaint you with the positions that health educators hold in your community and provide contacts for your first job search. In addition, health education students obtain a variety of skills, such as planning, behavior change, and evaluation, that are relevant to many different jobs. The career placement center at your college or university can help you to assess your interests, abilities, and work values and to prepare your résumé and begin your job search. Entry level health education positions may be advertised in the newspaper, listed in the job banks run by chapters of the Society for Public Health Education, or posted in health departments. In many cases, there is not widespread advertising of positions. Because of this, informal communication through local health education professional associations and with potential employers can be essential to learning of the availability of entry-level health education positions.

It is at this point that your self-assessment, course work, and field experience will pay off. When you graduate from an accredited institution of higher education with a health education emphasis, you will be eligible to sit for the examination for the Certified Health Education Specialist (CHES) certification. (For further information about the examination, contact the National Commission for Health Education Credentialing, Professional Examination Service, 475 Riverside Drive, Suite 740, New York, New York, 10115). The examination is based on the seven areas of responsibility and their competencies with application to the major settings where health educators are employed. Your becoming a CHES provides assurance to employers and consumers that you are qualified to practice as a health education specialist.

In addition to the specific skills in health education, employers look for a variety of other personal traits in job applicants. These include the ability to work with others in a team, motivation to work hard, a positive attitude toward work, leadership, maturity, flexibility, the ability to communicate well, intelligence, the ability to solve problems, integrity, tolerance for stress, honesty and organizational ability (Woods, 1987). Which traits do you possess already and which traits do you feel you need to work to improve? The internship offers you an opportunity to demonstrate that you possess these traits, and your field supervisor's assessment of your performance should include the demonstration of these traits as well as the specific health education competencies. Assessments such as these will be an important basis for letters of reference for future employment.

The first job gives the health educator the chance to show what he or she can do; it provides the opportunity to garner experience and make contacts; not infrequently it gives major direction to the health educator's career. The new employee undergoes a process of enculturation to the employing organization, gaining an appreciation of the behavior, values, and traditions associated with it. Success at a new job will depend on having realistic job expectations, understanding your job description, orienting yourself to the workplace, developing good communication skills, managing time effectively, working as part of a team, benefiting from performance evaluations, understanding office politics, dressing appropriately, and demonstrating good manners (Woods, 1987).

The new health educator will receive much formal and informal training on-the-job. This allows for further development of specific health education competencies. Perhaps the most learning will come from observing experienced health educators and consulting with them on situations that arise in practice. Some health educators find that the professional arena offers all the education they need, while others find they need to add new skills and knowledge through graduate education in order to advance professionally. Learning does not end with the first job—it really just begins at that point. Informal or formal continuing education is an important part of the health educator's career. It enables the health educator to keep up with new knowledge, new techniques, and new issues in health education practice and provides for professional development and career enhancement.

Summary

In this chapter, we discussed the characteristics of a profession from a sociological perspective and described health education as an emerging profession. Health education has a system for voluntary credentialing, designed to ensure the quality of preparation and practice of health educators. There are seven responsibilities on which certification is based: (1) assessing individual and community needs for health education; (2) planning effective health education programs; (3) implementing health education programs; (4) evaluating the effectiveness of health education programs; (5) coordinating the provision of health education services; (6) acting as a resource person in health education; and (7) communicating health and health education needs, concerns and resources. Health education has a code of ethics to guide practitioners in making decisions about what is right and wrong in their professional practice. Health education undergraduate students are encouraged to excel in their classes, obtain field experience through course work and internships, become involved in health education activities in the department, and to join a professional association.

Chapter 15

Practice Settings

Health promotion is both multisectoral and interdisciplinary; it must not be compartmentalized or function in isolation. Rather, it needs to operate across the entire continuum of health and health services development and beyond the health sector as well. Agriculture, education, mass media, transportation, and housing are among the many sectors sharing health concerns.

—World Health Organization

Introduction

As you have seen in examples throughout this text, health education takes place in schools, worksites, health care settings, health departments, voluntary health agencies, and other community settings. The settings differ in their organizational structure, the mission of the organization, and the centrality of the mission to health education. The process of health education, however, is the same across settings, although the relative emphasis on specific competencies, the primary content areas, and the target population for health education will differ. In some organizations, there will be many health educators employed, while in others there may be only one.

In this chapter, we will compare and contrast four important settings for health education: schools, worksites, health care organizations, and community organizations. We will take an ecological approach, looking at how health education within each setting addresses each of the four intervention levels (individual, interpersonal, organizational, and governmental) and also how they work together to improve the health status of the communities they serve. As you read each section, try to imagine yourself working in the setting, think about what problems you would be addressing, and what skills and competencies you would most need.

Comparison of Settings

First, we will compare the mission and the primary customer being served for several types of organizations within the four general settings (see table 15.1). For schools and worksites, health education is less central to the primary mission of the organization than it is in health-related organizations. In schools, the

Table 15.1 Mission and Primary Customers for Various Settings

Setting	Primary Mission	Who is served?
School	Education	Children/ adolescents
Worksite	Produce goods and services; Make a profit (if applicable)	Consumers of products and services
Hospital	Treat illness and trauma	Patients
Community primary care setting	Prevent, detect, and treat illness and trauma	Patients
Health Department	Chronic and infectious disease prevention and control	Public
Voluntary health agency	Prevention and control targeted disease/condition	Public

primary focus is on students' cognitive performance and educational achievement. Health education and health promotion support the central mission of the school in that a healthy, well-nourished child is better able to learn. In worksites, the supportive role of health education and health promotion is similar: an employee who is fit and healthy is more productive and uses fewer health care services, thus contributing to the "bottom line."

A consideration of the mission and the primary consumer suggests topic areas that will be important for health education. For school-based programming, adolescent risk-taking behaviors related to sexuality, alcohol and drug use, and smoking, as well as the primary prevention of chronic disease are key topics. Linking children to health care services and to nutrition programs as needed is also important. For worksites, primary prevention programming in the areas of fitness, nutrition, tobacco use, drug and alcohol use, and stress management are central.

Patient education in hospitals is typically concerned with adherence to medical regimens, self-management of chronic disease, informed consent, and pretreatment instruction and is often carried out by the patient's medical care provider. Hospitals may also offer community health education programming on a variety of topics related to health and fitness. The latter activity has often been conceived as a public relations program to increase community awareness and to influence choice of a hospital when in-patient care is necessary.

In primary care settings, the emphasis is on clinical preventive services in addition to adherence and other topics associated with treatment. Specific services, such as taking a risk-factor history; counseling related to exercise, tobacco, alcohol and drug use, and sexual activity; screening for breast, cervical, prostate, and colon cancer; and hypertension screening have been recommended for specific age and sex groups. Educational materials and services are needed to support these clinical activities.

The public health education effort in voluntary health agencies, such as the American Heart Association, is focused on public information related to the prevention, detection, and treatment of their disease. Besides direct communication through the media, voluntary agencies disseminate their programs to school districts, worksites, physicians' offices, and community organizations for use with students, employees, patients, and other consumers.

These settings can be considered channels for the delivery of health education and health promotion to senior citizens, adults, adolescents, and young children in a community. Each of the settings has an important role to play in accomplishing the goals set forth in *Year 2000 Objectives for the Nation*.

Table 15.2 lists the Year 2000 educational and community-based program objectives by setting. Comprehensive programming in health education, health promotion, and patient education is called for within each setting as appropriate. The community objectives include culturally sensitive health promotion programs, community-wide programming, partnerships with the media, and an emphasis on senior citizens. Another community objective is that health promotion topics be discussed within families. In addition to these broad program objectives, objectives for each setting are included within each of the Year 2000 health content areas.

Often organizations from various settings coordinate their activities through coalitions and task forces. For example, a coalition on smoking may include the American Cancer Society, the American Heart Association, the American Lung Association, the health department, the department of education, the medical society, anti-tobacco advocacy groups, and other interested groups that seek to increase and maintain smoking prevention and control activities and policies. To accomplish this, the coalition could engage in legislative and policy advocacy; distribute program materials and provide training for teachers, physicians, cessation group leaders, and worksite health promotion coordinators; and conduct community awareness campaigns. Such tobacco control coalitions are active in almost every state (Marconi and Bennett, 1990).

We will now examine each setting more closely. For each setting, we will show its role in accomplishing the Year 2000 objectives, present a typical organizational chart, discuss the role of health education within the organization, and describe a multilevel program common to that setting.

Table 15.2 Objectives for Educational and Community-Based Programs by Setting

Setting	Objectives
School	1. Increase to at least 75% the proportion of the nation's elementary and secondary schools that provide planned and sequential kindergarten through twelfth-grade quality school health education.
Worksite	1. Increase to at least 50% the proportion of postsecondary institutions with institution-wide health promotion programs for students, faculty, and staff.
	2. Increase to at least 85% the proportion of workplaces with 50 or more employees that offer health promotion activities, preferably as part of a comprehensive employee health promotion program.
	3. Increase to at least 20% the proportion of hourly workers who participate regularly in employer-sponsored health promotion activities.
Health care provider	1. Increase to at least 90% the proportion of hospitals, health maintenance organizations, and large group practices that provide patient education programs, and to at least 90% the proportion of community hospitals that offer community health promotion programs addressing the priority health needs of their communities.
Community	1. Increase to at least 90% the proportion of people aged 65 and older who had the opportunity to participate during the preceding year in at least one organized health promotion program through a senior center, lifecare facility, or other community-based setting that serves older adults.
	2. Establish community health promotion programs that separately or together address at least three of the *Healthy People 2000* priorities and reach at least 40% of each state's population.
	3. Increase to at least 50% the proportion of counties that have established culturally and linguistically appropriate community health promotion programs for racial and ethnic minority populations.
	4. Increase to at least 75% the proportion of people aged 10 and older who have discussed issues related to nutrition, physical activity, sexual behavior, tobacco, alcohol, other drugs, or safety with family members on at least one occasion during the preceding month.
	5. Increase to at least 75% the proportion of local television network affiliates in the top 20 television markets that have become partners with one or more community organizations to address one of the health problems outlined by the *Healthy People 2000* objectives.
	6. Increase to at least 90% the proportion of people who are served by a local health department that is effectively carrying out the core functions of public health.

Source: *Healthy People 2000*, USDHHS, 1990.

Schools

School-based health promotion is receiving wide attention from both public health and educational agencies and advocates. Twenty-five reports published between 1989 and 1991 were reviewed by the Harvard School Health Education Project (Lavin, Shapiro and Weill, 1992). They identified five themes crucial to the development of effective health education:

1. Education and health are interrelated.
2. The biggest threats to health are "social morbidities."
3. A more comprehensive, integrated approach is needed.
4. Health promotion and education efforts should be centered in and around school.
5. Prevention efforts are cost-effective; the social and economic costs of inaction are too high and still escalating.

First, if the well-being of children and adolescents is to be improved, a comprehensive approach is needed that links health and education. Second, social morbidities—threats to health from the social environment or behavior—must be addressed. These include unintentional injuries, homicide, suicide, child abuse and neglect, lead poisoning, substance abuse, sexually transmitted diseases, unintended pregnancy, and HIV infection. Third, an integrated system of prevention and education activities, including social, family and health services as well as classroom education, is recommended to stop the downward spiral experienced by high-risk youth. Fourth, schools are the only institutions that involve all children and their families and thus are the natural hub for community services directed to this population. Fifth, an emphasis on *prevention* is crucial. Innovative school-based health and social service programs have been adopted in many states and are expected to continue to expand as the United States reforms its health care system.

The *Healthy People 2000* general objectives for schools are to increase the high school graduation rate and to offer a quality comprehensive K-12 health education program. Schools are also targeted for such specific health education topics as nutrition, tobacco-use prevention, alcohol and drug prevention, human sexuality (through school, religious or youth programs), age-appropriate HIV education, sexually transmitted disease prevention, nonviolent conflict resolution, and injury prevention and control. Specific policies and programs include a healthful lunch and breakfast program; daily physical education that is oriented to lifetime physical activities; a tobacco-free environment; and requirements for effective head, face, eye, and mouth protection for sports and recreation events.

The *Healthy People 2000* objectives must be considered within the context of a comprehensive school health program. In chapter 3, comprehensive school health programs were described as having eight components: school health services, school health education, school health environment, integrated school and community health promotion efforts, school physical education, school food service, school counseling, and school health promotion programs for faculty and staff. Such a program requires coordination of services across various administrative units of a school district.

School districts typically have a decentralized organizational structure. The district central office houses the superintendent, personnel director, curriculum coordinators, school health services director, school food service director, and other administrative personnel. There has been a recent trend to site-based management and decision-making, with determination of goals, implementation activities, and allocation of resources at the campus level (Texas Association of School Administrators, 1992). Principals are accountable for their schools and the staff and students within them. Teachers must follow curricular guidelines from the state and district, but may choose supplementary materials suitable for their classes. Figure 15.1 provides a typical school district organizational chart, indicating where the different components of comprehensive school health are located. Health educators may work as classroom teachers or within a faculty-staff health promotion program or school health services. Classroom teaching requires state teaching certification. Health educators may also work with schools through their positions in local health departments or voluntary health agencies.

Figure 15.1 Organizational Chart for a School District

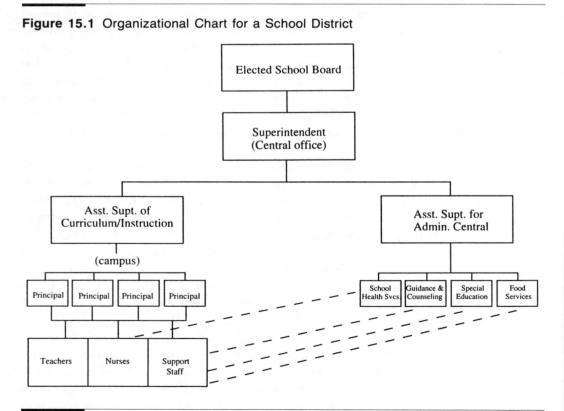

Classroom Instruction

Classroom health instruction has three goals. The first is that health be embraced as a value, along with responsibility, honesty, worthy citizenship, and quality of life. Second is that students be provided with the knowledge, skills, and empowerment needed to choose and maintain healthful personal behaviors. The third goal relates to students as lifetime learners, that they be able to obtain, evaluate, and use new information for future health-related decisions (Lohrmann, Gold and Jubb, 1987).

These goals are carried out through a planned sequential curriculum that emphasizes motivation for health maintenance, development of decision-making competencies, and health-related knowledge in ten content areas. Categorical content areas are community health, consumer health, environmental health, family life, growth and development, nutritional health, personal health, prevention and control of diseases and disorders, safety and accident prevention, and substance use and abuse (Seffrin, 1990).

Curriculum development must address the needs of growing and developing children over a thirteen-year period. The topics to be presented at each grade level and the educational activities must be selected with care. This involves consideration of scope and sequence. **Scope** refers to the breadth of content that might be covered during any given year and is related to the educational needs of children of that age. **Sequence** considers how best to meet these needs in view of past learning and how best to build up complex concepts and attitudes over a period of years. Instructional methods found to be effective include the use of discovery "hands-on" approaches; small, cooperative learning, student work groups; cross-age and peer teaching; positive approaches that emphasize normal growth and development; and opportunities to build self-esteem and self-efficacy (Seffrin, 1990). Figure 15.2 shows a typical page of a curriculum guide used to plan individual lessons. These guides may be developed by a school district or state or by national educational organizations.

At the elementary grade level, health education is provided by teachers certified to teach grades K-8 in most states. These teachers are generalists and only a few states require preservice education in health for elementary certification. The majority of states have certification standards in health instruction for secondary school teachers, although many teachers have dual certification to teach health and another subject (often physical education).

Faculty-Staff Programs

Health educators may also work within faculty-staff health promotion programs. These programs are a relatively new addition to school-site programming and have often begun with volunteer committees providing the coordination. Schools have a variety of resources for worksite health promotion: personnel (e.g., health education teachers, nurses, nutritionists, physical education teachers, counselors) and facilities/equipment (e.g., gymnasiums, tracks and fields, blood pressure cuffs,

Figure 15.2

Unit of study: Understanding others: social communication—Grade 6

Behavioral objective: Given a description or a dramatization of a social situation in which a person attempts to hide his or her true feelings, the learner will identify the underlying emotion and present a logical motive for its concealment.

Content	Methods and resources	Evaluation

I. Motives for suppression
  A. Embarrassment
  B. Fear of retaliation
  C. Social customs
  D. Concern for others
	1. Find situations in which feelings are concealed in appropriate children's fiction; read these to the class and discuss them.	1. Present in a multiple-choice format short narrations that require identification of feelings.

II. Methods of suppression
  A. Conscious self-control
  B. Displaying opposite emotion (love-hate)
  C. Fooling one's self
    1. Sour grapes
    2. Blaming others
	2. Ask each learner to write a short story in which a feeling is concealed; allow children to read their stories to the class if they wish. Discuss.
	
	3. Ask for volunteers to dramatize appropriate situations in which feelings are concealed.
		2. Observe class responses to the situations; be alert for emotions that were commonly misconstrued.

Typical page of a curriculum guide. Such general guides serve as resources for the development of lesson plans for specific classroom groups.

Source: Frank H. Jenne and Walter H. Greene, *Turner's School Health and Health Education*. St. Louis: C.V. Mosby Co., 1976. Used by permission.

---

scales, audiovisual equipment, computers). Schools are a major employer, representing 5% of employed persons or nearly 6.4 million employees in 1990 (U.S. Bureau of the Census, 1994). Evaluations of school-site health promotion programs have demonstrated benefits in fitness level, life-style behavior, general well-being, and absenteeism (Blair, Tritsch, and Kutsch, 1989). It is anticipated that these programs will increase in importance within a comprehensive school health program. The next section of this chapter discusses worksite health promotion programs in more detail and the health educator's role within them.

School Health Services

School health services are in the midst of great change, moving from a traditional program of acute care for minor illnesses and injuries and mandated screenings to an emphasis on primary care services, health education, and linkages to mental health and substance abuse programs, social services, and other community services, such as nutrition and recreation. School-based delivery of primary care services has been shown to be an effective way to reach children and adolescents at risk, and school-based clinics are increasing in number. As schools move toward more comprehensive primary programs that address social morbidities, the role of health education will increase in importance. Although health educators have rarely been employed within school health services, this may change as these services function more like those in primary health care settings.

Comprehensive School Health

Comprehensive school health provides a natural focus for ecological programming. The "Go for Health" program was described in relationship to the MATCH framework in chapter 6, and interventions at the individual, interpersonal, organizational, and community levels were outlined. Table 15.3 provides an ecological model of programming for alcohol misuse prevention. The primary objectives are to promote abstinence from alcohol, discourage driving while intoxicated, delay initiation of alcohol use, discourage riding with a driver who has been drinking, and to promote social norms for abstinence. These behaviors and norms are facilitated and reinforced through the involvement of students, parents and teachers.

Table 15.3 Ecological Programming in Schools for Alcohol Misuse Prevention

Level	Program Strategy
Individual	Information and discussion on alcohol as a risk provided in classroom; Articles in student newspaper.
Interpersonal	Discussion groups on norms and behaviors related to alcohol use by teens; Student groups plan strategies to prevent misuse of alcohol; Students make commitments to each other for support in responsible behavior related to alcohol use and driving; Parents contract with students to call if they need rides from social events.
Organizational	Policies banning alcohol at school events; Promotion of alcohol-free social events; Provision of rides to and from events.
Community	Alcohol-free gathering places for teenagers; Media campaigns, focused on teenagers, on risks from alcohol and benefits from not misusing alcohol.

Comprehensive school health programs address sensitive issues—sex education, HIV/AIDS prevention education, values clarification, and the provision of health services on campuses—that have caused controversy in many communities. A National School Board Association publication stated that "managing controversy is one of the most difficult and critical aspects of implementing a truly effective program; however, a health program that does not honestly address controversial issues in an age and culturally appropriate manner is, at best, ineffectual in helping children make appropriate choices and avoid risky behaviors" (cited in *All Well News*, Texas Association of School Administrators, 1994). Health educators in schools must work with their communities to foster open discussion, freedom of thought, and reasoned debate on school curricula and services. The focus must remain on improving the health and well-being of youth.

Worksites

In addition to comprehensive employee health promotion programs, *Healthy People 2000* objectives specifically encourage worksites to offer programs in physical activity and fitness, nutrition and weight control, stress reduction, worker safety and health, blood pressure and/or cholesterol education and control, and back protection; to have mandated vehicle occupant protection systems; and to have policies for smoking, alcohol, and other drugs, and for hiring of people with disabilities. This coordinates worksite programming with that in other settings to assure coverage of the national goals.

Compared to the other settings, worksite health promotion programs are of relatively recent origin, with most starting after the mid-1970s. However, there has been rapid expansion of health promotion at the worksite. The 1992 National Survey of Worksite Health Promotion Activities (USDHHS, 1993) found that 81 percent of worksites with 50 or more employees offered at least one health promotion activity, in comparison to 66 percent in 1985. Activities reported by at least one-third of the worksites were job hazards/injury prevention (64 percent of sites), exercise/physical fitness (41 percent), smoking control (40 percent), stress management (37 percent), and alcohol/other drugs (36 percent).

O'Donnell (1994) cites three primary motivations for employers to invest in health promotion programs: to reduce medical care costs, to enhance productivity, and to enhance the image of the company. Programming that improves the health of participants (particularly those at high risk), that addresses injuries and accidents on the job, and that encourages more appropriate utilization of health care services will impact health care costs. Productivity is improved by health status, but perhaps more importantly by employee attitudes, including job satisfaction, respect for employer, and concentration on the job. Access to a health promotion program is perceived by employees as a benefit, increasing their satisfaction with the company. Utilization of the program will lead to both improved employee attitudes and health. Corporate image is enhanced by awareness of the program within the community. This increases the company's general visibility and demonstrates that it is a concerned employer.

The scope and organization of a worksite health promotion program vary by size of the company, available resources, management preferences, and industry type. For example, fitness facilities are typically found in large companies with a white-collar workforce, often the home office of a large corporation. The programs offered in these companies may be primarily fitness-oriented or may be more comprehensive. Companies without fitness facilities may contract with community facilities for services.

A broad worksite program will include fitness, nutrition and weight control, stress management, smoking cessation, and preventive health (screening and education). The other program dimension is depth, with levels ranging from communication and awareness (e.g., newsletters, health fairs, screening without feedback), behavior and life-style change (e.g., offering weight-loss or smoking-cessation programs), and the creation of supportive environments for health promotion (e.g., physical setting, corporate policies, corporate culture). Obviously, small programs with few resources will be better able to offer low-intensity programming.

Figure 15.3 illustrates a typical organizational structure for a large in-house program. The health promotion manager is at mid-level and reports to the Vice President for Human Resources. An employee advisory committee, composed of employees from all levels, provides a link to the employee population.

Staff Selection and Program Design

The staffing of the health promotion program depends on the services offered. For fitness assessment and exercise leadership, a fitness professional should be hired. The American College of Sports Medicine provides certification for these individuals. A health educator, trained in planning, coordinating, and delivering programs, would be responsible for the health education programs. If the health promotion program is built around a fitness facility, the program should be headed by a fitness professional; conversely, if it does not, the program should be headed by a health educator.

Smaller programs may be managed by an employee volunteer as part of his or her other job duties, with services provided through contractual arrangements with community professionals, or by using volunteers from the worksite or community. Again, an employee advisory committee is a key resource and could spearhead the program. Committee members could be selected to provide services needed by the program, for example, graphic design, marketing, data processing, accounting, and training.

As with all programs, the sequence of program activities is through needs assessment, planning, implementation, and evaluation. Surveys and focus groups indicate employee interest and needs. Based on the findings and the resources available, a program mix is developed. This includes which topics will be covered

Figure 15.3 Organizational Chart for a Worksite Program

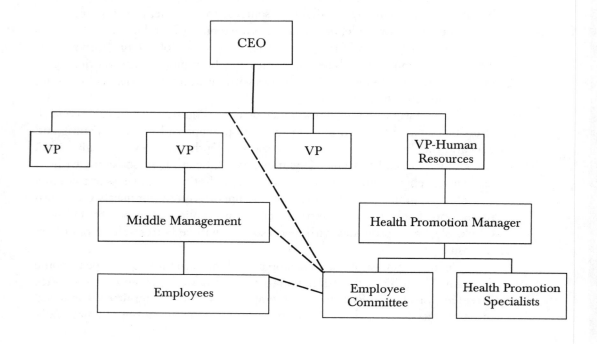

and the level or intensity of the programming for each area. Corporate events should be coordinated with national campaigns, e.g., National Heart Month in February and the Great American Smoke-out in November. A program calendar of events is laid out and responsibilities for promoting, conducting and evaluating the event assigned.

Table 15.4 provides an ecological model for an emphasis on nutrition at a worksite. The primary objective at the individual level is to increase the individual's nutrition awareness, knowledge, motivation, and behavior. This can be done using low-intensity activities, such as newsletter stories, posters, payroll stuffers, a library of books or videos, or through high-intensity classes. Interpersonal support for behavior change comes through the involvement of buddies, families, and coworkers. Competitions, interactive group behavior change programs, and instructions to choose a friend for contracting behavior change goals are strategies to foster interpersonal support. Environmental supports offered by the organization include providing healthful food options in vending machines and cafeterias and incentives through subsidization. To provide healthful food on-site, the worksite health promotion coordinator must target

Table 15.4 Ecological Model for Nutrition Programming at a Worksite

Level	Program Strategy
Individual	Nutrition information available through newsletters, books, and video; Nutrition behavior-change programs.
Interpersonal	Healthful food cooking contests; Nutrition classes for families; Buddy programs for weight loss; Competitions for weight loss.
Organizational	Cafeteria offers low-fat and low-calorie choices; Labeling of nutritional content of foods in cafeteria; Subsidized healthful foods; Vending machines with healthful foods.
Community	Institutional food service vendors offer low-fat and low-calorie foods; Nearby restaurants offer low-fat and low-calorie foods; A community campaign focuses on good nutrition.

the institutional food service vendors and vending machine companies to provide the appropriate foods. Another target in the community could be owners and chefs of near-by restaurants where employees eat to encourage them to offer more healthful menu selections and nutrition information. Companies could also work with voluntary agencies and other groups to develop community media campaigns on nutrition.

Coordination with Other Units

A health promotion program alone cannot accomplish the *Healthy People 2000* objectives for the worksite or provide a comprehensive approach to health promotion. It must coordinate with other programs within the company or link to community resources. The occupational safety and health program within an organization is responsible for monitoring environmental hazards, controlling them through engineering, training workers in safety practices, and informing them of risks they may encounter in their work. **Ergonomics**, the science of adapting the workplace to the needs of the individual and the task to be done, has grown in importance. Repetitive-motion injuries and conditions caused by postural problems are leading causes of workers' compensation claims. Medical departments have traditionally offered employee physical examinations and screening programs and linked employees to physicians within the community as needed.

Employee assistance programs offer short-term counseling and referral to community providers for employees and consultation to supervisors, personnel representatives, and union stewards regarding employee job performance problems. Originally focused around alcohol and drug problems, employee assistance programs are now usually "broad-brush," addressing such employee concerns as family, financial, and work problems. In addition, management practices, such as employee involvement, cross-functional team building, and job redesign influence the well-being of employees.

Coordination among these programs is necessary to provide individual-centered services. This includes easy referral of employees from one program to another and comprehensive programming to ensure that prevention, screening, and treatment are available and that both environmental and individual approaches to risk reduction are used. In reality, this may be difficult to accomplish. Within an organization, these programs may compete for scarce resources. Boundaries between the programs are fuzzy, and professionals within each program sometimes become territorial. For example, smoking cessation is treated within health promotion, while other addictive behaviors are the province of the employee assistance programs. Should employee assistance programs offer primary prevention programs in stress management, family-work conflicts, and other mental health issues? Should postural training and exercises to prevent back problems be provided by physical therapists, ergonomists, or the health promotion program? It is in the clear interest of the company and the employee that these efforts be coordinated. Creating cross-functional teams with members from these programs and placing them within a single unit of the organization, such as human resources, will facilitate shared programming.

Health Care Settings

In the hospital, direct patient education is part of ongoing patient care and is typically delivered by nurses and physicians. In addition, group classes may be offered separate from the patient's hospital unit (e.g., diabetes education, prenatal classes), and instruction may be delivered through closed-circuit television. A patient education manager is responsible for the planning and coordination of a hospital-wide patient education program, the design and evaluation of specific programs, and the acquisition, development and distribution of educational materials (Giloth, 1993). In the health care setting, perhaps more than any other, the health educator functions as a team member, providing consultation to other providers. For direct providers of services, skills are needed in patient/family assessment, interpersonal communication, group dynamics, the tailoring and delivery of interventions, and documentation in the medical record (Villejo, 1993).

Figure 15.4 provides a typical organization chart for a hospital. Note the separation of the medical staff and the nursing and administrative units of the hospital. In this hospital, health education is located in corporate development, along with human resources, employee health, public affairs, and volunteer services. In other hospitals, health education may be located within patient

Figure 15.4 Organizational Chart for a Hospital

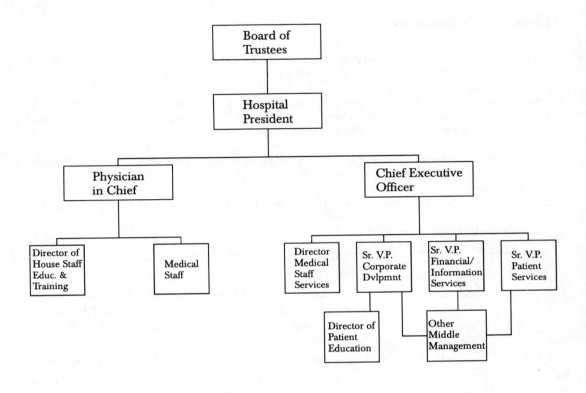

services. This chart clearly shows the importance of coordinating the patient education function across different organization units. Joint planning committees are essential and policies and procedures for the overall program must be developed.

Table 15.5 provides an ecological model for self-management of cystic fibrosis in a clinical setting and is based on the work of Bartholomew and colleagues (1991). The program has self-paced modules for parents and patients aged 3–6 years, 7–12 years, and 13 years to adulthood. It is designed to be incorporated into the provision of health care. Intervention objectives at the individual level are the knowledge, beliefs, and attitudes of patients and parents targeted through the self-paced modules. At the interpersonal level, interaction occurs with family members among themselves and with the health care team. This interaction is encouraged through activities suggested by the modules and in health care team training. Organization level interventions are the adoption

Table 15.5 Ecological Programming for Self-Management of Cystic Fibrosis (CF) in a Clinical Setting

Level	Strategies
Individual	Educational modules including feature stories, information about the disease process, skills, and self-monitoring.
Interpersonal	Interaction with health care team members about patient concerns related to CF and goals for self-management; Family discussion and practice of self-management behaviors and symptom monitoring.
Organizational	Primary care physician refers family to program; CF Family Education Program provided by CF Center.
Community	School nurses and teachers assist child and family in self-management of CF.

Source: Bartholomew et al., 1991.

and implementation of the Cystic Fibrosis Family Education Program. Outside the health care setting, schoolteachers and nurses are involved in special education of children with cystic fibrosis and assist families and patients with CF self-management at school.

In addition to in-hospital patient education, hospitals often sponsor health promotion programs for their employees, for the general public, and for corporations. The focus of these programs is on life-style health behaviors and risk assessment. The role of the health educator in these programs is similar to that described for the worksite health promotion setting.

Primary Care

For primary care settings, the emphasis is on the implementation of clinical preventive services. Specific *Healthy People 2000* objectives are to increase, among primary care physicians, routine assessment and counseling regarding physical activity; nutrition; tobacco use; alcohol; preconception care; cognitive, emotional, and behavioral functioning (for children and adults); safety precautions to prevent unintentional injury; occupational health exposures; use of prescribed and over-the-counter medications (with older adults); and cancer screening recommendations. Other objectives for primary care providers include ensuring the receipt of HIV and bacterial sexually transmitted disease treatment and counseling, prenatal care, infant care, immunizations, blood pressure screening and treatment, cholesterol screening and treatment, and breast, cervical, colon, oral and skin cancer screening. As in the hospital setting, the primary responsibility for patient education resides with nurses and physicians. However, for health maintenance organizations, clinics, and large practices, a patient education manager may function as coordinator of the program.

Community Health Settings

Public, tax-supported health agencies and private voluntary health agencies provide a variety of health services to the public. At the national level, government agencies provide health protection, health promotion, health services (for certain underserved populations), and research. The Department of Health and Human Services includes the National Institutes of Health; the Centers for Disease Control and Prevention; the Food and Drug Administration; the Indian Health Service; the Alcohol, Drug Abuse and Mental Health Administration; and the Health Care Finance Administration. Direct health-related services are provided to citizens through state and local health departments.

In the voluntary sector, such organizations as the American Cancer Society, the American Heart Association, the American Lung Association, and the March of Dimes Birth Defects Foundation provide public health education, grants for research, and some patient support activities. These organizations obtain funds through donations from citizens and organizations in a community. Their work is done through volunteers, who link the organization to schools, worksites, and health care sites and provide direction for the organization. Health educators employed in voluntary organizations provide staff support to volunteer committees and boards, manage the organization's outreach to the delivery channels (schools, worksites, health care, and community sites), and manage the public health education function. In chapter 12, we presented a case study of a voluntary agency worksite health promotion program. This provided an organizational chart and a description of voluntary agency staff activities.

Health Departments

State and local health departments work collaboratively to provide health protection and health promotion services to the public. Direct health services are offered by the local agencies, with planning, consultation, vital statistics, laboratory services, regulation, and coordination functions occurring at the state, as well as the local, levels.

Health educators work as consultants for the educational component of programs within such diverse areas as family planning, nutrition, dental health, tobacco control, chronic disease, AIDS, immunizations, and communicable diseases. They may work on the design of print and video materials for programs and educational campaigns, develop plans for community organization and outreach, and provide training in adult education. At the local level, they may be involved in the direct delivery of health education services in a public health clinic or in the health department's outreach to schools and worksites.

Figure 15.5 provides an organizational chart for a typical state health department. Health promotion provides staff services to a variety of programs and the director reports to the Deputy Commissioner for Programs. In this case, the health promotion department is centralized and participates on task-related teams with other units. The health promotion activities may be decentralized, and, in some health departments, the health educators are located as staff within the program area they serve. In this case, coordination of the health promotion program may be weak.

Table 15.6 contains strategies at the individual, group, organizational, and community level for a health department program to deliver breast cancer screening services to low-income women and is based on the work of Gottlieb and Dignan (1994). To accomplish these strategies, the health educator must develop brochures, press releases, and television and radio spots and coordinate a communications campaign with community media and local organizations. Interpersonal interaction is facilitated through a volunteer outreach program, using women drawn from the population being served. This requires working with local leaders to identify and train volunteers, develop materials, and

Figure 15.5 Organizational Chart for a State Health Department

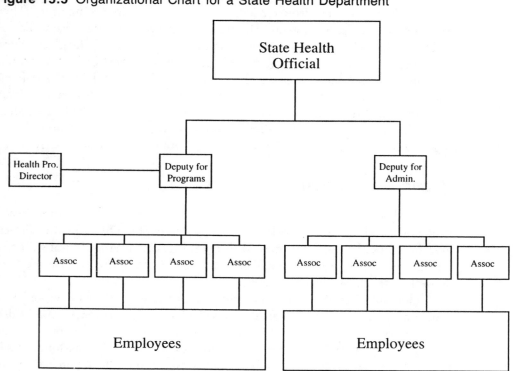

Table 15.6 Ecological Programming for a Health Department Intervention to Increase Breast Cancer Screening among Low-Income Women

Level	Strategies
Individual	Mass media campaigns to increase knowledge of the risks of breast cancer, the benefits of screening, and how to obtain screening services.
Interpersonal	Use of community volunteers to alert women to the importance of breast cancer screening and how to obtain information; Encourage discussion of breast cancer screening and benefits through small group educational programs and through feature stories in media.
Organizational	Provider referral of women already enrolled in health department programs; Outreach activities directed to worksites, senior centers and churches to alert women about the program.
Community	Create coalitions of providers to offer coordinated screening, referral, diagnostic, and treatment services; Provide community-wide social services including transportation, financial assistance, and home health services.

coordinate the program. The health educator must work with the provider community to establish coordinated services, so that women referred by the health department obtain all services needed at high quality. This will require negotiations for reimbursement, arrangements for care for indigent women, and a tracking system for referral and feedback. As you can see, facilitating and coordinating services provided by others is a significant part of the health educator's role.

Management of Health Promotion Programs

We conclude this chapter with a brief discussion concerning the management of health promotion programs. This is generic to all settings, although specific work settings vary in management role due to program size and scope, authority relationships, and organization type. Baun (1994) has described five key areas of responsibility for a health promotion director: human resources management, health promotion programming management, marketing management, management of budget and financial control, and facility and equipment management.

The management of human resources includes developing a plan to determine the staffing level and types of staff needed to carry out the program and the processes needed for recruitment, hiring, training, replacing, and evaluating employees. Job descriptions are written to list the duties and responsibilities of the job, requisite experience and skill, working conditions, and authority-responsibility relationships (i.e., to whom the job reports and who is supervised). Current management practices emphasize employee involvement and are centered around work teams, in which team members share a common purpose and each member contributes to the accomplishment of the team goals. Staff development and training enables individuals to meet their work responsibilities and personal and professional goals. Performance of both teams and individuals is evaluated by the manager on a formal and informal basis. Coaching by managers is a continuous process, while formal performance reviews (including both self- and supervisor-appraisal) occur at intervals (usually semi-annually or annually) specified by the organization.

The process of planning, organizing, implementing, and maintaining health promotion programs has been discussed in Part II (chapters 5–8) of this book. Planning and organization involve needs and resources assessment; development of a mission statement, goals and objectives, and priorities; choice of program strategies and activities to achieve the objectives; task assignments for staff; and identification of necessary resources. Program implementation and maintenance includes materials development or acquisition, promotional activities, delivery of the intervention (e.g., individual counseling, classes, communication campaign, policy change), and evaluation of the process and impact of the intervention. Maintaining the program requires feedback from the evaluative process and "recharge" of the program to make it more effective.

Marketing may be described as finding out what people want and providing it for them. It is an integral part of the program planning process. In health promotion settings, there are multiple targets or "customers" of intervention. These include the target population for the behavior change and persons at the interpersonal, organizational, community, and government levels whose actions would support the behavior change (see chapter 6 for a review of the MATCH model). For example, customers include community members, students, employees, patients; family members, friends, coworkers, teachers, nurses, physicians; administrators, newspaper and television community affairs personnel, community leaders, and elected officials. For any program, the market is segmented into groups with similar characteristics, wants, and needs. Then the market mix—including the program or service offered, the price (including time, other opportunities lost, and money), the place or location, and promotion to encourage participation—is designed for specific market segments.

Financial control and budgeting bring the program process to life and are crucial for quality control. Budgets are the formal financial plan of the organizational goals and objectives. A budget reflects the costs, revenues, and volume of health promotion programs and services and also how the health promotion unit fits within the larger organization. Health promotion managers prepare a line-item operating budget, showing expenditures required for carrying out the department's goals and objectives, and a capital budget, showing expenditures for equipment and facility improvements. Some of the costs within categories are fixed, e.g., rent or personnel, while others are variable, e.g., printing, materials, temporary personnel. Three columns are to be completed for each line-item: budgeted expenditures, actual expenditures, and variance. Projections are made across the months of the budget for all categories, reflecting plans for hiring of personnel or use of supplies. Each month, the manager compares what was budgeted and what was actually expended for that month and for the year to date. The variance between budgeted and expended amounts flags potential management problems with the program and is a powerful tool for keeping programs on course. Maintaining records of expenditures and revenues is essential, and each organization will have policies and procedures for purchasing, travel, reimbursements, and personnel expenses.

All programs include facilities and equipment, including office furniture, audiovisual equipment, communications equipment, computers, and information systems. Fitness facilities include exercise equipment, specific exercise space (e.g., basketball, racquetball courts), and showers. The planning and management of such facilities will be a key part of the manager's job. A written facility and equipment plan with program justification, written policies and procedures for purchasing and maintenance, and inventory control are necessary, and each employing organization will have its own system for accomplishing these responsibilities.

Summary

Health education is carried out in schools, worksites, health care organizations, and community agencies. The process of health education is the same across settings, although the content areas covered, the target populations, and the competencies required will differ with the organization mission and structure. Each setting provides a channel for accomplishing the Year 2000 health objectives for the nation. Common management functions across the settings are human resources management, health promotion programming management, marketing management, management of budget and financial control, and facility and equipment management. Health education students should focus on obtaining the general knowledge and competencies required across settings and then concentrate on content and skills specific to the setting in which they are most interested.

From Past to Present to Future

I shall be telling this with a sigh
Somewhere ages and ages hence:
Two roads diverged in a wood, and I—
I took the one less traveled by,
And that has made all the difference.

—Robert Frost, *"The Road Not Taken"*

Introduction

Considering the many difficulties involved both in finding relevance in historical events and in developing a clear picture of the realities of the present, it may seem audacious to speculate on the future. But a moment's reflection reveals this process as necessary to the making of most important decisions. College and university students, for example, frequently must make decisions that commit them to courses of action that have profound effects on their professional careers. What school to enter? What degree programs? What specialty? Later on choices are made as to what job to take. Once on the job, one soon encounters opportunities to participate in decisions that affect the future success of the organization. All of these challenges require that assumptions be made as to how conditions may or may not change over time.

The Forecasting Process

Admittedly, the common advice to "live in the here and now" seems quite valid. Much of life consists of handling tasks that obviously must be done and thus offer us little choice. But now and then we come to a "fork in the road," and it becomes exceedingly useful to take a hard look toward the future—even though the view may be quite foggy and indistinct. Alvin Toffler (1989:xx–xxi), who has written three quite influential books on this subject, describes both the pitfalls and the values of such an endeavor.

> It hardly seems necessary to add that the future is not "knowable" in the sense of exact prediction. Life is filled with surrealistic surprise. . . . Statistics change. New technologies supplant older ones. Political leaders rise and fall. Nevertheless, as we advance into the terra incognita of tomorrow, it is better to have a general and incomplete map, subject to change and correction, than to have no map at all.

The key point here is the value of a map, even if crude. Exact prediction is impossible, but probabilities can often be estimated with a fair degree of accuracy and over time will give the thoughtful decision maker a definite edge. Futurists such as Toffler, as well as many other observers of the American scene, have developed many tools useful for the construction of their futuristic maps. Demographic trends, for example, are relatively easy to plot and often provide useful information for the advanced planning of health education programs, as well as other health services that must be tailored to the needs of specific age groups. Currently, in the 1990s, we have a smaller proportion of people in their sixties, compared with earlier decades, because of the lower birth rate prevailing during the depression decade of the 1930s; it takes no great skill to predict that there will also be a smaller proportion of people in their seventies as the new century begins, although the estimate requires an adjustment for the steadily increasing survivability of older Americans.

Innovations, such as cellular telephones, generally go through a predictable sequence of technological refinement, improvement of production methods with consequent reduction of costs, establishment of marketing and distribution systems, and eventual widespread adoption. Managers of mutual funds and other investors regularly stake large sums of money on their ability to gauge the pace of this cycle. Although the stages may vary in length, the whole process is generally measured in years rather than months. Both penicillin and the Pap smear were discovered in the 1920s but were not widely used until the late 1940s. And this lag between invention and application doesn't appear to be shortening. Air bags, for example, were conceived in the 1950s and are now just beginning to gain widespread acceptance. One obvious implication that arises from these observations is that if the solution to some current problem is in the theory or early developmental stage, such as genetic engineering for example, don't expect much relief in the next few months.

One common mistake in estimating the future consequences of current trends is to ignore the probability of some sort of societal reaction. Too often some self-styled expert will simply plot some measurable trend on a sheet of graph paper and then extend the line along its average slope to support some doomsday or Pollyanna scenario. Whether or not it is ethical to use such tactics to jolt the general public out of its apathy and precipitate the desired societal reaction is arguable; however, health educators as professionals should always seek the most accurate assessment of health related situations. During the late 1960s and early 1970s, for example, many predicted that the world's population would outpace food production and that petroleum would be exhausted by the turn of the century, thus raising the threat of massive famines, energy shortages, and subsequent economic chaos. More astute observers could foresee that people would not stand idly by as these problems intensified. World food production increased as the so-called "green revolution" accelerated; population growth was moderated by both the natural result of increased urbanization and industrialization and the deliberate intervention of various programs of population control; and the rising prices of gasoline, heating oil, and other petroleum products initiated a wave of conservation measures. These responses did not provide a complete solution to these threatening problems; however, as so often happens, they prevented the dramatic tragedy and reduced the problems to manageable levels.

With the various limitations of the prognostication process in mind, the approach selected for this chapter includes an effort to identify the most durable trends which appear relevant to health education, to anticipate any major changes in these trends, and to suggest through cautious speculation what the implication will be for health education as a professional field. The trends are categorized into those occurring within (1) society at large, (2) health-related organizations and institutions, and (3) health education itself. (See figure 16.1.)

Figure 16.1

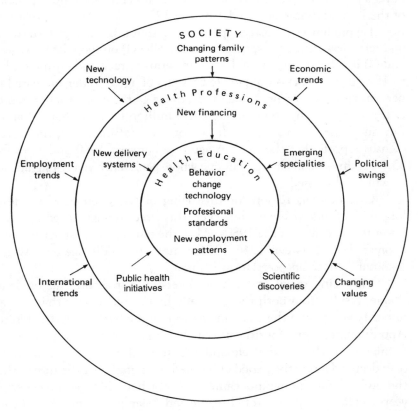

Sources of change. The future of health education is affected by external influences from society at large and the other health professions, along with its own internal changes.

Societal Trends

Modern societies tend to be highly interdependent; consequently, individuals and organizations frequently are affected by events that are seemingly unrelated to their welfare. The more successful leaders in business and industry, and among various professional groups, generally try to stay informed about broad societal trends as well as happenings within their own field. In the following pages the more prominent trends related to demographic, economic, political, and cultural factors will be reviewed and discussed in terms of their implications for health education.

Demographic Trends

After a period of rapid growth during the 1950s and 1960s the population growth of the United States slowed during the 1970s and 1980s to a relatively steady rate of approximately 1 percent per year. Within this stable pattern two important and relentless trends are apparent, specifically: (1) our population is getting older and (2) it is becoming more diverse in terms of race and ethnicity. From 1980 to 1991 the proportion of people 65 years of age or older increased from 11.3 percent to 12.6 percent, a small percentage gain but one that increases the size of this age group by approximately five million to more than 30 million (U.S. Bureau of the Census, 1992). In a more general indicator, the Bureau of the Census reports that the median age rose between 1980 and 1991 from 30 to 33.1. Again, a small change, but one whose persistence yields a significant impact, as will be discussed.

One obvious reason for this aging of the population is the increased longevity of older citizens; however, this effect is augmented by the generally lower fertility rates of the 1980s. Also, the nation's largest age group, the baby boomers born between 1946–1964, is now in middle age and its aging has a dominant effect on population statistics.

Increasing racial and ethnic diversity, our second major demographic theme, results from both the generally higher birth rates that prevail among minority groups and the changing pattern of immigration to the United States. Approximately one-fourth of our nation's population gain results from immigration whereas the remainder is internal growth, i.e., the net of births over deaths. During the period of heaviest immigration at the turn of the century, the bulk of our immigrants came from northern Europe; however, in recent years a greater proportion of Hispanic and Asian people make up the immigrant population. The percentage of black Americans in the United States increased modestly from 11.7 to 12.1 percent from 1980 to 1990; during the same period the percentage of Hispanics increased from 6.4 to 9.0 percent, Asian-Pacific Islanders from 1.5 to 2.9 percent, and Native Americans from 0.6 to 0.8 percent. In terms of race, these increases together bring the proportion of minorities in our population from 16.8 percent to 19.7 percent over a 10-year period;

encompassed within this pattern is the aforementioned growth of the Hispanic population (6.4 percent to 9.0 percent) who may be of any race. These trends seem destined to continue into the foreseeable future. The U.S. Bureau of the Census (1993) provides low, middle, and high range estimates of projected changes in the size of the various population groups for the coming years. The middle range forecasts suggest that, by the year 2000, blacks will comprise 12.9 percent of the population, Hispanics 11.1 percent, Asian-Pacific Islanders 4.5 percent, and Native Americans 0.9 percent. This steady increase in the minority group proportion of the population appears important and substantial but in no way overwhelming in view of our cultural tradition of diversity and assimilation.

Figure 16.2 Growth of Minority Populations in the U.S., 1980–1990

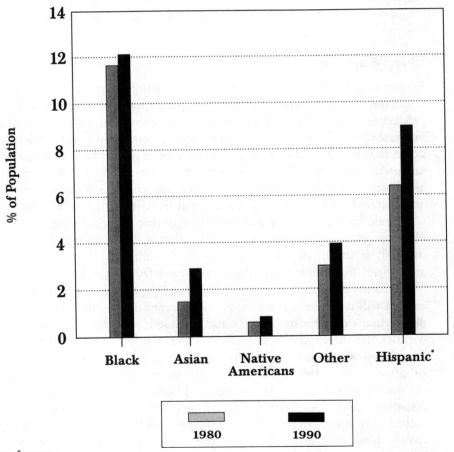

*May be of any race

Source: U.S. Bureau of the Census, *Statistical Abstract of the United States: 1992* (112th Edition). Washington, DC, 1993.

Economic Trends

As noted in chapter 2, the health status of individuals is closely related to their economic status; poverty appears as a powerful determinant of a wide variety of health problems. The general strength of the nation's economy is related to the poverty problem in two important ways. A strong economy creates both a greater number of jobs and more higher paying jobs; this situation prevents many people from falling into poverty because of unemployment and provides the opportunity for others to escape from their low-income status by their own efforts. A second effect of a strong economy is the creation of added revenues for publicly-funded targeted programs so that the residual "hard-core" poverty problem can be attacked. As corporate profits and individual incomes increase, tax revenues automatically increase; and even if additional tax increases seem necessary to solve social problems, such actions are less burdensome and meet less resistance in an expanding economy. The middle- and upper-income classes can contribute more to the cause and still pursue their own versions of the "American dream." As will be discussed, the prospects for this positive scenario are not encouraging.

Slow Wage Growth

Economic growth among mature industrial nations such as our own generally fluctuates within a relatively narrow range, with anything below 2 percent producing considerable economic pain in the form of unemployment and business failures. On the other hand, a 5 percent rate represents a veritable economic boom that is seldom sustainable for more than a year or two. During the 1800s and early 1900s, these fluctuations were often extreme, taking the form of "boom and bust" cycles which provided financial opportunities for nimble traders but considerable pain for most other participants. Fortunately, several factors have combined to reduce economic volatility during the past couple of decades, although economists frequently caution that it could return. At this writing in 1995, we are in an economic recovery that offers to provide growth in the area of a 3 percent annual rate for the next few years. The widely followed Value Line (1995) investment service, for example, predicts that annual GDP growth will range between 2.7 and 3.4 percent during 1995–98. Such a pace pleases many economists and investors because it provides a modicum of growth without the inflationary pressures that eventually produce a recession.

But while many upscale Americans are content with the current economic situation of the 1990s, there are aspects unique to this period that put considerable pressure on the average middle-income worker and create a near disastrous situation for those lacking the specialized skills that college or advanced technical training can provide. This modest, less than robust, economic growth has combined with other changes in the workplace to create what many pundits have termed "jobless prosperity," a phrase which identifies the focal point of the problem but distorts its nature. Americans are finding jobs; even in the recession year of 1991, 118 million people or approximately 62 percent of our population were employed (U.S. Bureau of the Census, 1992). However, a disproportionate number of these jobs tended to be in the lower paying service sector rather than the manufacturing sector; moreover, several factors have combined to restrict pay raises in virtually all forms of employment, regardless of sector. After adjustments for inflation, the hourly earnings for U.S. workers have been stagnant since 1973, a contradiction of the American tradition of each generation achieving a better life than the previous one (Cyert and Mowery, 1989).

International Competition

The added pressure on the American worker results in part from the advent of international competition. In the 1950s and 1960s the economies of most nations were largely self-contained; they created and served their own markets; their respective wealth or poverty tended to be retained within their borders. More so than today, the economic welfare of workers depended on what nation they happened to be born in; relatively unskilled workers in rich countries could earn a living wage, whereas even skilled workers in poor countries might live in poverty. Beginning perhaps in the 1970s this situation largely changed. Communication satellites and other technology broke down many of the cultural barriers to international trade. It was easier to determine consumer preferences and target overseas markets, which in any event were becoming more similar as people watched the same television programs, listened to the same music, and wore the same clothes. Global transportation networks made it easier to deliver goods in remote locations; and government trade restrictions eased because of a combination of motives such as changing ideologies, the need for reciprocal access to markets, and the demands of domestic consumers.

On balance the advent of international competition has yielded several benefits. The American consumer, for example, has enjoyed lower prices, a broader selection of products and, in some cases, better quality; moreover, many overseas markets became available to American business firms and many heretofore poor nations were able to improve their living standards. But the opening of world markets exposed many American companies to competitive pressures that prompted them to streamline their operations to reduce labor costs. Although the process took longer than expected, the efficient use of computers reduced the size of clerical staffs and eliminated many middle management positions. Within manufacturing operations, the pace of automation was greatly accelerated. The net effect of all this was that many workers lost their jobs and many companies were able to expand their business without expanding their labor force.

Not surprisingly, both American workers and business firms have generally proven themselves to be flexible, resilient, and adaptable in the face of new global challenges. Although there have been widespread layoffs, many small firms have been started and many former middle managers have found new economic life as private consultants.

Technical Demands on Workers

Back in the 1960s when most manufacturing jobs required relatively simple skills, many young men could drop out of high school at age sixteen and go to work in steel mills or automobile factories with good prospects of soon earning more than the teachers they left behind. Since that time, most jobs that offer the chance to earn good wages have become much more complex, technically demanding, and rapidly changing. Prospects are still good for those with specialized training and the ability to adapt to the changing demands of the workplace. However, the outlook is bleak for entry level workers with poor basic skills. They frequently find employment—but in jobs paying minimum or near minimum wages. As Cyert and Mowery (1989:59) point out:

> Even if technological progress were to stop tomorrow, the employment prospects for labor force entrants who lack strong fundamental skills would be dismal. Those same skills will be even more important in finding and retaining quality jobs in the future.

Currently 21 percent of American children live in families with incomes below the poverty line; among Hispanics and African American children a shocking 39 and 46 percent, respectively, find themselves in a similar situation (National Center for Health Statistics, 1994). These poverty-level families are frequently headed by a single parent who may be ill equipped in terms of time, energy, and ability to provide the help and support children need to do well in school; and where poverty rates are high, school districts often lack funds and are thus unable to meet the special needs of economically disadvantaged children. These children often enter adulthood with poor employment opportunities and higher risks of crime, drug abuse, early pregnancies, and other health liabilities.

Medical Care Inflation

The very high and ever increasing costs of medical care also impact directly on the American employment situation. Large employers in particular have traditionally been expected to provide health insurance as a benefit to their employees. Moreover, with the constant threat of new government legislation on health care, many small businesses fear that they may have to bear the cost of health insurance for any worker they may add to their payrolls. In an effort to control or avoid this major cost factor, employers faced with the need for more output have often opted to work their current employees overtime, hire temporary or part-time workers, or increase their efforts at automation; obviously, none of these actions help the prospects of those seeking full-time employment.

Even when employers decide to add workers to their payroll and provide full benefits, the individual employee's economic welfare is diminished by the current high costs of health care. Every dollar paid for employee health insurance is one less dollar available for employee take-home pay. In order to keep their cost structures low enough to compete with foreign firms, who pay uniformly lower rates either in taxes or premiums for health insurance, employers must keep wages and other benefits low. In the United States during 1991 an average of $2,868 was spent on each citizen as compared with $1,659 in Germany and $1,267 in Japan (National Center for Health Statistics, 1994). This suggests that American business firms pay more than twice as much for medical care as their major international competitors, and there is little indication that their work force is any healthier despite this added expenditure. Moreover, every dollar lost to excessive health care costs is one less available for more modern machinery, in-service training, or research and development, all of which can add to worker productivity.

Government and Corporate Debt

The high level of debt of the federal government, as well as many states, municipalities, and corporations, impacts negatively on the average citizen in several ways. The need for governments to service their debt requires them to maintain high rates of taxation and thus restrain economic growth. Every additional dollar employers spend for taxes is one less available for expansion of their company, upgrading of their production equipment, or improvement of worker compensation. Also, the tax dollars collected which could be spent on things that increase economic growth such as better schools, highways, and basic research, now mostly go to pay interest on government bonds. Although many corporations and state and local governments appear to be avoiding or reducing their indebtedness, the federal government, with its approximate four trillion dollar debt, seems destined to be a drag on our overall economic well-being for the foreseeable future.

Political Trends

Within the United States political trends have shown a historic tendency to cycle between liberal and conservative periods of dominance. The presidential administrations of Theodore Roosevelt and Woodrow Wilson of the early 1900s were periods of progressive reform which were followed by 12 years of conservatism during the Coolidge and Hoover administrations. The Franklin D. Roosevelt and Harry Truman administrations of the 1930s and 1940s were characterized by very proactive governmental policies directed at social and economic problems, followed by the two terms of Dwight D. Eisenhower and a greatly reduced role for government. The Kennedy-Johnson "Great Society" period of the 1960s represented perhaps the last major effort at liberal reform. Since that time the cycle has continued, but within a context many would describe as having a long-term secular trend toward a more conservative society. These trends are important to the work of most health educators, whose programs are typically supported by public funds. Liberals are more prone to establish and support government programs to attack social and economic problems. The social security program, Medicaid and Medicare, the Peace Corps, and the

Headstart program, for example, were all established when the more liberal Democratic party held power. Liberals also tend to be distrustful of large corporations and see the need for more government regulation of business to avoid excessive economic power and to protect workers and threats to the environment. Conservatives, however, tend to distrust both governmental regulations and tax-supported programs. They tend to challenge individuals to pull themselves up by "their own bootstraps" and seek to create economic environments that are more rewarding to the ambitious and less kind to the lazy or unskilled. Each of these major political philosophies has its strong points but, historically, both public health and health education tend to receive more support during periods of liberal dominance.

At this writing, we are in the third year of President Clinton's Democratic administration, and there is thus a general expectation of a more active role for government in the attack on various social and economic problems. Yet, any policy initiatives will surely be hampered by both financial and political restraints. The overhanging national debt with its 200- to 300-billion-dollar annual interest charge, together with the current federal budget deficit which keeps adding to this debt, necessitate the channeling of tax revenues into debt service rather than into social programs. Even if these financial realities could be surmounted, in the current political climate the general public shows little appetite for any new government solutions to our problems. Political candidates must generally promise to "hold the line" or cut taxes and reduce government spending to get elected. School bond elections are being regularly defeated in all parts of the nation; both Republican and Democratic candidates alike seek to avoid the liberal image.

At some point a reaction may occur and swing the political pendulum back toward the liberal end of the scale; however, at the current time the conservative philosophy seems likely to prevail; any change may be slow in coming and the liberal reaction may be weak. Two major demographic trends support this prognosis. It has long been observed that age tends to make one more conservative. According to folklore, "Anyone who is not a liberal at twenty has no heart—and anyone who is not a conservative at forty has no head"; consequently, the aforementioned aging of the general population tends to promote a conservative bias to the American scene. Moreover, older citizens tend to be more attentive to the political process; a greater proportion register and vote, thus they tend to have more political power than mere numbers would suggest. One political humorist recently characterized the members of the American Association of Retired Persons as the "Geezers from Hell" because of their very effective performance in the political arena.

People in lower income groups tend to be more liberal whereas the affluent tend to be more conservative. There are many exceptions to this rule; however, on balance the poor tend to look to government to provide some assistance, provide some training, or otherwise help them improve their lot. The more affluent are naturally reluctant to change the status-quo. Although hourly wage rates have not increased appreciably during the past decade, the typical family has managed to increase its income by putting more of its members to work; the principal breadwinner's spouse and often older children now bring in paychecks. At this writing, an estimated 35.7 million or 14.2 percent of the American people have income levels below the official poverty line (U.S. Bureau of the Census, 1993). This is a large group of people who represent a serious national problem; however, it is considerably smaller than was the case when the last period of liberal dominance began in 1960. At that time more than 22 percent of the population was below the poverty line and thus represented a proportionately larger source of liberal support. It appears to be somewhat of a political paradox that as more people escape from poverty it becomes politically more difficult to help those who remain behind.

Cultural Trends

Shifting the view from the narrower economic and political arenas to society at large, two durable trends are found which have important implications for health education. The first of these, greater health consciousness within the general public, is a very positive factor that is the result, at least in part, of the fruits of our past efforts. The second, added stress on the family unit, is a serious health liability which seems to intensify despite the many efforts directed at its control.

Health Consciousness

Throughout history people have displayed a high degree of concern for health, and this characteristic was very much in evidence in the United States during the first half of the century when great progress was made against infectious diseases. However, during the decades of the 1950s and 1960s it became apparent that this threat was largely under control and risk factors for the major chronic diseases were not yet very well identified. The general public tended to remain oblivious to the effects of life-style factors on health status and, among other consequences, saw its middle-aged members suffer twice the mortality rate from heart disease than prevails among their more aware counterparts of the present day.

During the latter part of the 1960s cigarette smoking began to decrease, fish and poultry began to gain favor over beef, and aerobic exercise started to become popular. Although the rate of improvement has slowed recently with occasional backsliding, this pattern still displays the characteristics of a strong trend rather than a mere fad. Annual per capita consumption of red meat has shown a persistent decline from 132 to 112 pounds between 1970 and 1990; during the same period egg consumption declined from 309 to 233, whereas fresh fruits rose from 79 to 92 and fresh vegetables from 89 to 111 pounds (U.S. Bureau of the Census, 1993). Rates of cigarette smoking among adults declined from 33.3 percent in 1979 to 25.4 percent in 1990; also, the proportion of the population reporting heavy use of alcohol dropped from 12 percent to

Figure 16.3 Food Consumption Trends in the U.S., 1970–1990

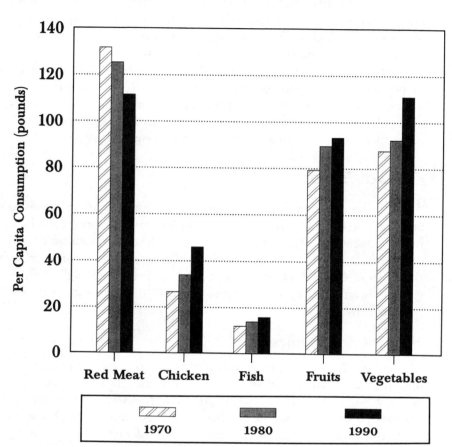

Source: U.S. Bureau of the Census, *Statistical Abstract of the United States: 1992* (112th Edition). Washington, DC, 1993.

9 percent between 1985 and 1990, thus reducing this risky category by almost two million (National Center for Health Statistics, 1994). Seat belt and children's car seat use continues to increase, and air bags have become a desired feature among new-car buyers. The demand for nutritional labeling of packaged foods has increased, and salad bars are more in evidence among fast-food establishments.

On balance this durable trend has very positive implications for most programs of health education and health promotion; people are generally more receptive to new campaigns and more likely to participate in the programs offered. However, at times the zeal for "clean living" has a negative effect on some programs, particularly in school settings when school boards seek to stifle full discussion of sensitive topics in the drug, alcohol, and sexuality area. As Engs (1991:158) notes, ". . . some school personnel are not allowed to discuss, much less demonstrate, techniques for low-risk and responsible drinking or sexuality." Fortunately, there are many other examples of school-based programs wherein the teachers have the freedom to function effectively in the classroom. In others, however, the struggle continues and much of the resistance comes from parents who are finding it increasingly difficult to cope with family responsibilities.

Family Stress

On balance, conditions appear to have improved considerably for the American family throughout the current century. Because of easier access to contraceptives, the availability of abortion, and the increased social acceptance of unmarried parents, fewer forced marriages result from unplanned pregnancies. Once a marriage or cohabitation partnership is formed, childbearing is frequently delayed; thus fewer dysfunctional marriages are held together out of concern for children. Employment opportunities for women, although lacking full equality, have been steadily improving; wives are more frequently equal contributors to the family income. A loss of job by either partner is still a serious economic blow, but not as devastating as in former times when the husband was frequently the sole breadwinner.

The net effect of these modern changes has been to provide more options, more latitude to partnerships tailored to the individual characteristics of the two people involved, and far less tendency to trap people in dead-end situations as so often occurred during the early years of the century when children usually came early, women were dependent on their husbands for economic survival, divorce laws were more restrictive, and divorce itself carried a heavy stigma. This added freedom, however, has not come without cost; society appears to be in a painful period of transition between the old and new family patterns. As noted, wages when adjusted for inflation have not increased since the early 1970s; thus, for most families, the garnering of two paychecks has become the only way to meet reasonable expectations for their family income. But while the expectation is very real, the various social and economic mechanisms needed to implement this expectation have been slow in coming.

The frequent lack of affordable day-care services for children places a severe burden on many families. Even in the intact family this problem is often more stressful to women who, because of tradition or the secondary status of their job, still assume more responsibility for childrearing. Women are also seven times more likely than men to be single parents, a situation which compounds the difficulties. But whether there be one parent or two, the challenges are severe. The common struggle to find suitable care, the transportation arrangements that are often required, the adjustments for changing work schedules, the frequent reliance on relatives or friends, create emotional stress for all involved. Even parents with good incomes frequently have difficulties;

for low-income parents the choice is often poor care or no care, a situation that frequently puts the children at risk. Naisbit and Aburdene (1990) note that the number of companies that provide day-care as an employee benefit has increased by 40 percent since 1984 and optimistically predict that it will become increasingly common, although they also note that 90 percent of firms with 10 or more employees still provide no assistance. Legislation was recently enacted requiring employers to provide day-care facilities for their employees; however, small businesses were excluded and larger employers now have a motive to discriminate against women in their hiring practices. Tax supported programs would appear to provide a more complete solution, but the political climate is currently not very accommodating to such proposals.

A more intractable problem is posed by the common need to change jobs either out of necessity because of layoffs or transfers or because a desirable opportunity opens up elsewhere. Such a situation may arise when one's spouse is comfortably settled into a hard earned, secure, and satisfying job. A frequent result is the restriction of one career to accommodate the other, long distance commuting, or separate living arrangements. The attendant stress these demands may place on the couple's relationship is obvious. Perhaps when we move further beyond the industrial era into the new "information age" that is so frequently projected, a job change will only require that we program a different phone number into the modem of our computer; but for most of us, that day is not yet in sight.

The stress that these and related modern pressures are placing on the family unit are reflected in a number of adverse results. The prevalence of divorced persons in the United States continues to soar; the rate per 1000 married persons increased from 47 in 1970, to 100 in 1980, to 142 in 1990. The percentage of children living with two parents continues to decline from 85.2 percent in 1970, to 76.7 percent in 1980, to 72.5 percent in 1990. Although data related to child abuse and neglect are difficult to obtain and interpret, it appears that children are suffering serious consequences from the pressures on the family unit. The suicide rate for children 15 through 19 years of age increased from 3.5 per 100,000 in 1960 to 11.1 in 1990, while homicide rates for this age group increased from 4.0 to 11.7 in the same period (National Center for Health Statistics, 1993). Rising rates for child abuse and continuing disappointments with school performance also suggest that all is not well in the family unit.

Implications of Current Societal Trends

Certain groups within our society typically are more at risk for health problems than the general population. These include the elderly, racial and ethnic minorities, and those newly immigrating to the country. In general these groups are increasing in size and are destined to become ever larger proportions of the total population. Another high-risk group, the poor, although not increasing significantly, are not diminishing and seem trapped in poverty because of their low educational level and poor job skills. Meanwhile, in mainstream society the family unit is under considerable stress as young couples often must cope with demands of two careers while raising children. These trends create ever increasing demands for all forms of health services, including programs for health education/promotion. During the foreseeable future, at least, this challenge must be addressed within the context of a generally conservative political climate and a federal government hampered by a historically high level of debt.

Trends within Health-Related Organizations

The health professions, with all their attendant activities, form a social and economic component so broad and diverse as to almost defy description. In terms of sheer size the health care industry with its various practitioners, hospitals and clinics, drug companies, and other vendors is by far the dominant segment. The public health establishment, with its broad array of federal, state, and local organizations, is the philosophical home for most community health educators, even though they may be employed by any of a variety of voluntary health organizations, private foundations, or private sector business firms. The public schools, with their programs of health services and education, form another major health related organization whose problems, activities, and future prospects have direct bearing on the overall future of health education/promotion.

Health Care Industry

An increasingly large share of public attention seems destined to be directed toward health care issues throughout the 1990s. In economic terms, it is America's premier growth industry with drug, medical supply, and health service stocks being some of the most durable performers on Wall Street. It is one of the most promising sources of new jobs, with most employment specialties expanding and entirely new ones created every year as new technology becomes available. In terms of human interest it is a consistent focus of media attention, as promising innovations in drug therapy or surgical techniques are reported.

Many positive aspects of health care in the United States can be noted: American high-tech medicine is undoubtedly the world's best; former Surgeon General C. Everett Koop often maintained that the approximate two-thirds of Americans with good health insurance receive the best medical care in the world. In selected cases it can save lives and prevent disability; even when it fails it often provides comfort and relieves suffering. However, as noted in chapter 3, there are a number of problems associated with health care that directly or indirectly have a negative impact on society's overall health status. Its overblown reputation as preserver and restorer of health tends to distract public attention from more important issues related to life-styles and living standards; it tends to neglect primary care and prevention in favor of narrow specialization and after-the-fact treatment; it attracts a disproportionate amount of the nation's talented people into its ranks, much to the detriment of other professional fields.

Serious Problems

These particular complaints will probably be discussed and debated for decades without forcing any substantial change, but two other closely related issues have considerable potential for driving events during the current decade. First, health care costs are rising faster than the general inflation rate and, in several ways, are causing economic pain and indirect health liabilities to large segments of the population. Secondly, at this writing approximately 35 million Americans have no health insurance and thus frequently go without essential services. The details of the cost problem are complex; however, any careful analysis reveals that (1) the sums are vast, (2) they are increasing faster than the nation's gross income, and (3) the proposed solutions are fraught with political difficulties.

For years we have lamented over the amount of money that is spent on national defense and worried about the interest payments on our growing national debt. The $752 billion spent on health care in 1991 would cover the $273 billion defense budget and the $286 billion interest on the debt, with enough left over to fund at least one-third of the nation's public schools. During the period 1980–91 the annual rate of increase for these costs was 10.6 percent as compared with a 5.4 rate for the overall economy. During 1991, health care costs comprised over 14 percent of our gross national product, which means that 14 percent of all the goods and services we produced that year were devoted to health care. This is a substantially higher rate than the 10 percent posted by Canada, who is our nearest rival for such expenditures, and who incidentally has a much healthier population than ours when measured in terms of infant mortality, longevity, and most other accepted criteria.

The effects of these high costs on the average citizen have been heavy and pervasive. They have been a major factor in the failure of real hourly wages to increase since the early 1970s as employers have struggled to provide employees with ever more expensive health insurance; they have been reflected in higher prices for virtually all products; they have thus made American exports less competitive in overseas markets; they have increased both state taxes for Medicaid programs for the poor and federal taxes for both the federal contribution to Medicaid and the full funding of Medicare for senior citizens. They have pressured both governmental agencies and employers to restrict benefits and tighten eligibility requirements to the extent that many of the poor no longer qualify for Medicaid, employers are increasingly reneging on their commitment to cover family members and retirees, and Medicare recipients find they must purchase supplemental policies if they are to retain good coverage.

Feeble Response

But while the effects on the public have been profound, the reaction has been relatively mild, diffuse, and unfocused. As noted, the approximate two-thirds of the population who are either working for or supported by someone working in a large- or middle-sized business firm or governmental organization are receiving good health care. These reasonably content recipients are actually paying an exorbitant price for this care, but much of the costs are hidden and indirect. During the past 25 years the proportion of health care costs paid directly by households has steadily diminished from 60.5 percent in 1965 to 36.9 percent in 1989; meanwhile the share for business firms has risen from 17.0 percent to 29.7 percent and government's share also rose from 20.7 percent to 30.6 percent (Levit et al., 1991). As a result of this shift, most people's out-of-pocket costs have been sheltered from the worst of the health care increases. The bulk of the impact on their situation has been in the form of minimal wage increases, higher prices, and reduced government services as tax revenues are redirected into health care. Wage earners, in general, have found it tough to get ahead; they know that something is wrong and have finally begun to realize that health costs are involved; however, they appear to have little understanding of the complexities of the problem. Meanwhile, employers with their presumably clearer view of these trends find the situation tolerable because they have been largely successful in passing the costs on to employees in the form of lower wages. As the chief executive officer of Alcoa Aluminum Corporation said in an interview ". . . most people believe that employers are covering those costs now, but that is not accurate. That money really belongs to employees and would be provided in cash compensation if it weren't being provided in health insurance" (Iglehart, 1991:82).

In regard to governmental costs, the federal government's Medicare costs are producing some strain; but thus far the bulk of the inflation in this area has been successfully passed on to the beleaguered worker in the form of a special Medicare tax which thus far has engendered less public resistance than other tax increases. The most visible part of the problem has been the strain on the various state Medicaid programs which are funded jointly by federal and state governments out of general tax revenues. State governments, in response to increasing costs and taxpayer resistance, have tended to reduce eligibility requirements as their major strategy. Consequently, the ranks of those with no health insurance, or with inadequate coverage, have grown and placed a strain on hospitals and individual health practitioners, who find themselves burdened with increasing amounts of uncompensated care. Their response to this loss of revenue has been to try, with varying success, to shift costs to other patients in the form of higher fees for per diem costs for hospital rooms or office visits, and other procedures.

Policy Gridlock

There are a number of powerful factors that mitigate against a solution to our nation's health care muddle anytime soon. The bulk of the costs are indirect and hidden from the general public; the huge sums involved tend to paralyze action even among knowledgeable persons who fear that any change will shift more of the burden in their direction; very powerful political lobbying groups from the health insurance industry, the drug industry, and health care practitioners have a strong interest in maintaining the status quo; those who are uninsured and suffering the most from the situation are generally poor and without political power; and, finally, all of this is taking place against a backdrop of heavy government debt and a less than robust economy that discourage bold initiatives.

Among the proposed solutions, a very strong case can be made for the adoption of a Canadian style program of national health insurance. In a country that is very similar to the United States both culturally and economically, the Canadian program serves its total population for a per capita cost approximately 33 percent less than ours, based on 1991 figures of $1,915 versus $2,868 (National Center for Health Statistics, 1993). The Canadian system is more popular among its users than the American system; 56 percent of Canadians agreed with the statement that, "On the whole the health care system works pretty well and only minor changes are needed to make it better," as compared with only 10 percent of Americans (Blendon and Taylor, 1989). Finally, as a society, Canadians appear to be healthier than Americans by most accepted measures; infant mortality in 1989, for example, was 7.1 per 1,000 births in Canada as compared with 9.8 in the United States; life expectancy for both males and females was longer in Canada whether measured at birth or at age 65 (National Center for Health Statistics, 1993).

Despite these persuasive considerations, there is little evidence of broad support for this or any other comprehensive proposal. As Paul Starr (1982) points out in his review of the historical aspects of this issue, national health insurance has been proposed periodically since 1915 and routinely rejected. The only exception to this political trend took place in the liberal heyday of the 1960s when the Medicaid and Medicare programs were enacted for the poor and the elderly. Then, as now, the poor were viewed as appropriate recipients of subsidized health care and the elderly at that time were similarly regarded. In contrast to today, their poverty rate was higher, rather than lower, than the general population, thus they appeared as another economically vulnerable group whose medical needs might otherwise go unmet. When considered in this light, the 1994 defeat of the ambitious reform plan proposed by President Clinton was consistent with the public's traditional reluctance to expand the government's role in the provision of health care to the average, economically viable citizen.

This defeat was both a serious political setback for the president and a severe disappointment for many serious students of this issue who note that no other modern, industrialized nation has been able to contain health costs without significant government intervention. The reform movement did manage, however, to focus the nation's attention on cost containment to an extraordinary degree. Employers have been particularly aggressive in their implementation of co-pay provisions while enticing or forcing more of their employees into health maintenance or managed care programs. Due in part to this initiative and perhaps in fear of the threat of government controls, drug companies, hospitals, and health-care providers in general held cost increases to relatively low levels. Congress now seems content to let the private sector bear the burden of cost containment with little or no governmental assistance or interference. At most there may be a bit more regulation of private insurance companies and adjustments in the tax code to provide incentives for efficient programs. Optimistically, this course may lead to the development of a unique, efficient, market-based American system; however, similar efforts in the past have resulted in more complexities, more paperwork, and expensive dislocations and evasions on the part of health-care providers. In any event, health care costs seem destined to be a major issue for Americans over the next several years.

Public Health Agencies

As a distinct professional field, health education's future, particularly that of community health education, is closely intertwined with the broader area of public health. Generally the prospects for its support, funding, public recognition, and so forth parallel that of its larger parent. Although the field of public health in the 1990s is sailing into political and economic headwinds, it is nonetheless making progress along a carefully charted course.

Historical Transition

Public health in the United States probably reached its high point of public support in the "glory days" of the fight against infectious diseases which took place in the first half of the present century. Much of this support waned during the 1950s and 1960s as the concern for infectious diseases receded and clinical medicine captured the public eye and sought to claim the field of chronic disease as its own private preserve. Rogers (1974), for example, noted that "in the last decade we have seen the progressive weakening of local, county and state public health departments." Although support began to increase during the 1970s and 1980s, a committee report of the prestigious Institute of Medicine in 1988 still judged the situation to be poor and suggested ". . . that this nation has lost sight of its public goals and has allowed the system of public activities to fall into disarray" (Institute of Medicine, 1988; as found in Breslow, 1990). This assessment seems overly harsh in view of the notable projects that were underway; it probably reflects concern over the obvious gap between then-current achievements and what was possible, given optimal support.

Goals Movement

One of the most visible means of promoting the public health movement in recent years as been the goals movement. Breslow (1990) credits the Lalone Report (1974), which established a goal-setting approach as a guide to Canadian public health policy, with providing the inspiration for a similar effort in the United States. In 1978 the Institute of Medicine of the National Academy of Sciences sponsored a conference on health promotion and disease prevention which led to a request by the Surgeon General of the U.S. Public Health Service to review current health progress. This review culminated in the publication of *Healthy People: The Surgeon General's Report on Health Promotion and Disease Prevention* (1979). As noted in chapter 1, this report attracted widespread public attention because of its quite positive assessment of the overall health of the American public and its establishment of goals to be attained by 1990.

This initial effort at goal setting provided useful guidance for the allocation of resources and in a number of instances, including a widely publicized mid-course review included in *Health, United States 1987* (National Center for Health Statistics, 1988), brought media attention to both notable examples of health progress and continuing problems. This experience prompted a more ambitious goal-setting effort for the 1990s which resulted in the publication of *Healthy People 2000* (USDHHS, 1990), a weighty document that provides a comprehensive national plan in a bit less than 700 pages. McGinnis (1990) points out a number of differences between these two national projects, some of which provide implications for health education while others offer help in the never ending task of attracting public funds. In regard to this latter purpose, the development process was very broad based, involving 300 organizations and more than 10,000 people—all of whom presumably have thus acquired a vested interest in the project. Secondly, throughout its development it was planned with a view towards implementation. "Careful planning was . . . undertaken early in the formulation process to identify strategies for translating the national objectives into health promotion program plans at many levels and within many sectors" (McGinnis, 1990:247).

In features that directly apply to health education, the greater number of problems addressed has resulted in many more objectives that are directly expressed in behavioral terms rather than in health status. Also, McGinnis (1990:244) noted that "a social consensus is emerging that our national goals ought not to be based on mortality reductions alone, but also on principles of reduced disability and improved quality of life. . . ." This appears to represent a significant move toward full acceptance of the World Health Organization's concept of positive health.

One of the major criticisms of the *Healthy People 2000* project may pose something of a dilemma for health educators. As one of the major goals the framers of the report specified the reduction of the serious discrepancies between the total population and special groups, namely, the poor, some racial and ethic minority groups, and people with disabilities; this goal was well received by most health personnel. However, many of this group were quite critical when, upon reviewing the specific objectives, they found a strong emphasis on behavioral change and little emphasis on providing these disadvantaged populations with the material help needed to maintain healthy life-styles. Many viewed this as a "victim-blaming approach" emanating out of the then-strong conservative bias of the federal government. There is some risk here that health education may be viewed as the low-cost alternative to health improvement and used inappropriately to the neglect of improvements in food supplements, housing, and medical services.

Public Schools

The prospects for health education within the public schools for the 1990s present a muddled picture on several accounts. Because of unfavorable comparisons between the performance of American schoolchildren and those of other countries, both public officials and the popular press have been highly critical of the public schools in recent years. Although much of this criticism is probably unjustified, it nonetheless tends to undermine financial support and generate strong demands for changes in current practices. This situation has been further aggravated by demographic trends wherein an increasing proportion of the electorate, including older adults, childless young professionals, and parents who have sent their children to private schools, no longer have a direct, vested interest in the welfare of their local public school. This situation, together with continuing public disenchantment with tax-supported programs, has tended to undermine the financial support of public schools and thus makes it difficult to initiate or expand any program that is not currently well entrenched. Moreover, the prevailing educational philosophy encourages more emphasis on "hard" subject matter and less on "softer" areas such as art, music, home economics, and, unfortunately, health education. Means (1962:383) noted several years ago that "school health education made most rapid advances during periods of progressive educational philosophy as contrasted with periods of traditional educational emphasis."

The difficulties that currently exist within many school districts were illustrated quite dramatically in a recent study by Smith and others (1992) in which the eight districts that had participated in the School Health Curriculum Project (SHCP) from 1969 to 1974 were surveyed to determine the current status of their programs. These settings were selected originally because of the promising conditions they appeared to offer for this model curriculum which embodied the concept of comprehensive school health education and which has since undergone several successful evaluations and thus proven its effectiveness. The survey revealed that only two of the original eight districts continued to fully implement the program. The status of the program was reported as "questionable" in two other districts and dropped completely in four. As the investigators report:

> District issues such as limited instructional budgets, compatibility of the program with the mission of the district, training new teachers, curricular replacement materials, coordination of implementation, and the low priority generally assigned to health instruction, may make institutionalization of any health curricula difficult. (Smith, Redican and Olsen, 1992:86)

As this study illustrates, many school districts are willing to support comprehensive school health education programs as long as external funding is available but frequently drop or cut them back when such funding expires. These and other factors have made it difficult for public schools to fully realize their potential contribution to the nation's health. Currently, in many school districts it is difficult to get administrative or teaching positions established for staff members who are fully committed to health education. Consequently, much school health education is taught and administered by physical education teachers, science teachers, guidance counselors, and other such persons whose main professional interests lie elsewhere. These nonspecialists frequently do creditable, even outstanding jobs of teaching health education. The typical public school system, however, has a crowded curriculum and limited funds; in such an environment, the programs that thrive have strong, dedicated, internal advocates willing to lobby vigorously for time allotments, curriculum revision, and needed equipment and materials. Given current trends, it is difficult to get people with such feeling for health education placed in school districts where they do not presently exist.

On a more positive note, the public schools currently enjoy increasing attention from external groups, particularly community health educators based in other organizations who see the schools as attractive sites for reaching target populations. The recent expansion of the concept of the school health program, which calls for greater involvement of public schools with community programs of health education/promotion, should encourage this trend. The expanded comprehensive school health program concept is also augmented by the strong movement toward school worksite health promotion programs as initiated by Tritsch (1991). Thus far 25 states have invited their school districts to send "teams" of participants to state conferences designed to train leaders of school based programs of health promotion for school personnel. Although such programs do not always have direct impact on the school health program as provided for the students, they do seem to enhance the prospects for good employee programs and thus set the stage for future gains for the total program (Drolet and Fetro, 1991).

Voluntary Health Organizations and Private Foundations

In theory at least, the current public disfavor with tax-supported solutions to social problems should be counterbalanced by stronger support for local volunteerism and various forms of philanthropy which appear as more effective and efficient vehicles. Presumably the downward pressure on taxes frees more dollars for charitable contributions. Although it is very doubtful that increased support of charitable organizations has offset cuts in the public sector, total philanthropic contributions do appear to be rising. The total amount of such monies expended for health increased from $5.3 to $9.9 billion between 1980 and 1990 (U.S. Bureau of the Census, 1992). This increase appears to be only slightly faster than inflation; however, this near $10 billion total is substantial and represents an important source of support for health education. Although the level of their funding may be affected by short-term swings in our economy, private foundations and voluntary health organizations are not likely to lose funding during the remainder of the decade and may even see a modest increase in the growth of their revenues.

Voluntary health organizations such as the American Heart Association or the American Cancer Society are typically funded by individual contributions. They regard education of the public as one of their key responsibilities, along with research and provision of health services in selected situations. As their name implies, they rely heavily on volunteers; however, they also employ health professionals as administrators and organizers, a group which includes health educators.

Private foundations usually do not provide direct services but fund research and various projects which they deem worthy and within their area of interest. They are typically endowed with large amounts of cash, securities, or other forms of capital. Among organizations taking a special interest in health issues is the Robert Wood Johnson Foundation, which has assets of over $3 billion and throughout its history has awarded more than $1 billion in grants. The Metropolitan Life Foundation for many years has been an active supporter of school health projects. Such organizations are generally established by individuals or corporations as living memorials to favored persons or as a public relations vehicle. Although their type and source of funding vary, they are often established in perpetuity, meaning that they operate on the income generated by their capital. Health and medical projects are often selected as recipients of foundation support and, within this category, health education has benefited in the past and should do even better in the future.

Merlin Duval (1981) notes that while many foundations are sympathetic to the cause of medicine, they generally avoid the funding of direct medical services. This policy is prompted by the desire of many of the trustees and other decision makers to be on the leading edge of movements—to support innovations rather than spend money on causes that are already proven and thus commonly well supported by other sources. The strong relationship of unfavorable behaviors to modern health problems, the promising improvements in behavioral change technology, and the inadequate degree of support for health education from other sources, combine to make this field an appropriate target for foundational support.

Private Sector

Worksite Health Promotion

The steady increase in the proportion of business firms offering some type of worksite health education programs represents another very persistent and promising trend for the future of health education. Green and Kreuter (1991:308) note this remarkable growth and suggest it

> . . . has been influenced by four phenomena: (1) changing demographic profiles in most workplaces, (2) growing concern for the burden on industry of rising medical care costs, health insurance premiums, and costs of lost productivity in

unhealthy workers, (3) recognition of the greater influence of behavior and environment on health, and (4) emerging evidence that health education and health promotion strategies have been effective in altering the behavioral and environmental precursors of health.

In regard to changing demographic profiles Green and Kreuter noted the ever increasing proportion of adults who have joined the work force in recent years. During 1989, for example, among persons over age 16 years, 76 percent of all men and 57 percent of all women were either employed or looking for employment. Thus, in addition to the internal advantages to the employer to offer health education, the worksite with its high concentration of population is also popular among external groups, such as voluntary health organizations, who offer health education programs.

There are, of course, several factors that give the firm itself a vested interest in the health of its employees. For example, American industry is already losing several million dollars annually because of employee alcoholism and premature deaths, many of which result from heart disease. This, along with health education's continually improving effectiveness, represent incentives that promise to become more intense.

There are other ways to lose the services of valued employees than through illness or death. They can move to another firm, retire early or, in perhaps the worst case, continue in service as disgruntled and marginal performers. Fitness and wellness programs are proving to be one of the more important methods to develop employee loyalty and raise morale. It is one of the few "nice things" that can be done for employees that is also cost effective. Another incentive, which is not yet in place but seems imminent, is the possibility of reduced rates for employee medical, disability, and life insurance plans. Although the costs are generally passed along to the employee in the form of reduced wages and salaries, anything that reduces costs or improves profits puts more money into the negotiation process and makes it easier to achieve a mutually satisfying settlement.

The heightened interest in worksite health education/promotion programs has prompted the development of a National Resource Center on Worksite Health Promotion. It is the result of the cooperative efforts of the Office of Disease Prevention and Health Promotion of the U.S. Public Health Service and the Washington Business Group on Health (Birkel and Muchnick, 1990). This organization provides a national repository of information on current programs around the country and also conducts national forums to disseminate information and resolve issues that develop as this movement continues.

Fee-for-Service Health Promotion

One of the newest and most exciting of the modern opportunities for health educators is found in programs that sell health education services directly to the consumer on a fee-for-service basis. A number of strong demographic, cultural, and economic trends appear to be continually improving the prospects for strong growth in this area. The leading edge of the postwar population bulge has moved into its middle adult years, which are typically the best earning and spending years. This natural advantage is augmented by the prevalence of two-paycheck families with few or no children. As compared with past generations, this group is well educated, raised on high expectations, and has demonstrated a penchant for self-improvement. Beyond the positive concern for self-development lies the negative motivation to cope with stress and maintain health during a busy, sometimes crushing schedule. These dynamics create a good market for commercialized health education in the form of weight control, smoking cessation, and stress management programs. Also, a few wellness programs have developed into a comprehensive approach to life-styling. Finally, we find that fitness centers are tending to broaden their programs to include attention to nutrition and weight control.

Implications of Trends within Health-Related Organizations

As noted in this section, two major trends among health-related organizations are evident. Health care costs are increasing rapidly and are prompting strong, although only partially effective efforts at control. Meanwhile, the public health establishment has developed a comprehensive, widely endorsed, and extremely promising master plan for health promotion. This situation has produced an interesting pattern of conflicting forces. Rising health care costs generate the need for programs of prevention while at the same time usurping the funds such programs require. However, both the public sector, specifically Congress and the various state legislatures, and private sector business firms are experiencing such increasing levels of financial pain that prospects are good for improved levels of support for health education/promotion despite the funding difficulties.

Trends within Health Education

As we approach the turn of the century, there is clearly a crucial need for improvement both in individual health behavior and in the environmental conditions related to health, and it is equally clear that programs of health education/promotion have a demonstrated capability to effect these improvements. Current programs are indeed making strong contributions to the nation's quest for improved health; however, this important accomplishment is still only a fraction of what it could be if such efforts received a more adequate level of funding. Fortunately health educators are making steady progress along two important avenues in their efforts to improve this situation: (1) they are doing a better job of marketing their current capabilities, and (2) they are working internally to improve and enhance these capabilities.

Improved Research Base

For much of its history, health education was characterized by practitioners who necessarily were guided by intuition and trial-and-error as they developed their programs. Many of the more successful programs appeared to rely more on high levels of energy and enthusiasm rather than any technical expertise. Fortunately such energy and enthusiasm are now being channeled into programs whose development is based on good research grounded in valid theory. Historically speaking, this is a fairly recent development. The work of Hochbaum, Rosenstock, and others on the health belief model in the 1950s is generally regarded as the beginning of systematic, theory-based research in health behavior (Becker, 1974). The years since have been particularly fruitful as health educators have been both discriminating consumers and adapters of the works of such psychologists as Bandura and Skinner, and effective producers of new knowledge in their own right. This latter effort, while originally spearheaded by investigators recruited from other fields, is now carried forward by others who were trained within schools of public health. Moreover, many of the generic health education programs which grew out of the school health and physical education tradition are now training researchers who are able to make significant contributions to health education's body of knowledge. Health educators now have sound theoretical frameworks on which to plan their programs. As noted by Glanz and others (1990:3), "The body of research in health behavior and health education has grown rapidly over the past two decades, and health education is recognized increasingly as a way to meet public health objectives and improve the success of public health interventions."

Improved Techniques of Planning and Evaluation

As the research into the determinants of health behavior began to yield definitive results, a growing body of knowledge accumulated. This new resource, in turn, provided the basis for the development of systematic planning models designed to translate these new scientific principles into practical programs. Notable examples include the PRECEDE model which developed as a predominantly educational approach by Green and others (1980) and later evolved into the PRECEDE-PROCEED (Green and Kreuter, 1991) model with a heavier emphasis on health promotion, and the even more comprehensive MATCH model (Simons-Morton DG et al., 1988a) which is described in chapter 6. A third model, PATCH as developed by the Centers for Disease Control in the early 1980s (Kreuter, 1992), focuses more on community organization than on direct assaults on individual health behavior. Although not so directly based in theory, its pragmatic approach to political and economic factors makes it a useful addition to the health educator's alternatives.

Notable improvements are also evident in the ability of health educators to evaluate their programs. The importance of this task cannot be overemphasized. In the form of "needs assessment," evaluation provides an accurate guide to the initial process of program development; later, as "formative evaluation" it directs mid-course corrections. In its "summative form," it provides both clear evidence of the effectiveness of good programs and accurate diagnosis of the weaknesses of ineffective programs; the results thus make either a valid case for further support and/or a factual basis for improvement. Accurate and meaningful evaluation may be divided into two important aspects, namely, (1) the development of valid and reliable measuring instruments and/or processes and (2) use of good design in the development of evaluation programs and strategies. In this latter process one must decide what things to consider or measure and when in the overall process such observation should take place. Once these decisions are made, valid measurement is essential to a fair assessment. Here again progress is evident on both fronts. As Green and Lewis (1986:25) note:

> The gaps in our capacity for measurement and evaluation are being filled. Better training of practitioners in the use of and interpretation of measurement and evaluation; more research specialists who have experience in practice; and more effective translation of research and evaluation into theory and policy all have helped close the gap in recent years.

Health educators are thus learning to make accurate measures of things that matter, and this capability translates directly into more effective programs and better community support.

Improved Professional Unity

Historically, health education has suffered from the confusion of an ill-defined membership and the lack of a strong, central professional organization. Although this problem still exists to some degree, considerable progress has been made toward a unified profession, particularly in the past 10 years. Health educators still find themselves dispersed among a number of professional organizations including, for example, The Society for Public Health Education, The Association for the Advancement of Health Education, The American School Health Association, and the section for Public Health Education and Health Promotion of the American Public Health Association; however, in contrast to past decades when the various memberships existed as separate subcultures, considerable cross-fertilization has taken place because of multiple memberships, interorganizational projects, and better communication among the various organizations.

A prime example of this growing cohesiveness is the coalition of the major professional organizations formed to address the problem of common standards for professional preparation; as discussed in chapter 14, this coalition developed a uniform and widely endorsed set of competencies as a guide to the training of entry-level health educators (National Task Force, 1985). Following this major accomplishment, the coalition reconstituted itself as the National Commission for Health Education Credentialing and has recently developed the testing process and other criteria for designating Certified Health Education Specialists

(Patterson, 1992). At this writing the certification movement is at an early and crucial stage of development; however, it appears to be gaining wide acceptance and realizing its promise as a strong and positive influence on the professional preparation of health educators.

Improved Professional Training

One of the most striking developments in the professional preparation of health educators during the 1970s was the vigorous growth in the number of training programs. The Association for the Advancement of Health Education (AAHE) periodically publishes a directory of colleges and universities offering such programs in its *Journal of Health Education*. This source listed 294 schools in 1982, as compared with 104 in 1970 (AAHE Directory, 1982). The number of listed programs declined noticeably throughout the remainder of the 1980s to 215 in 1991 (AAHE Directory, 1991). This decrease probably resulted from the financial difficulties many colleges and universities experienced during this period together with the general swing to more traditional educational philosophies within many institutions which tend to favor traditional liberal arts, as opposed to more applied, programs.

Program quality is, of course, more difficult to assess than quantity. One might hope that the stronger programs survived the attrition of the 1980s while the weaker ones were lost. Comprehensive data on this point have not been gathered; however, informal observations suggest substantial improvements. The faculty of the various departments offering these programs include an increasing number of persons holding public health degrees, often in addition to a graduate degree in school health education. Although schools of public health have no monopoly on expertise in health education, they have much to contribute and this evidence of cross-fertilization is a hopeful sign. The increased emphasis on community, as opposed to school, health education as witnessed by reports in the various professional journals, suggests a constructive response to demographic trends and market realities. Also, the vigorous efforts within the profession to define more closely the body of knowledge and essential competencies of the field cannot help but strengthen the future development of these programs.

Workable Philosophy

On the face of it, the underlying rationale for health education/promotion is simple; life-style factors are important determinants of health status; health education/promotion can make favorable changes in such factors and thus improve individual levels of health. But once this concept is put into practice through the development of specific programs, some complex moral and philosophical issues soon arise. Although these issues are as old as the field itself, they have only recently begun to attract the interest of a significant proportion of health educators; their resolution is one of the important tasks of the current decade.

Victim Blaming

Throughout the relatively brief history of health education its practitioners have pretty much restricted their attention to the health behavior of individuals. Although they have long recognized the fact that poor environmental factors, such as poor working conditions and low economic status, are frequently of equal or greater import to individual health, their typical response has been to help the individual adjust to poor environmental factors. According to this strategy workers laboring under tight deadlines and heavy work loads are taught to go home after work and do relaxation exercises, listen to soothing audiotapes, get a good night's sleep, and come back to the same stressful conditions the next day; low-income parents without enough money to feed and care for their children are taught how to make the best of it with their meager dollars.

For obvious reasons, this way of responding to the needs of clients appeared unduly restricted to many health educators. Accordingly, as Minkler (1989) describes, during the mid-1980s an alternative view of health promotion emerged that sought to help people change poor conditions where possible and appropriate, rather than merely help them adapt passively to these conditions through behavior change. This newly proposed view of the role of health educators requires that they frequently become political activists and lobby city councils, legislators, boards of directors, and other such bodies for needed changes. Health educators who embrace this expanded role may find themselves in the uneasy position of criticizing the business firm or governmental organization that is providing their paycheck. Such cases pose another ethical dilemma, namely, who is the health educator's true client and primary concern? The employer? Or the employees? The urgency and importance of these questions vary considerably depending on the particular health educator's setting and target group; however, they appear destined to command much attention in the coming years.

Paternalism

Our society is based on the concept of individual freedom. Generally we oppose efforts to impose society's will on individuals unless such action is necessary to protect other people's rights. Any effort to protect adult citizens against any misguided personal behavior is termed "paternalism" and regarded by many as an unjust assault on individual autonomy. The Code of Ethics of the Society for Public Health Education, which is perhaps the most widely endorsed of such documents, states unequivocally:

> Health educators must protect the right of individuals to make their own decisions regarding health as long as such decisions pose no threat to the health of others. (Taub et al., 1987:85)

This principle is one of many such pronouncements that is easier to endorse in principle than to apply in actual practice. People may say they accept it and soon after find themselves signing a petition for a law to require all motorcyclists to wear helmets or, perhaps, to increase the criminal penalties for helping someone commit suicide.

Beauchamp (1988:89) argues for a more moderate position stating:

> . . . we must not permit a libertarian and absolute autonomy to be our reigning principle. Instead we must employ a standard of basic autonomy that permits reasonable, minimally intrusive restrictions that yield significant gains in the health and safety of the public.

As discussed throughout this text, there are a number of approaches to the task of behavior change. We can merely inform people as to the safest or healthiest practices; we can present persuasive, or perhaps, deceptive arguments; we can manipulate the environment to provide incentives or disincentives; or we can seek legislation compelling people to "do the right thing." Only the first of these, informing or educating in an unbiased manner, is acceptable to the educational purist. But many would argue that such a position is a philosophical luxury that we cannot afford. The resolution of this issue is a challenging task that has only just begun.

Health Education's Response

Despite the inconsistencies that health educators frequently confront, it should be noted that the bulk of the concern and criticism on ethical and philosophical matters comes from inside the profession itself. Most outsiders—physicians and other health professionals, legislators, business people, parents—expect us to make favorable changes in the behavior of our clients. Although our effectiveness may be criticized, our methods are seldom viewed as too aggressive. In a world of multimillion dollar advertising budgets and diabolically clever marketing ploys, the average health promotion program hardly seems threatening to anyone's autonomy. Our current efforts to improve our philosophical stance represent a response to our own sensitivities rather than to outside pressure. As such, it appears as one of the hallmarks of a strong profession.

Implications of Trends within Health Education

Health education appears to be rapidly evolving into a mature, clearly defined, and highly competent profession. Its programs are becoming more efficient and more predictable. Moreover, its practitioners are communicating more effectively both with other health professionals and with the general public. These positive developments suggest that support for program development and implementation, professional training, and research will continue to grow in the coming years and provide a solid basis for further growth.

Summary

The members of any occupation or professional field are well advised to keep an eye on the future as well as the present. Good decisions about the management of a program or one's personal career usually involve some prediction, estimate, or "best guess" as to the future course of events. Intuition and luck surely play a role in this difficult process, but more effective clues are provided by the assessment of current trends. The genesis of the future usually exists in concrete, visible form in the pattern of present events; the prognosticator's task is to distinguish trends that will endure and perhaps accelerate from mere fads. Within this chapter trends that appear destined to influence the future of health education were identified within (1) society at large, (2) health-related organizations, and (3) health education itself as a professional field.

In regard to the first category, both increased longevity and lower fertility rates among whites appear certain to continue increasing the size of the elderly component of our society. Also, because of both higher birth rates among minority groups and increased immigration, an increasing proportion of our population will be comprised of racial and ethnic minorities. The advent of a more global economy has brought American workers into close competition with their overseas counterparts; this factor together with the increasing technical demands of well-paying jobs has tended to reduce the prospects of the less well educated members of our society of acquiring meaningful employment and a "living wage." The growth of these population groups, who typically are more at risk, seem destined to create an increased demand for health services of all forms, including programs of health education/promotion.

The continuing problem of escalating health care costs appears to present mixed implications. It increases the need for programs of disease prevention and health promotion as cost-containment strategies while, at the same time, it absorbs an increasing proportion of the nation's resources, thus making it difficult to mount the needed programs. This problem is exacerbated by both the conservative political climate and the large national debt, which combine to discourage funding of tax-supported programs. However, the very persuasive case presented by the *Healthy People 2000* plan should insure some degree of increased support despite these difficult obstacles. The prospects also appear favorable for more employer-sponsored worksite programs as business leaders become increasingly aware of the financial benefits of a more healthy work force. Commercial health and fitness programs, as manifested by the growing number of successful health spas and wellness centers, also appear to represent a strong and durable trend.

Current trends within the field of health education appear uniformly positive. As the authors' review the years since the first edition of this text, we find that the field of health education/promotion has made steady progress and held to a remarkably consistent course. The historically fragmented array of professional organizations are communicating better with one another and joining together in joint projects. The earlier Role Delineation Project has progressed as planned into a full-fledged program to insure adequate training levels and professional standards; research has continued; programs have improved. The early tentative steps toward the expanded concept of health promotion are now taken decisively and are both improving program effectiveness and moving health educators closer to the center of the struggle to improve the health of our society. Now more than ever, it is a good time to be a health educator.

Definitions and Descriptions of Health Education and Health Promotion by Date of Publication

Date	Definition or Description	Reference
1943	Health education is a process of facilitating . . . desirable learning experiences through which people become more aware of health problems and actively interested in securing solutions.	American Public Health Association Statement
1949	Health education is a process of growth in an individual by means of which he alters his behavior or changes his attitudes toward health practices as a result of new experiences he has had.	Dorothy B. Nyswander. "Evaluation of Health Education Practice." *Public Health News* 30.
1961	Health education . . . may be defined as the process of providing learning experiences which favorably influence understandings, attitudes, and conduct in regard to individual and community health.	National Education Association and American Medical Association, Joint Committee on Health Problems in Education. *Health Education: A Guide for Teachers and a Text for Teacher Education.* Washington, DC.
1964	Health education cannot rest on knowledge alone; it must motivate the individual toward healthful living. What is taught in the schools must be so related to the daily lives of the students that they can act intelligently in matters of health. . . .	Elena M. Sliepcevich. *School Health Education: A Summary Report.* Washington, DC: School Health Education Study.

1965   Health education is guiding individuals or groups to perceive given healthful actions as being in line with their own values and goals.

Kasey McMahon and E. McMahon. "Education as a Living Process," in American Hospital Association, *Health Education in the Hospital*. Chicago.

1966   Health education is a process which effects changes in the health practices of people and in the knowledge and attitudes to such changes. Education is an internal process of the individual concerned. . . . Education thus places responsibility on the individual and is essentially different from a compliance approach. It involves motivation, communication, and decision-making.

"Professional Preparation in Health Education in Schools of Public Health." A report prepared for the 1965 Annual Meeting of the Association of Schools, *Health Education Monographs* 21.

1972   I am assuming that in health education we are talking about those processes by which people are not only better informed but actually change their attitudes and behavior in ways which will be increasingly beneficial to good personal and community health.

Robert L. Johnson. "Health Education: Ramifications and Consequences." *Health Education Monographs* 31.

1972   Health education attempts to close the gaps between what is known about optimum health practice and that which is actually practiced. The target groups comprise the focus for health education efforts; first, individuals who lack adequate health knowledge, and second, individuals who possess adequate knowledge but for many reasons do not practice recommended health behavior. In attempting to close this gap, health education is concerned not only with individuals and their families, but also with the institutions and social conditions that impede or facilitate individuals toward achieving optimum health.

W. Griffiths. "Health Education Definitions, Problems, and Philosophies." *Health Education Monographs* 31.

1972   While health education has many definitions and is practiced in many ways, it should be kept in mind that the real index of health education is behavior. The objective of all health education in the community, the schools or in the hospital is to "lead people to think, feel and act wisely on matters pertaining to health and illness."

L. L. Keyes. "Health Education in Perspective—An Overview." *Health Education Monographs* 31.

1973   [Health education is the] process that bridges the gap between health information and health practices. Health education motivates the person to take the information and do something with it—to keep himself healthier by avoiding

The Report of the President's Committee on Health Education. New York, 801 Second Avenue.

actions that are harmful and by forming habits that are beneficial.

1973   An effective health education program should concentrate on helping the individual better understand and appreciate himself, to know what makes him tick, to have self-respect. Such a program should help the individual feel right about other people and have a sense of responsibility to his neighbors and fellow human beings. These individuals would be better equipped to think for themselves, to make their own decisions, to set realistic goals.

J. J. Darden. "Once More Into the Breach—to the Defense of Health Education." *The Journal of School Health* 43, 8:573-575.

1973   [Health education is] a process with intellectual, psychological, and social dimensions relating to activities which increase the abilities of people to make informed decisions affecting their personal, family, and community well-being.

"New Definitions: Report of the 1972-1973 Joint Committee on Health Education Terminology." *Health Education Monographs* 33:03-70.

1974   The ultimate goal of health education is the improvement of the nation's health and the reduction of preventable illness, disability, and death. . . Health education is that dimension of health care that is concerned with influencing behavioral factors . . .

S. K. Simonds. "Health Education in the Mid-70's—State of the Art." Paper prepared for Task Force IV.

1974   Success in health education has to be measured in human term—lives saved, suffering and disability reduced, productivity and creativity enhanced, and something called the quality of life made more rewarding for everyone. That sounds like a tall order to lay at the doorstep of health education. And, certainly, it is, but, realistically, how could we be satisfied with less?

Charles Edwards. "Statement." *Federal Focus on Health Education: Conference Proceedings.* Department of Health, Education, and Welfare, Center for Disease Control, Atlanta.

1974   Health education is an integral part of high quality health care. . . The major emphasis . . . is health promotion, which includes health maintenance, disease and trauma management, and the improvement of the health care system and its utilization.

American Hospital Association. "Statement on the Role and Responsibilities of Hospitals." Chicago: American Hospital Association.

1976   Health education is concerned with the health-related behaviors of people.

Society of Public Health Education, *What Is a Public Health Educator?*

1976   Health educators are modern pioneers—ever seeking new understanding into human behavior, new ways to apply this knowledge in solving individual and community health problems.

Society of Public Health Education, *What Is a Public Health Educator?*

1978   The goal of health education is to provide information that individuals can use to enhance health status . . . the person who is educated

Nicholas Galli. *Foundations and Principles of Health Education.* New York: John Wiley and Sons, Inc.

about health is not only well-informed, but uses this information in daily life ideally resulting in higher levels of well-being.

1979	Health promotion begins with people who are basically healthy and seeks the development of community and individual measures which can help them to develop lifestyles that can maintain and enhance the state of well-being.	USDHHS. *Healthy People: The Surgeon General's Report on Health Promotion and Disease Prevention*. Washington, DC: USDHHS (PHS).
1980	An individual prepared to assist individuals, acting separately or collectively, to make informed decisions regarding matters affecting their personal health and that of others.	Bureau of Health Education and the Office of Health Information, Health Promotion and Physical Fitness and Sports Medicine. "Role Delineation Project." *Focal Points*. Washington, DC: USDHEW (CDC).
1980	Health education is any combination of learning experiences designed to facilitate voluntary adaptations of behavior conducive to health.	Lawrence W. Green, Marshall W. Kreuter, Sigrid G. Deeds, and Kay B. Partridge. *Health Education Planning: A Diagnostic Approach*. Palo Alto: Mayfield Publishing Co.
1980	The process of advocating health in order to enhance the probability that personal (individual, family and community), private (professional and business), and public (federal, state and local government) support of positive health practices will become a societal norm. The process of advocating health may be conducted by a variety of modalities, including but not limited to health education.	R. B. Dwore and Marshall W. Kreuter. "Reinforcing the Case for Health Promotion." *Family and Community Health* 2:103–119.
1983	Any combination of educational, organizational, economic, and environmental supports for behavior conducive to health.	Lawrence W. Green and K. W. Johnson. "Health Education and Health Promotion," Chapter 33 in *Handbook of Health, Health Care, and the Health Professions*, E. Mechanic (ed.). New York: Macmillan.
1991	Health promotion and disease prevention is the aggregate of all purposeful activities designed to improve personal and public health through a combination of strategies, including the competent implementation of behavioral change strategies, health education, health protection measures, risk factor detection, health enhancement and health maintenance.	Joint Committee on Health Education Terminology. "Report of the Joint Committee on Health Education Terminology." *Journal of Health Education* 22 (2): 97–108.

The health education field is that multidisciplinary practice which is concerned with designing, implementing, and evaluating educational programs that enable individuals, families, groups, organizations, and communities.

to play active roles in achieving, protecting, and sustaining health.

The health education process is that continuum of learning which enables people, as individuals and as members of social structures, to voluntarily make decisions, modify behaviors, and change social conditions in ways which are health enhancing.

A health educator is a practitioner who is professionally prepared in a field of health education, who demonstrates competence in both theory and practice, and who accepts responsibility to advance the aims of the health education profession.

1995   Health promotion refers to a set of processes that can be employed to change the conditions that affect health.

Health education is the profession principally devoted to employing health education and health promotion processes to foster healthful behavior and alter the conditions that affect health behavior and health directly.

Bruce G. Simons-Morton, Walter H. Greene, Nell Gottlieb. *Introduction to Health Education and Health Promotion, 2nd Edition*. Prospect Heights, IL: Waveland Press.

Self-Assessment for Health Educators

RESPONSIBILITY I: The health educator, working with individuals, groups, and organizations is responsible for:

Assessing individual and community needs for health education.

The health educator can:

Competency A: Obtain health related data about social and cultural environments, growth and development factors, needs, and interests.

	not competent		very competent	
1. Select valid sources of information about health needs and health knowledge.	1	2	3	4
2. Utilize computerized sources of health-related information.	1	2	3	4
3. Employ or develop appropriate data-gathering information.	1	2	3	4
4. Apply survey techniques to acquire health data.	1	2	3	4

Competency B: Distinguish between behaviors that foster and those that hinder well-being.

	not competent		very competent	
1. Investigate physical, social, emotional, and intellectual factors influencing health behaviors.	1	2	3	4
2. Identify behaviors that tend to promote or compromise health.	1	2	3	4
3. Recognize the role of learning and affective experiences in shaping patterns of health behavior.	1	2	3	4

465

Competency C: Infer needs for health education on the basis of obtained data.

	not competent		very competent	
1. Examine needs assessment data.	1	2	3	4
2. Determine priority areas of need for health education.	1	2	3	4

RESPONSIBILITY II: The health educator, working with individuals, groups, and organizations is responsible for:

Planning effective health education programs.

The health educator can:

Competency A: Recruit community organizations, resource people, and potential participants for support and assistance in program planning.

	not competent		very competent	
1. Communicate need for the program to those whose cooperation will be essential.	1	2	3	4
2. Obtain commitments from personnel and decision makers who will be involved in the program.	1	2	3	4
3. Seek ideas and opinions of those who will affect or be affected by the program.	1	2	3	4
4. Incorporate feasible ideas and recommendations into the planning process.	1	2	3	4

Competency B: Develop a logical scope and sequence plan for a health education program.

1. Determine the range of health information requisite to a given program of instruction.	1	2	3	4
2. Organize the subject areas comprising the scope of a program in logical sequence.	1	2	3	4

Competency C: Formulate appropriate and measurable program objectives.

1. Infer educational objectives facilitative of achievement of specified competencies.	1	2	3	4
2. Develop a framework of broadly stated operational objectives relevant to a proposed health education program.	1	2	3	4

Competency D: Design educational programs consistent with specified program objectives.

1. Match proposed learning activities with those implicit in the stated objectives.	1	2	3	4
2. Formulate a wide variety of alternative educational methods.	1	2	3	4
3. Select strategies best suited to implementation of educational objectives in a given setting.	1	2	3	4
4. Plan a sequence of learning opportunities building upon and reinforcing mastery of preceding objective.	1	2	3	4

RESPONSIBILITY III: The health educator, working with individuals, groups, and organizations is responsible for:

Implementing health education programs.

The health educator can:

Competency A: Exhibit competence in carrying out planned educational programs.

	not competent		very competent	
1. Employ a wide range of educational methods and techniques.	1	2	3	4
2. Apply individual or group process methods as appropriate to given learning situations.	1	2	3	4
3. Utilize instructional equipment and other instructional media effectively.	1	2	3	4
4. Select methods that best facilitate practice objectives.	1	2	3	4

Competency B: Infer enabling objectives as needed to implement instructional programs in specified settings.

1. Pretest learners to ascertain present abilities and knowledge relative to proposed program objectives.	1	2	3	4
2. Develop subordinate measurable objectives as needed for instruction.	1	2	3	4

Competency C: Select methods and media best suited to implement program plans for specific learners.

1. Analyze learner characteristics, legal aspects, feasibility, and other considerations influencing choices among methods.	1	2	3	4
2. Evaluate the efficacy of alternative methods and techniques capable of facilitating program objectives.	1	2	3	4
3. Determine the availability of information, personnel, time, and equipment needed to implement the program for a given audience.	1	2	3	4

Competency D: Monitor educational programs, adjusting objectives and activities as necessary.

1. Compare actual program activities with the stated objectives.	1	2	3	4
2. Assess the relevance of existing program objectives to current needs.	1	2	3	4
3. Revise program activities and objectives as necessitated by changes in learner needs.	1	2	3	4
4. Appraise applicability of resources and materials relative to given educational objectives.	1	2	3	4

RESPONSIBILITY IV: The health educator, working with individuals, groups and organizations is responsible for:

Evaluating effectiveness of health education programs.

The health educator can:

Competency A: Develop plans to assess achievement of program objectives.

	not competent		very competent	
1. Determine standards of performance to be applied as criteria of effectiveness.	1	2	3	4
2. Establish a realistic scope of evaluation efforts.	1	2	3	4
3. Develop an inventory of existing valid and reliable tests and survey instruments.	1	2	3	4
4. Select appropriate methods for evaluating program effectiveness.	1	2	3	4

Competency B: Carry out evaluation plans.

1. Facilitate administration of the tests and activities specified in the plan.	1	2	3	4
2. Utilize data collecting methods appropriate to the objectives.	1	2	3	4
3. Analyze resulting evaluation data.	1	2	3	4

Competency C: Interpret results of program evaluation.

1. Apply criteria of effectiveness to obtained results of a program.	1	2	3	4
2. Translate evaluation results into terms easily understood by others.	1	2	3	4
3. Report effectiveness of educational programs in achieving proposed objectives.	1	2	3	4

Competency D: Infer implications from findings for future program planning.

1. Explore possible explanations for important evaluation findings.	1	2	3	4
2. Recommend strategies for implementing results of evaluation.	1	2	3	4

RESPONSIBILITY V: The health educator working with individuals, groups, and organizations is responsible for:

Coordinating provision of health education services.

The health educator can:

Competency A: Develop a plan for coordinating health education services.

	not competent		very competent	
1. Determine the extent of available health education services.	1	2	3	4
2. Match health education services to proposed program activities.	1	2	3	4
3. Identify gaps and overlaps in the provision of collaborative health services.	1	2	3	4

Competency B: Facilitate cooperation between and among levels of program personnel.

1. Promote cooperation and feedback among personnel related to the program.	1	2	3	4
2. Apply various methods of conflict reduction as needed.	1	2	3	4
3. Analyze the role of health educator as liaison between program staff and outside groups and organizations.	1	2	3	4

Competency C: Formulate practical modes of collaboration among the health agencies and organizations.

1. Stimulate development of cooperation among personnel responsible for community health education programs.	1	2	3	4
2. Suggest approaches for integrating health education within existing health programs.	1	2	3	4
3. Develop plans for promoting collaborative efforts among health agencies and organizations with mutual interests.	1	2	3	4

Competency D: Organize inservice training programs for teachers, volunteers, and other interested personnel.

1. Plan an operational, competency oriented training program.	1	2	3	4
2. Utilize instructional resources that meet a variety of inservice training needs.	1	2	3	4
3. Demonstrate a wide range of strategies for conducting inservice training programs.	1	2	3	4

RESPONSIBILITY VI: The health educator, working with individuals, groups and organizations is responsible for:

Acting as a resource person in health education.

The health educator can:

Competency A: Utilize computerized health information retrieval systems effectively.

	not competent		very competent	
1. Match an information need with the appropriate retrieval system.	1	2	3	4
2. Access principal online and other data-based health information resources.	1	2	3	4

Competency B: Establish effective consultative relationships with those requesting assistance in solving health-related problems.

1. Analyze parameters of effective consultative relationships.	1	2	3	4
2. Describe special skills and abilities needed by health educators for consultation activities.	1	2	3	4
3. Formulate a plan for providing consultation to other health professionals.	1	2	3	4
4. Explain the process of marketing health education consultative services.	1	2	3	4

Competency C: Interpret and respond to requests for health information.

1. Analyze general processes for identifying the information needed to satisfy a request.	1	2	3	4
2. Employ a wide range of approaches in referring requesters to valid sources of health information.	1	2	3	4

Competency D: Select effective educational resource materials for dissemination.

1. Assemble educational material of value to the health of individuals and community groups.	1	2	3	4
2. Evaluate the worth and applicability of resource materials for given audiences.	1	2	3	4
3. Apply various processes in the acquisition of resource materials.	1	2	3	4
4. Compare different methods for distributing educational materials.	1	2	3	4

RESPONSIBILITY VII: The health educator, working with individuals, groups, and organizations is responsible for:

Communicating health and health education needs, concerns, and resources.

The health educator can:

Competency A: Interpret concepts, purposes, and theories of health education.

	not competent		very competent	
1. Evaluate the state of the art of health education.	1	2	3	4
2. Analyze the foundations of the discipline of health education.	1	2	3	4
3. Describe major responsibilities of the health educator in the practice of health education.	1	2	3	4

Competency B: Predict the impact of societal value systems on health education programs.

1. Investigate social forces causing opposing viewpoints regarding health education needs and concerns.	1	2	3	4
2. Employ a wide range of strategies for dealing with controversial health issues.	1	2	3	4

Competency C: Select a variety of communication methods and techniques in providing health information.

1. Utilize a wide range of techniques for communicating health and health education information and education.	1	2	3	4
2. Demonstrate proficiency in communicating health information and health education needs.	1	2	3	4

Competency D: Foster communication between health care providers and consumers.

1. Identify the significance and implications of health care providers' messages to consumers.	1	2	3	4
2. Act as liaison between consumer groups and individuals, and health care provider organizations.	1	2	3	4

National Task Force on the Preparation and Practice of Health Educators. *A Framework for the Development of Competency-Based Curricula for Entry-Level Health Educators.* New York: National Task Force on the Preparation and Practice of Health Educators, 1985. Reprinted by permission of the National Commission for Health Education Credentialing, Inc.

Food Allergy News
  703-691-3179
        Food Allergy Network
$24 Sub.   10400 Eaton Pl., Ste.107
            Fairfax, VA 22030

SOPHE Code of Ethics (1983)

Preamble

Health educators, in using educational processes to influence human well being, take on profound responsibilities. Their professional situation is varied and complex; they work with people of different backgrounds, in diverse settings, and have varying responsibilities in this country as well as overseas. Health educators are involved with their discipline, their colleagues, their employers, their constituents, their government's position, other interest groups, and processes and issues affecting the general welfare of people, locally, nationally, and internationally.

In a field of complex involvements, value conflicts generate ethical dilemmas. It is a prime responsibility of health educators to anticipate and to resolve them in such a way as not to do damage either to the constituency with whom they work or their profession. Where these conditions cannot be met, the health educator would be well advised not to be involved.

The health educator must be committed to the principles of self-determination and liberty. Ethical precepts which guide the design of strategies and methods must ultimately reflect a respect for the right of individuals and communities to affirm their own ways of living.

The following principles are deemed fundamental to health educators' responsible ethical pursuit of their profession:

Article I: Relations with the Public

Health educators' ultimate responsibility is to the general public. When there is a conflict of interest among individuals, groups, agencies, or institutions, health educators must consider all issues and give priority to those whose goals are closest to the principles of self-determination and enhancement of freedom of choice.

Section 1 _____

Health educators must protect the right of individuals to make their own decisions regarding health as long as such decisions pose no threat to the health of others.

Section 2 _____

Health educators should be candid and truthful in their dealings with the public.

Section 3 _____

Health educators should not exploit the public by misrepresenting or exaggerating the potential benefits of services or programs with which they are associated.

Section 4 _____

As people who devote their professional lives to improving people's well being, health educators bear a responsibility to speak out on issues which would have a deleterious effect upon the public's health.

Section 5 _____

In all dealings, health educators should be honest about their qualifications and the limitations of their expertise.

Section 6 _____

In a world where privacy is frequently threatened, health educators should protect the physical, social, and psychological welfare of the public and ensure their privacy and dignity.

Section 7 _____

Health educators should involve clients actively in the entire educational change process so that all aspects are clearly understood by clients.

Section 8 _____

Health educators affirm an egalitarian ethic. Believing that health is a basic human right, they act to ensure that neither the benefits nor the quality of their professional services are denied or impaired to all people to whom they are responsible.

Article II: Responsibility to the Profession

Health educators are responsible for the good reputation of their discipline.

Section 1 _____

They should maintain their competence at the highest level through continuing study and training, for example:

1. Active membership in professional organizations.
2. Review of professional, technical, and lay journals.
3. Previewing of new products and media materials.
4. Creation and distribution of new programs and materials including the publication of professional and lay papers.
5. Involvement in economic and legislative issues related to public health.
6. Assumption of a leadership or participative role in cooperative endeavors.

Section 2

When they participate in actions related to hiring, promotion, or advancement, they should ensure that no exclusionary practices be enacted against individuals on the basis of sex, marital status, color, age, social class, religion, sexual preference, ethnic background, national origin, or other origin, or other non-professional attributes.

Section 3

Health educators should protect and enhance the integrity of the profession by responsible discussion and criticism of the profession.

Article III: Responsibility to Colleagues

Section 1

Health educators should maintain high standards of professional conduct as recommended by the Code of Ethics, and should encourage health education colleagues to do likewise.

Section 2

Health educators should make no critical remarks about colleagues in situations where possible conflicts of interest exist, especially where their own personal gain is involved or the personal gain of close friends.

Section 3

Health educators should take action through appropriate channels against unethical conduct by any other member of the profession.

Article IV: Responsibility in Employing Educational Strategies and Methods

In designing strategies and methods, health educators must not compromise their professional standards, nor reduce the trust in health education held by the general public. They should be sensitive to the prevailing community standard and existing cultural or social norms. Health educators should also be aware of the possible impact of their strategies and methods upon the community and other health professionals.

The strategies and methods must not place the burden of change solely on the targeted population but must involve other appropriate groups to bring about effective change.

In the design/implementation of strategies and methods, health educators have an obligation to two principles: First, the people have a right to make decisions affecting their lives. Second, there is a moral imperative to provide them with all relevant information and resources possible to make their choice freely and intelligently.

Section 1

To protect public confidence in the profession, health educators should avoid strategies and methods that are clearly in violation of accepted moral and legal standards.

Section 2

In conducting programs, the health educator's responsibility is not only to the participants, but also to the community at large.

Section 3

The selection of strategies and methods should include the active involvement of the people to be affected.

Section 4

The potential outcomes, both positive and negative, that can result from the proposed strategies should be communicated to all the appropriate individuals who will be affected.

Section 5

Health educators should implement strategies and methods which direct change whenever possible by choice, rather than by coercion. However, where a community is being harmed, or would be harmed by others, actions which limit the freedom of the harm-producing agents are justified. Where voluntary action has not succeeded in producing a desired outcome, coercive strategies and methods may be necessary but should be employed most cautiously.

Article V: Responsibilities to Employers

In their relations with employers, health educators should:

Section 1

Be honest about their qualifications (education, experience, training), capabilities, and aims.

Section 2

Reflect seriously upon the goals of the organization for which they are to work and consider with great care their employer's stated aims and their past behavior, prior to entering any commitment.

Section 3

Act within the boundaries of their professional competence.

Section 4 _____

Accept responsibility and accountability for their areas of practice, including responsibility for maintenance of optimum standards.

Section 5 _____

Exercise informed judgment and use professional standards and guidelines as criteria in seeking consultation, accepting responsibilities, and delegating health education activities to others.

Section 6 _____

Maintain competence in their areas of professional practice.

Section 7 _____

Be careful not to promise outcomes or to imply acceptance of conditions contrary to their professional ethics.

Section 8 _____

Avoid competing commitments, conflict of interest situations, secret agreements, and endorsement of products.

Article VI: Responsibility to Students

The preparation and training of prospective health educators entails serious responsibilities affecting the well being of the profession, the public, and the students. All those involved in such preparation and training, including teachers, administrators, and practicum supervisors, have an obligation to accord students the same respect and treatment accorded all other client groups and to provide the highest quality education possible.

Educators should be receptive and seriously responsive to student's interests, opinions, and desires in all aspects of their academic work and relationships. The principles and methods of health education that are taught should be practiced in the education of future professionals. Teachers and educators should share their passions, convictions, commitments, and visions as well as their knowledge and skills with their students. Personal and professional honesty and integrity are the essential qualities of a good teacher.

Section 1 _____

Selection of students for professional preparation programs should preclude discrimination on any grounds other than ability and potential contribution to the profession and the public health.

Section 2 _____

The ethical dimensions of the practice of health education should be stressed at all levels of professional preparation.

Section 3 _____

The educational environment—physical, social, and emotional—should, to the greatest degree possible, be conducive to the health of all involved.

Section 4 _____

The responsibilities of all teachers to their students include careful preparation; presentation of material that is accurate, up-to-date, and timely; providing reasonable and timely feedback; having and stating clear and reasonable expectations; and fairness in grading and evaluation.

Section 5 _____

Faculty owe students a reasonable degree of accessibility. Other demands, such as research and administration, must be kept in balance with responsibilities to students.

Section 6 _____

Students should receive counseling regarding career opportunities and assistance securing professional employment upon completion of their studies.

Section 7 _____

Field work and internships should be based upon the professional interests and needs of the student and should provide meaningful opportunities to gain useful experience and adequate supervision.

Article VII: Responsibility in Research and Evaluation

The health educator engaged in research and evaluation studies should:

Section 1 _____

Consider carefully its possible consequences for human beings.

Section 2 _____

Ascertain that the consent of participants in research is voluntary and informed, without any implied deprivation or penalty for refusal to participate, and with due regard for participant's privacy and dignity.

Section 3 _____

Protect participants from unwarranted physical or mental discomfort, distress, harm, danger, or deprivation.

Section 4 _____

Treat all information secured from participants as confidential.

Section 5 _____

Take credit only for work actually done and credit contributions made by others.

Section 6 _____

Provide no reports to sponsors that are not also available to the general public and, where practicable, to the population studied.

Section 7 _____

Discuss the results of evaluation of services only with persons directly and professionally concerned with them.

References

1. Clark K. The implications of developing a profession-wide code of ethics. *Health Educ Quart* 10(2):120–125, 1983.
2. Daniels A. How free should professions be? E. Friedson (ed), *The Professions and Their Prospects.* Beverly Hills: Sage, 1977.
3. Hollander R. Ecologists, ethical codes, and the struggles of a new profession. *Hastings Center Report*, February, 1976:45–46.
4. Penland L., Beyrer M. Ethics and health education: Issues and implications. *Health Education*, July/August 1981, 6–7.
5. Rachels J. Can ethics provide answers? *Hastings Center Report*, June 1980, pp. 32–40.
6. Reamer F. Ethical dilemmas in social work practice. *Social Work*, January/February 1983, 31–35.
7. Richardson G., Jose N. Ethical issues in school health: A survey. *Health Education*, March/April 1983, 5–9.
8. Veatch R. Professional ethics: New principles for physicians? *Hastings Center Report*, June 1980, 16–19.
9. American College Health Association: *Recommended Standards and Practices for a College Health Program, 1984.* Rockville, MD: American College Health Association, 1984.
10. Bayles M. *Professional Ethics.* Belmont, CA: Wadsworth, 1981.

Bibliography

AAHE directory of institutions offering specialization in undergraduate professional preparation programs in health education. *Health Education* 13:31–39, 1982.

AAHE directory of institutions offering specialization in undergraduate and graduate professional preparation programs in school, community, and public health education. *Health Education* 22:365–382, 1991.

Abrams DB, Elder JP, Carleton RA, Lasater TM, Artz LM. Social learning principles for organizational health promotion: An integrated approach. In *Health Behavior and Industry: A Behavioral Medicine Perspective*, Cataldo MF, Coates TJ (eds). New York: John Wiley, 1986.

Ajzen I. *Attitudes, Personality, and Behavior*. Chicago: The Dorsey Press, 1988.

Ajzen I, Fishbein M. *Understanding Attitudes and Predicting Social Behavior*. Englewood Cliffs, NJ: Prentice-Hall, 1980.

Aldrich HE. *Organizations and Environments*. Englewood Cliffs, NJ: Prentice-Hall, 1979.

Allen J, Allen RF. From short term compliance to long term freedom: Culture-based health promotion by health professionals. *Am J Health Promot* 1(1): 39–47, 1986.

Allen J, Bellingham, R. Building supportive cultural environments. In *Health Promotion in the Workplace, 2nd Edition*, O'Donnell MP, Harris JS (eds). Albany, NY: Delmar Publishers, 1994.

Allen RF, Allen J. A sense of community, a shared vision and a positive culture: Core enabling factors in culture-based health promotion efforts. *Am J Health Promot* 1(3): 40–47, 1987.

Allen RF, Kraft C, Allen J, Certner B. *The Organizational Unconscious*. Burlington, VT: Human Resources Institute Press, 1987.

Allensworth DD, Kolbe LJ. The comprehensive school health program: Exploring an expanded concept. *J School Health* 57:409–412, 1987.

Ambler RW, Dull BH (eds). *Closing the Gap: The Burden of Unnecessary Illness*. New York: Oxford, 1987.

American Medical Association. *Statement on Patient Education*. Chicago: AMA, 1975.

American Public Health Association. *Making Health Education Work*. Washington, DC, 1976.

Antonovsky A. Social class, life expectancy and overall mortality. *Milbank Memorial Fund Quarterly* 45:31–73, 1967.

Association of Schools of Public Health. *Organizational Listing*. ASPH, 1015 15th St. NW, Suite 405, Washington, DC 20005, mimeo, 1994.

Augustyn MC, Simons-Morton BG. Adolescent drinking and driving: Etiology and intervention. *Journal of Drug Education*, 1995.

Bandura A. *Social Learning Theory*. Englewood Cliffs, NJ: Prentice-Hall, 1977.

Bandura A. *Social Foundations of Thought and Action: A Social Cognitive Theory*. Englewood Cliffs, NJ: Prentice-Hall, 1986.

Bandura A, Walters RH. *Social Learning and Personality Development*. New York: Holt, Rinehart, & Winston, 1963.

481

Baranowski T. Beliefs as motivational influences at stages in behavior change. *Internat Quart Comm Health Educ* 13(1): 3–29, 1992.

Baranowski T, Henske J, Simons-Morton BG, Palmer J, Tiernan K, Hooks P. Dietary change for CVD Prevention Among Black American Families. *Health Educ Res* 5(4): 433–443, 1990.

Baranowski T, Simons-Morton BG, Hooks P, Henske J, Tiernan K, Burkhalter H, Harper H, Palmer J. A center-based program for exercise change among Black-Americans. *Health Educ Quart* 17(2): 179–196, 1990.

Bartholomew LK, Parcel GS, Seilheimer DK, Cqyzewski D, Spinelli SH, Congdon B. Development of a health education program to promote the self-management of cystic fibrosis. *Health Educ Quart* 18(4): 429–444, 1991.

Bartlett EE, Windsor RA, Lowe JB, Nelson G. Guidelines for conducting smoking cessation programs. *Health Educ* 17:31–37, 1986.

Baun WB. Program management. In *Health Promotion in the Workplace, 2nd Edition*, O'Donnell MP, Harris JS (eds). Albany, NY: Delmar, 1994.

Beauchamp DE. *The Health of The Republic.* Philadelphia: Temple University Press, 1988.

Becker MH. *The Health Belief Model and Personal Health Behaviors.* Thorofare, NJ: Charles B. Slack, 1974.

Beery W, Schoenbach VJ, Wagner EH, et al. *Health Risk Appraisal.* Rockville, MD: DHHS Publ No PHS 86-3396, 1986.

Bender GA. *Great Moments in Medicine.* Detroit: Parke-Davis, 1961.

Bennis WG, Benne KD, Chin R. *The Planning of Change, 2nd Edition.* New York: Holt, Rinehart, & Winston, 1979.

Bettinghaus EP. Health promotion and the knowledge-attitude-behavior continuum. *Prev Med* 15:475–491, 1986.

Bingham E, Meader WV. Governmental regulation of environmental hazards in the 1990s. *Annu Rev Public Health* 11:419–434, 1990.

Birkel R, Muchnick S. The national resource center on worksite health promotion. *Health Educ* 21: 49–50, 1990.

Blair SN, Kohl HW, Gordon NF, Paffenbarger RS, Jr. How much physical activity is good for health? *Annu Rev Public Health* 13:99–126, 1991.

Blair SN, Tritsch L, Kutsch S. Worksite health promotion for school faculty and staff. *J School Health* 57(10): 469–473, 1987.

Blendon RJ, Taylor H. Views on health care: Public opinion in three nations. *Health Affairs* 8:149–157, 1989.

Block P. *Flawless Consulting: A Guide to Getting Your Expertise Used.* Austin: Learning Concepts, 1981.

Blomquist KB. Modeling and health behavior: Strategies for prevention in the schools. *Health Educ* 17:8–11, 1986.

Bloom BS, et al. *Taxonomy of Educational Objectives: The Classification of Educational Goals. Handbook I: Cognitive Domain.* New York: David McKay Company, 1956.

Bonk DJ, Bensky JM. Current involvement of hospitals in health promotion. In *Hospital Health Promotion,* Sol N, Wilson PK (eds). Champaign, IL: Human Kinetics Books, 1989.

Borich GD. *Program Evaluation: Models and Techniques.* Department of Educational Psychology, The University of Texas at Austin, TX 78712, mimeo, 1993.

Bouchard CR, Shephard J, Stephens T, Sutton JR, McPherson BD (eds). *Exercise, Fitness, and Health: A Consensus of Current Knowledge.* Champaign, IL: Human Kinetics Books, 1990.

Bower GH, Hilgard ER. *Theories of Learning, 5th Edition.* Englewood Cliffs, NJ: Prentice-Hall, 1981.

Boyle RH, and The Environmental Defense Fund. *Malignant Neglect.* New York: Alfred A. Knopf, 1979.

Bracht N (ed). *Health Promotion at the Community Level.* Newbury Park, CA: Sage Publications, 1990.

Bracht N, Kingsbury L. Community organization principles in health promotion: A five-stage model. In *Health Promotion at the Community Level,* Bracht N (ed). Newbury Park, CA: Sage Publications, 1990.

Brager GA, Holloway S. *Changing Human Service Organizations: Politics and Practice.* New York: Free Press, 1978.

Brager GA, Specht H, Torczyner JL. *Community Organizing, 2nd Edition.* New York: Columbia University Press, 1987.

Breckon DJ, Harvey JR, Lancaster RB. *Community Health Education: Settings, Roles, and Skills.* Rockville, MD: Aspen Publishers, 1989.

Brenner MH. Mortality, social stress, and the modern economy: experiences of the United States, Britain, and Sweden, 1900–1970. Paper presented at the Annual Meeting of the American Association for the Advancement of Science, Boston, Feb. 21, 1977.

Breslow L. The future of public health: Prospects in the United States for the 1990s. *Annu Rev Public Health* 11:1–28, 1990.

Brown JL, Allen D. Hunger in America. *Annu Rev Public Health* 9:503–526, 1988.

Brownell KD. *Behavior Therapy for Obesity: A Treatment Manual*. Philadelphia: University of Pennsylvania, 1979.

Brownell KD, Cohen RY, Stunkard AJ, Felix MR, Cooley NB. Weight loss competitions at the work site: Impact on weight, morale, and cost effectiveness. *Am J Public Health* 74:1283–1285, 1984.

Burdine JN, McLeroy KB, Gottlieb NH. Ethical dilemmas in health promotion: An introduction. *Health Educ Quart* 14(1): 7–9, 1987.

Bureau of Health Education. Health education and credentialing: The role delineation. *Focal Points*. USDHHS, July 1980.

Callahan D. Health and society: Some ethical imperatives. In *Doing Better and Feeling Worse*, Knowles JH (ed). New York: W. W. Norton, 1977.

Cardenas MP, Simons-Morton BG. The effect of anticipatory guidance on mother's self-efficacy and behavioral intentions to prevent burns caused by hot tap water. *Patient Educ and Couns* 21:117–123, 1993.

Carlaw R, Middelmark MB, Bracht NF, et al. Organization for a community cardiovascular health program: Experiences from the Minnesota Heart Health Program. *Health Educ Quart* 11(3): 243–252, 1984.

Challenges in Health Care. Princeton, NJ: The Robert Wood Johnson Foundation, 1991.

Clark NM, Zimmerman BJ. A social cognitive view of self-regulated learning about health. *Health Educ Res* 5:371–379, 1990.

Cleary HP. Issues in the credentialing of health education specialists. *Advances in Health Education and Promotion*, Vol. 1, Part A: 129–154.

Coalition of National Health Education Organizations. *CNHEO Directory*. Chapel Hill, NC, 1990.

Cockerham WC. *Medical Sociology, 4th Edition*. Englewood Cliffs, NJ: Prentice-Hall, 1989.

Colsher PL, Wallace RB. Is modest alcohol consumption better than none at all? *Annu Rev Public Health* 10:503–526, 1989.

Connel DB, Turner RR, Mason EF. Summary of findings of the school health education evaluation: Health promotion effectiveness, implementation, and costs. *J School Health* 55:316–321, 1985.

Cortese PA. Credentialing—an idea whose time has come. *Health Educ Quart* 17(3): 247–251, 1990.

Council for Education in Public Health. *Organizational Listing*. CEPH, 1015 15th St. NW, Suite 403, Washington, DC 20005, mimeo, 1994.

Cummings TG, Worley CG. *Organization Development and Change, 5th Edition*. Minneapolis/St Paul: West Publishing, 1993.

Cunningham WP, Saigo BW. *Environment Science: A Global Concern*. Dubuque, IA: William C. Brown, 1992.

Cyert RM, Mowery DC. Technology, employment and U.S. competitiveness. *Scientific Amer* 260:54–62, 1989.

Dawber TR. *The Framingham Study*. Cambridge: Harvard University Press, 1980.

Deal TE, Kennedy AA. *Corporate Cultures: The Rites and Rituals of Corporate Life*. Reading, MA: Addison Wesley, 1982.

Deeds, Sigrid G. *The Health Education Specialist*. Loose Canon Publications, 1992.

DeFriese GH, Crossland CL, Pearson CE, Sullivan CJ (Special Issue eds). Comprehensive school health programs: Current status and future prospects. *J School Health* 60(4): 123–190, 1990.

DeFriese GH, Fielding JE. Health risk appraisal in the 1990s. *Annu Rev Public Health* 11:1–28, 1990.

DiClemente CC, Prochaska JO, Fairhurst S, Velicer WF, Velasquez MM, Rossi JS. The processes of smoking cessation: An analysis of precontemplation, contemplation, and preparation stages of change. *J Consult and Clin Psych* 59:295–304, 1991.

Dignan MB. *Measurement and Evaluation of Health Education, 2nd Edition*. Springfield, IL: Charles C Thomas, 1989.

Dinkmeyer D, McKay GD. *Parenting Teenagers: Systematic Training for Effective Parenting of Teens*. Circle Pines, MN: American Guidance Service, 1990.

Doak CC, Doak LG, Root JH. *Teaching Patients with Low Literacy Skills*. Philadelphia: J.B. Lippincott, 1985.

Doak LG, Doak CC. Lowering the silent barriers to compliance for patients with low literacy skills. *Amer Hosp Assoc* 1987.

Dolfman ML. The concept of health: An historic and analytic examination. *J School Health* 48:491, 1973.

Doll R. Health and environment in the 1990s. *Am J Public Health* 82:933–940, 1992.

Doll R, Peto R. *The Causes of Cancer*. Oxford: Oxford University Press, 1981.

Drolet JC, Fetro JV. State conference for school worksite wellness: A synthesis of research and evaluation. *J Health Educ* 22:76–79, 1991.

Dubos R. *Mirage of Health.* New York: Harper & Row, 1959.

Dubos R. *Man Adapting.* New Haven: Yale University Press, 1965.

Dunn HL. What high-level wellness means. *Health Values* 1:9–16, 1977.

Durant W. *The Life of Greece.* New York: Simon & Schuster, 1936.

Duval MK. Advancing and financing health education in the 1980s. *Health Educ* 12:27, 1981.

Dwore RB, Kreuter MW. Update: Reinforcing the case for health promotion. *Family Comm Health* 2:103–119, 1980.

Ebert RH. The medical school. *Scientific Amer* 229:138–148, 1973.

Education Policy Commission. *The Central Purpose of Education.* Washington, DC: National Education Association and the American Association of School Administrators, 1961.

Eisen M, Zellman GL, McAlister AL. A health belief model approach to adolescents' fertility control: Some pilot program findings. *Health Educ Quart* 12:185–210, 1985.

Elder JP, McGraw SA, Abrams PB, et al. Organizational and community approaches to community-wide prevention of heart disease: The first two years of the Pawtucket Heart Health Program. *Prev Med* 15(2): 107–117, 1986.

Elder JP, Melbourne FH, Lasater TM, Wells BL, Carleton RA. Applications of behavior modification to community health education: The case of heart disease prevention. *Health Educ Quart* 12:151–168, 1985.

Elder JP, Neef NA. Behavior modification and the primary and secondary prevention of cancer. *Family Comm Health* 9:14–24, 1986.

Engs RC. Resurgence of a new "clean living" movement in the United States. *J School Health* 61:155–159, 1991.

Enstrom JE. Cancer mortality among Mormons. *Cancer* 36:825, 1975.

Farquhar JW, Fortmann SP, Maccob N, et al. The Stanford Five City Project: Design and methods. *Amer J of Epidem* 122:323–334, 1985.

Fielding JE. Smoking: Health effects and control. In *Maxcy-Rosenau Public Health and Preventive Medicine, 13th Edition*, Last J, Wallace RB (eds). Norwalk, CT: Appleton and Lange, 1991.

Fingerhut LA, Wilson RW, Feldman JJ. Health and disease in the United States. *Annu Rev Public Health* 1:1–36, 1980.

Fodor JT, Dalis GT. *Health Instruction: Theory and Application, 4th Edition.* Philadelphia: Lea & Febiger, 1989.

Ford ME. *Motivating Humans: Goals, Emotions, and Personal Agency Beliefs.* Newbury Park, CA: Sage Publications, 1992.

Frederiksen LW, Solomon LJ, Brehony KA (eds). *Marketing Health Behavior: Principles, Techniques, and Applications.* New York: Plenum Press, 1984.

Freudenberg N. Shaping the future of health education: From behavior change to social change. *Health Education Monographs* 6(4): 372, 1978.

Freudenberg N. Health education for social change: A strategy for public health in the U.S. *Internat J Health Educ* 24(3): 138, 1981.

Freudenberg N. *Not in Our Backyards.* New York: Monthly Review Press, 1984.

Freudenberg N. Training health educators for social change. *Internat Quart Comm Health Educ* 5(1): 37–52, 1984–85.

Freudenberg N, Golub M. Health education, public policy and disease prevention: A case history of the New York City Coalition to End Lead Poisoning. *Health Educ Quart* 14(4): 387–401, 1987.

Gilmore GD, Campbell MD, Becker BL. *Needs Assessment Strategies for Health Education and Health Promotion.* Indianapolis: Benchmark Press, 1989.

Giloth BE (ed). *Managing Hospital-based Patient Education.* Chicago: American Hospital Publishing, 1993.

Giloth BE. Developing effective patient education management structures. In *Managing Hospital-based Patient Education*, Giloth BE (ed). Chicago: American Hospital Publishing, 1993.

Glanz K, Lewis FM, Rimer BK (eds). *Health Behavior and Health Education.* San Francisco: Jossey-Bass, 1990.

Goldstein AP, Kanfer FH. *Maximizing Treatment Gains: Transfer Enhancement in Psychotherapy.* New York: Academic Press, 1979.

Goodloe NR, Arreola PM. Spiritual health: Out of the closet. *J Health Educ* 23:221–226, 1993.

Goodman RM, Steckler AB. Mobilizing organizations for health enhancement: Theories of organizational change. In *Health Behavior and Health Education*, Glanz K, Lewis FM, Rimer BK (eds). San Francisco: Jossey-Bass, 1990.

Gottlieb, NH. Treading across the shoals of professionalism: Challenges for SOPHE and health education in the 1990s. *Health Educ Quart* 19:149–155, 1992.

Gottlieb NH, Dignan M. Training and experience qualifications for public health education in breast and cervical cancer control programs. Atlanta: Division of Chronic Disease Prevention and Control, Centers for Disease Control, 1994.

Gottlieb NH, Lovato CY, Weinstein R, Green LW, Eriksen MP. The implementation of a restrictive worksite smoking policy in a large decentralized organization. *Health Educ Quart* 19(1): 77–100, 1992.

Gough M. Estimating "environmental" carcinogenesis: A comparison of divergent approaches. (Discussion Paper) CRM 89–01. Washington, DC: Resources for the Future, 1988.

Graham S, Reeder LG. Social epidemiology of chronic diseases. In *Handbook of Medical Sociology, 3rd Edition*, Freeman HE, Levine S, Reeder LG (eds). Englewood Cliffs, NJ: Prentice-Hall, 1979.

Green LW. *Community Health, 6th Edition*. St. Louis: Times Mirror/Mosby, 1990.

Green LW, Johnson KW. Health education and health promotion. In *Handbook of Health, Health Care, and the Health Professions*, Mechanic E (ed). New York: Macmillan, 1983.

Green LW, Kreuter MW, Deeds SG, Partridge KB. *Health Education Planning: A Diagnostic Approach*. Palo Alto, CA: Mayfield, 1980.

Green LW, Kreuter MW. *Health Promotion Planning: An Educational and Environmental Approach, 2nd Edition*. Mountain View, CA: Mayfield, 1991.

Green LW, Lewis FM. *Measurement and Evaluation in Health Education*. Palo Alto, CA: Mayfield, 1986.

Green LW, McAlister AL. Macro-interventions to support health behavior: Some theoretical perspectives and practical reflections. *Health Educ Quart* 11:322–339, 1984.

Green LW, Simons-Morton DG. Education and life-style determinants of health and disease. In *Maxcy-Rosenau Public Health and Preventive Medicine, 13th Edition*, Last J, Wallace RB (eds). Norwalk, CT: Appleton and Lange, 1991.

Greenwald P. Assessment of risk factors for cancer. *Prev Med* 9:260, 1980.

Grimley DM, Riley GE, Bellis JM, Prochaska JO. Assessing the stages of change and decision-making or contraceptive use for prevention of pregnancy, sexually transmitted disease, and acquired immunodeficiency syndrome. *Health Educ Quart* 20(4): 455–470, 1993.

Gross SJ. *Of Foxes and Henhouses*. Westport, CT: Quorum Books, 1984.

Haddon W. Advances in the epidemiology of injuries as a basis for public policy. *Am J Public Health* 95:411–421, 1980.

Haily BJ, Lalor KM, Byrne HA, Starling LM. The effects of self-reinforcement and peer-reinforcement on the practice of breast self-examination. *Health Educ Res* 7:165–174, 1992.

Hall RH. *Dimensions of Work*. Beverly Hills: Sage, 1984.

Hanlon JS. *Public Health Administration and Practice, 6th Edition*. St. Louis: C. V. Mosby, 1974.

Hanson WB, Graham JW. Preventing alcohol marijuana, and cigarette use among adolescents: Peer pressure resistance training versus establishing conservative norms. *Prev Med* 20:414–430, 1991.

Hosper HJ, Kok G, Strecher VJ. Attributions for previous failures and subsequent outcome in a weight reduction program. *Health Educ Quart* 17(4): 409–415, 1990.

Hoyman, H. Rethinking an ecologic system model of man's health, disease, aging, death. *J School Health* 45:509, 1975.

Huxley A. *Brave New World*. New York: Bantam Books, 1946.

Iglehart, JK. Health care and American business: One CEO's view. *Health Affairs* 10:76–86, 1991.

Institute of Medicine Committee for the Study of the Future of Public Health. *The Future of Public Health*. Washington, DC: National Academy Press, 1988.

IOX Program Associates. *Program Evaluation Handbook: Drug Abuse Education*. Atlanta: Centers for Disease Control, 1988.

Jacobs EE. *Creative Counseling Techniques: An Illustrated Guide*. Odessa, FL: Psychological Assessment Resources, 1992.

Janis IL, Mann L. *Decision Making: A Psychological Analysis of Conflict, Choice, and Commitment*. New York: The Free Press, 1977.

Janz NK, Becker MH. The health belief model: A decade later. *Health Educ Quart* 11(1): 1–47, 1984.

Joint Committee on Health Education Terminology (JCHET). *Report of the Joint Committee on Health Education Terminology*. Reston, VA: Association for the Advancement of Health Education, 1990.

Jones PD, Wigley TM. Global warming trends. *Scientific Amer* 263:84–91, 1990.

Kalish HI. *From Behavior Science to Behavior Modification*. New York: McGraw-Hill, 1981.

Kanfer FH, Goldstein AP (eds). *Helping People Change: A Textbook of Methods*. New York: Pergamon Press, 1986.

Karoly P, Harris A. Operant methods. In *Helping People Change: A Textbook of Methods*, Kanfer FH, Goldstein AP (eds). New York: Pergamon, 1986.

Kazdin AE. *Behavior Modification in Applied Settings*, 3rd Edition. Homewood, IL: The Dorsey Press, 1984.

Kazdin AE. *Behavior Modification in Applied Settings*, 4th Edition. Pacific Grove, CA: Brooks/Cole, 1989.

Kettner PM, Moroney RM, Martin LL. *Designing and Managing Programs: An Effectiveness-Based Approach*. Newbury Park, CA: Sage Publications, 1990.

Kilwein JH. No pain no gain: A puritan legacy. *Health Educ Quart* 16(1): 9-12, 1989.

Kitagawa EM, Hauser PM. *Differential Mortality in the United States: A Study in Socioeconomic Epidemiology*. Cambridge: Harvard University Press, 1973.

Klein JD, Sadowski LS. Personal health services as a component of comprehensive school health programs. *J School Health* 60(4): 164-169, 1990.

Knowles M. *The Modern Practice of Adult Education*. Chicago: Follett, 1980.

Kok G, de Vries H, Mudde AN, Strecher VJ. Planned health education and the role of self-efficacy: Dutch research. *Health Educ Res* 6:231-238, 1991.

Koskela K, Puska P, Tuomilehto J. The North Karelia project: A first evaluation. *Internat J Health Educ* 19(1): 59, 1976.

Kotler P. *Marketing for Nonprofit Organizations*. Englewood Cliffs, NJ: Prentice-Hall, 1982.

Kotler P. Social marketing and health behavior. In *Marketing Health Behavior: Principles, Techniques, and Applications*, Frederiksen LW, Solomon LJ, Brehony KA (eds). New York: Plenum Press, 1984.

Kreuger RA. *Focus Groups: A Practical Guide for Applied Research*. Newbury Park, CA: Sage Publications, 1988.

Kreuter MW. PATCH: Its origin, basic concepts, and links to contemporary public health policy. *J Health Educ* 23:135-139, 1992.

Lalone MA. *New Perspectives on the Health of Canadians*. Ottawa, Canada: Ministry of National Health and Welfare, 1974.

LaRosa JH, Haines CM. *It's Your Business: A Guide to Heart and Lung Health at the Workplace*. National Heart, Lung and Blood Institute, National Institutes of Health, USDHHS, NIH Pub. No. 86-2210, 1986.

Larson MS. *The Rise of Professionalism*. Berkeley: University of California Press, 1977.

Last J, Wallace RB (eds). *Maxcy-Rosenau Public Health and Preventive Medicine*, 13th Edition. Norwalk, CT: Appleton and Lange, 1991.

Lave LB, Ennever FK. Toxic substances control in the 1990s. *Annu Rev Public Health* 11:69-87, 1990.

Lavin AT, Shapiro GR, Weill KS. Creating an agenda for school-based health promotion: A review of 25 selected reports. *J School Health* 62(6): 212-228, 1992.

Leape LL. Unnecessary surgery. *Annu Rev Public Health* 13:363-383, 1992.

Lefebvre RC, Flora JA. Social marketing and public health intervention. *Health Educ Quart* 15(3): 299-315, 1988.

Levit KR, Lazenby HC, Letsch SW, Cowan CA. Data watch: National health care spending, 1989. *Health Affairs* 10:117-130, 1991.

Lewin K. *Field Theory in Social Science*. New York: Harper and Brothers, 1951.

Lohrmann DK, Gold RS, Jubb WH. School health education: A foundation for school health programs. *J School Health* 57(10): 420-425, 1987.

MacMillan DL. *Behavior Modification in Education*. New York: Macmillan, 1973.

Magner LN. *A History of Medicine*. New York: Marcel Dekker, 1992.

Mahler H. Present status of WHO's initiative, "health for all by the year 2000." *Annu Rev Public Health* 9:71-97, 1988.

Marconi KM, Bennett GC. State coalitions for prevention and control of tobacco use. *MMWR* 39:476-485, 1990.

Marmot MG, Kogevinas M, Elston MA. Social economic status and disease. *Annu Rev Public Health* 8:111-135, 1987.

Maslow A. *Motivation and Personality*. New York: Harper & Row, 1970.

Mayer RR. *Social Science and Institutional Change*. Washington, DC: DHEW Pub. No. (ADM) 78-627, 1979.

McAlister AL, Puska P, Orlandi M, Bye LL, Zbylot P. Behavior modification: Principles and illustrations. In *Oxford Textbook of Public Health*, Holland WW, Detals R, Knox EG (eds). London: Oxford Medical Publications, 1989.

McGinnis JM. Recent history of federal initiatives in prevention policy. *Amer Psych* 41(2): 205-212, 1985.

McGinnis LM. Setting objectives for public health in the 1990s. *Annu Rev Public Health* 11:231–250, 1990.

McGuire WJ. Behavioral medicine, public health and communication theories. *Health Educ* May/June, 1981.

McGuire WJ. Public communication as a strategy for inducing health promoting behavior change. *Prev Med* 13:299–313, 1984.

McKeachie WJ. *Teaching Tips: A Guidebook for the Beginning College Teacher, 8th Edition.* Lexington, MA: D.C. Heath, 1986.

McKenzie JF, Jurs JL. *Planning, Implementing and Evaluating Health Promotion Programs.* New York: Macmillan, 1993.

McKeown T. Determinants of health. *Human Nature.* April, 1978.

McKinlay JB, McKinlay S. Medical measures and the decline of mortality. In *The Sociology of Health and Illness*, Conrad P, Kern R. (eds). New York: St. Martin's Press, 1986.

McLeroy KR, Bibeau D, Steckler A, Glanz K. An ecological perspective on health promotion programs. *Health Educ Quart* 25:351–377, 1988.

McLeroy KR, Gottlieb NH, Burdine JN. The business of health promotion: Ethical issues and professional responsibilities. *Health Educ Quart* 14(1): 91–109, 1987.

McLeroy KR, Steckler AB, Goodman RM, Burdine JN. Health education research, theory, and practice: Future directions. *Health Educ Res* 7:1–8, 1992.

McLeroy KR, Steckler AB, Simons-Morton BG, Goodman RM, Gottlieb N, Burdine JN. Social science theory in health education: Time for a new model? *Health Educ Res* 8(3): 305–312, 1993.

Means RK. *A History of Health Education.* Philadelphia: Lea & Febiger, 1962.

Means RK. *Historical Perspectives on School Health.* Thorofare, NJ: Charles B. Slack, 1975.

Middelmark MB, Luepker RV, Jacobs DR, et al. Community-wide prevention of cardiovascular disease: Education strategies of the Minnesota Heart Health Program. *Prev Med* 15:1–17, 1986.

Minkler M. Health education, health promotion and the open society: An historical perspective. *Health Educ Quart* 16:17–30, 1989.

Minkler M. Improving health through community organizaton. In *Health Behavior and Health Education: Theory, Research, and Practice*, Glanz K, Lewis FM, Rimer BK (eds). San Francisco: Jossey-Bass, 1990.

Minkler M, Cox K. Creating critical consciousness in health: Applications of Freire's philosophy and methods to the health care setting. *Internat J Health Serv* 10(2): 311–323, 1980.

Moberg DP. *Evaluation of Prevention Programs: A Basic Guide for Practitioners.* The Prevention Committee of the Division of Community Services, Wisconsin Department of Health and Social Services, 1984.

Mullan F. *Plagues and Politics.* New York: Basic Books, 1989.

Nadakavukaren A. *Our Global Environment: A Health Perspective, 4th Edition.* Prospect Heights, IL: Waveland Press, 1995.

Nadler L. *Designing Training Programs: The Critical Events Model.* Reading, MA: Addison-Wesley, 1982.

Naisbitt J, Aburdene P. *Megatrends 2000: Ten Directions for the 1990s.* New York: William Morrow, 1990.

National Center for Health Education. *Initial Role Delineation for Health Education.* Washington, DC: USDHHS, HRA Publication No. 80–44, April, 1980.

National Center for Health Statistics. *Health, United States, 1987.* Hyattsville, MD: Public Health Service, 1988.

National Center for Health Statistics. *Health, United States, 1990.* Hyattsville, MD: Public Health Service, 1991.

National Center for Health Statistics. *Health, United States, 1991.* Hyattsville, MD: Public Health Service, 1992.

National Center for Health Statistics. *Health, United States, 1992.* Hyattsville, MD: Public Health Service, 1993.

National Center for Health Statistics. *Health, United States, 1993.* Hyattsville, MD: Public Health Service, 1994.

National Research Council: Committee on Diet and Health. *Diet and Health: Implications for Reducing Chronic Disease Risk.* Washington, DC: National Academy Press, 1989.

National Task Force on the Preparation and Practice of Health Educators: *A Competency-based Curriculum Framework for the Professional Preparation of Entry-Level Health Educators.* National Task Force on the Preparation and Practice of Health Educators, 30 East 29th St., New York, NY, 10016, 1985.

Novelli WD. Applying social marketing to health promotion and disease prevention. In *Health*

Behavior and Health Education, Glanz K, Lewis FM, Rimer BK (eds). San Francisco: Jossey-Bass, 1990.

Nyswander D. The open society: Its implications for health educators. *Health Educ Mono* 1:3–13, 1967.

O'Donnell MP, Harris JS (eds). *Health Promotion in the Workplace, 2nd Edition*. Albany, NY: Delmar, 1994.

O'Donnell MP. Employers' financial perspective on health promotion. In *Health Promotion in the Workplace, 2nd Edition*, O'Donnell MP, Harris JS (eds). Albany, NY: Delmar, 1994.

Office on Smoking and Health. *Smoking and Health: A Report of the Surgeon General*. Washington DC, Public Health Service, DHHS Pub. No. (PHS) 79–50066, 1979.

Orwell, G. *Nineteen Eighty-four*. New York: New American Library, 1949.

Ottoson JM, Green LW. Reconciling concept and context: Theory of implementation. *Advances in Health Educ and Prom* 2:353–382, 1987.

Ouichi WG. *Theory Z: How American Business Can Meet the Japanese Challenge*. Reading, MA: Addison-Wesley, 1981.

Ouichi WG, Wilkins AL. Organizational culture. *Annu Rev Soc* 11:457–483, 1985.

Parcel GS, Baranowski T. Social learning theory and health education. *Health Educ* 12:14–18, 1981.

Parcel GS, Simons-Morton BG, Kolbe LJ. School health promotion: Integrating organizational change and student learning strategies. *Health Educ Quart* 15(4): 435–450, 1988.

Parcel GS, Simons-Morton BG, O'Hara NM, Baranowski T, Wilson B. School promotion of healthful diet and physical activity: Impact on learning outcomes and self-reported behavior. *Health Educ Quart* 16(2): 181–199, 1989.

Parcel GS, Simons-Morton BG, O'Hara NM, Kolbe LJ, Baranowski T, Bee DE. School health promotion and cardiovascular health: An integration of institutional change and social learning theory intervention. *J School Health* 57(4): 150–156, 1987.

Patrick DL, Bergner M. Measurement of health status in the 1990s, *Annu Rev Public Health* 11:165–184, 1990.

Patterson SM. Historical perspective of selected professional preparation conferences that have influenced credentialing for health education specialists. *J Health Educ* 23:101–108, 1992.

Perry C, Baranowski T, Parcel G. How individuals, environments, and health behavior interact:

Social learning theory. In *Health Behavior and Health Education*, Glanz K, Lewis FM, Rimer BK (eds). San Francisco: Jossey-Bass, 1990.

Phillips RL. The role of life-style and dietary habits in risk of cancer among Seventh-Day Adventists. *Cancer Res* 35:3513, 1975.

Pincus T, Callahan LF, Burkhauser RV. Most chronic diseases are reported more frequently by individuals with fewer than 12 years of formal education in the age range 18-64 United States population. *J Chronic Dis* 40:865, 1987.

Pollock M. *Planning and Implementing Health Education in Schools*. Palo Alto: Mayfield, 1987.

Porter IH. Control of hereditary disorders. *Annu Rev Public Health* 3:277–319, 1982.

Powles J. On the limits of modern medicine. In *The Challenges of Community Medicine*, Kane RL (ed). New York: Springer, 1974.

Prochaska JO, DiClemente CC. *The Transtheoretical Approach: Crossing the Traditional Boundaries of Therapy*. Homewood, IL: Dow-Jones/Irwin, 1984.

Rappaport J. Studies in empowerment: Introduction to the issue. *Prev in Human Serv* 3:1–7, 1984.

Ratcliffe J. Introduction. In *Assessing the Contributions of the Social Sciences to Health*. AAAS Selected Symposium 26, Brenner MH, Mooney A, Nagy TJ (eds). Boulder, CO: Westview Press, 1980.

Raths LE, Merrill HM, Simon SB. *Values and Teaching*. Columbus, OH: Charles E. Merrill, 1978.

Reichgott M, Simons-Morton BG. Strategies to improve compliance with anti-hypertensive therapy. *Primary Care* 10(1): 21–28, 1983.

Report of the Working Group on Concept and Principles of Health Promotion. *Health Promotion* 1(1): 73–76, 1986.

Richardson MA, Simons-Morton BG, Annegers JF. Effect of perceived barriers on compliance with anti-hypertension medication. *Health Educ Quart* 20(4): 489–504, 1993.

Roberts H. *Community Development: Learning and Action*. Toronto: Univer. of Toronto Press, 1979.

Roemer M. The value of medical care for health promotion. *Am J Public Health* 74:243–248, 1984.

Rogers CR. *On Becoming A Person*. Boston: Houghton Mifflin, 1961.

Rogers DE. A private sector view of public health today. *Am J Public Health* 64:529–533, 1974.

Rogers DE. Report card on our national response to the AIDS epidemic—some A's, too many D's. *Am J Public Health* 82:522–524, 1992.

Rogers EM. *Diffusion of Innovations, 3rd Edition*. New York: The Free Press, 1983.

Rokeach M. *Understanding Human Values: Individual and Societal*. New York: The Free Press, 1979.

Rosen G. *A History of Public Health*. New York: MD Publications, 1958.

Rosenstock IM. The health belief model: Explaining health behavior through expectancies. In *Health Behavior and Health Education*, Glanz K, Lewis FM, Rimer BK (eds). San Francisco: Jossey-Bass, 1990.

Rosenstock IM, Strecher VJ, Becker MH. Social learning theory and the health belief model. *Health Educ Quart* 15:175-183, 1988.

Rosow JM, Zager R. *Productivity through Work Innovations*. New York: Pergamon Press, 1982.

Ross HS, Mico PR. *Theory and Practice in Health Education*. Palo Alto, CA: Mayfield, 1980.

Rothman J. Three models of community organization practice. In *Strategies of Community Organization: A Book of Readings*, Cox FM, et al., (eds). Itasca, IL: Peacock, 1970.

Rotter JB. *Social Learning and Clinical Psychology*. Englewood Cliffs, NJ: Prentice-Hall, 1954.

Rotter JB, Chance JE, Phares EJ. *Applications of a Social Learning Theory of Personality*. New York: Holt, Rinehart, & Winston, 1972.

Ruzek SB. Towards a more inclusive model of women's health. *Am J Public Health* 83:6-7, 1993.

Schinke SP, Botvin GJ, Orlandi MA. *Substance Abuse in Children and Adolescents: Evaluation and Intervention*. Newbury Park: Sage Publications, 1991.

Schull WJ, Hanis CL. Genetics and public health in the 1990s. *Annu Rev Public Health* 11:105-125, 1990.

Schuster RC, Kilbey MM. Prevention of drug abuse. In *Maxcy-Rosenau Public Health and Preventive Medicine, 13th Edition*, Last J, Wallace RB (eds). Norwalk, CT: Appleton and Lange, 1991.

Schein EH. Organizational culture. *Amer Psych* 45(2): 109-119, 1990.

Seffrin JR. The comprehensive school health curriculum: Closing the gap between state-of-the-art and state-of-the-practice. *J School Health* 60(4): 151-156, 1990.

Selye H. *Stress Without Distress*. Philadelphia: J. B. Lippincott, 1974.

Sethia NK, von Glinow MA. Arriving at four cultures by managing the reward system. In *Gaining Control of the Corporate Culture*, Killmann RH et al. (eds). San Francisco: Jossey-Bass, 1985.

Simons-Morton BG, Brink SG, Bates D. The effectiveness and cost effectiveness of persuasive communications and incentives in increasing safety belt use: The safety belt connection project. *Health Educ Quart* 14(2): 167-179, 1987.

Simons-Morton BG, Brink SG, Lee R, Bunker J. Unsafe in any season: Injury control in beach-front communities. *Family and Community Health* 11(1): 17-27, 1988.

Simons-Morton BG, Brink SG, Parcel GS, McIntyre RM, Chapman M, Longoria J. *Preventing Acute Alcohol-related Health Problems Among Adolescents and Young Adults: A CDC Handbook for Community Intervention*. Atlanta, GA: Centers for Disease Control, 1991a.

Simons-Morton BG, Brink SG, Simons-Morton DG, Parcel GS, McIntyre RM, Chapman M, Longoria J. An ecological approach to preventing injuries due to drinking and driving. *Health Educ Quart* 16(3): 397-411, 1989.

Simons-Morton BG, Coates TJ, Saylor KE, Sereghy E, Barofsky I. Great Sensations: A program to encourage heart healthy snacking by high school students. *J of School Health* 54(8): 288-291, 1984.

Simons-Morton BG, Parcel GS, Barnanowski T, O'Hara N, Forthofer R. Promoting a healthful diet and physical activity among children: Results of a school-based intervention study. *Am J Public Health* 81(2): 986-991, 1991b.

Simons-Morton BG, Parcel GS, O'Hara NM. Implementing organizational changes to promote healthful diet and physical activity at school. *Health Educ Quart* 15(1): 115-130, 1988.

Simons-Morton BG, Simons-Morton DG. Controlling Injuries Due to Drinking and Driving: The Context and Functions of Education. *Surgeon General's Workshop on Drunk Driving: Background Papers*. Rockville, MD: Office of the Surgeon General (PHS) USDHHS, 1989.

Simons-Morton DG, Brink SG, Parcel GS, et al. *Promoting physical activity Among Adults: A CDC Community Intervention Handbook*. Centers for Disease Control: Atlanta GA, 1988b.

Simons-Morton DG, Mullen PD, Mains DA, Tabak ER, Green LW. Characteristics of controlled studies of patient education and counseling for preventive health behaviors. *Patient Educ and Couns* 19:175-204, 1992.

Simons-Morton DG, Parcel GS, Brink SG. *Smoking Control among Women: A CDC Community*

Intervention Handbook. Atlanta, GA: Centers for Disease Control, 1987.

Simons-Morton DG, Simons-Morton BG, Parcel GS, Bunker JF. Influencing personal and environmental conditions for community health: A multilevel intervention model. *Family and Community Health* 11(2): 25–35, 1988.

Skinner BF. *Beyond Freedom and Dignity.* New York: Alfred A. Knopf, 1971.

Skinner BF. *About Behaviorism.* New York: Alfred A. Knopf, 1974.

Sliepcevich EM. *School Health Education Study: A Summary Report.* Washington, DC: School Health Education Study, 1964.

Smith GS, Falk H. Unintentional injuries. In *Closing the Gap: The Burden of Unnecessary Illness,* Ambler RW, Dull HB (eds). New York: Oxford University Press, 1987.

Smith D, Redican KJ, Olsen LK. The longevity of growing healthy: An analysis of the eight original sites implementing the school health curriculum project. *J School Health* 62:83–87, 1992.

Society for Public Health Education (SOPHE). *What Is A Public Health Educator?* Berkeley: CA: Society for Public Health Education, 1976.

Society for Public Health Education. *SOPHE Code of Ethics.* Berkeley: CA: Society for Public Health Education, 1983.

Sol N, Wilson PK (eds). *Hospital Health Promotion.* Champaign, IL: Human Kinetics Books, 1989.

Starr P. *The Social Transformation of American Medicine.* New York: Basic Books, 1982.

Steckler A, Dawson, Goodman RM, Epstein N. Policy advocacy: Three emerging roles for health education. *Advances in Health Education and Promotion, Vol 2.* Greenwich, CT: JAI Press, 1987.

Steckler A, Goodman RM, McLeroy KR, Davis S, Koch G. Measuring the diffusion of innovative health promotion programs. *Am J Health Promot* 6(3): 214–224, 1992.

Steele F. *The Role of the Internal Consultant.* Boston: CBI Publishing, 1982.

Steuart, GW. Psycho-sociological bases of behaviour change. *Communications and Behavior Change: Proceedings of the VII International Conference on Health and Health Education.* Buenos Aires: International Union for Health Education, 1969.

Strecher VJ, DeVellis BM, Becker MH, Rosentock IM. The role of self-efficacy in achieving health behavior change. *Health Educ Quart* 13:73–91, 1986.

Stuart RB. Case work treatment of depression viewed as an interpersonal disturbance. *Social Work* 12:27–36, 1967.

Sullivan D. Model for comprehensive, systematic program development in health education. *Health Educ Report* 1 1:4–5, 1973.

Syme SL. Social determinants of disease. In *Maxcy-Rosenau Public Health and Preventive Medicine, 13th Edition,* Last J, Wallace RB (eds). Norwalk, CT: Appleton and Lange, 1991.

Taub A, Kreuter M, Parcel G, Vitello E. Report from the AAHE/SOPHE joint committee on ethics. *Health Educ Quart* 14:79–90, 1987.

Terris M. Approach to an epidemiology of health. *Am J Public Health* 65:1037–1045, 1975.

Terris M. Public health policy for the 1990s. *Annu Rev Public Health* 11:39–51, 1990.

Texas Association of School Administrators. A vision all its own. *Insight,* Winter: 15–16, 1992.

Texas Association of School Administrators. *All Well News,* Spring, 1994.

Thomas L. *The Lives of a Cell.* New York: Bantam Books, 1975.

Thomas L. *The Medusa and the Snail.* New York: Bantam Books, 1980.

Toffler A. *Power Shift: Knowledge, Wealth, and Violence at the Edge of the 21st Century.* New York: Bantam Books, 1990.

Trice HM, Beyer JM. *The Cultures of Work Organizations.* Englewood Cliffs, NJ: Prentice-Hall, 1993.

Tritsch L. A look back on the seaside conference. *J Health Educ* 22:70–72, 1991.

Trollope A. *An Autobiography.* New York: Oxford University Press, 1980.

U.S. Bureau of the Census. *Statistical Abstract of the United States: 1991. 111th Edition.* Washington, DC, 1991.

U.S. Bureau of the Census. *Statistical Abstract of the United States: 1992. 112th Edition.* Washington, DC, 1992.

U.S. Bureau of the Census. *Statistical Abstract of the United States: 1993. 113th Edition..* Washington, DC, 1993.

USDHEW. *Smoking and Health.* Washington, DC: USDHEW, 1964.

USDHEW. *Report on Licensure and Related Personnel Credentialing.* Washington, DC: DHEW Pub. No. (HSM) 72-11, 1971.

USDHEW. *The Health Consequences of Smoking.* Washington, DC: USDHEW, 1972.

USDHHS. *Healthy People: The Surgeon General's Report on Health Promotion and Disease Prevention.* Washington, DC: USDHEW (PHS), 1979.

USDHHS. *Promoting Health—Preventing Disease: Objectives for the Nation*. Washington, DC: PHS, 1980.

USDHHS. *Healthy People 2000. National Health Promotion and Disease Prevention Objectives*. Washington, DC: PHS, 1990.

USDHHS. *Promoting Health—Preventing Disease: Year 2000 Objectives for the Nation*. Washington, DC: PHS, 1991.

USDHHS. *Healthy Communities 2000: Model Standards, Guidelines for Community Attainment of the Year 2000 National Health Objectives*. Washington, DC: DHHS Publication No. (PHS) 91-502-12, 1991.

USDHHS. *1992 National Survey of Worksite Health Promotion Activities Summary Report*. Washington, DC: PHS, 1993.

U.S. Preventive Services Task Force. *Guide to Clinical Preventive Services*. Baltimore, MD: Williams & Wilkins, 1989.

U.N. Development Programme. *Human Development Report 1991*. New York: Oxford University Press, 1991.

U.N. Development Programme. *Human Development Report 1993*. New York: Oxford University Press, 1993.

Value Line Investment Survey: Part 2, Selection and Opinion. The quarterly economic review 1995; 24:8225.

Verbrugge LM. Recent, present, and future health of American adults. *Annu Rev Public Health* 10:333-361, 1989.

Villejo LA. Designing patient education programs for target populations. In *Managing Hospital-based Patient Education*, Giloth BE (ed). Chicago: American Hospital Publishing, 1993.

Wallace HM, Patrick K, Parcel GS, Igoe JB (eds). *Principles and Practices of Student Health, Vol. Two: School Health*. Oakland, CA: Third Party Publishing, 1992.

Wallack L, Dorfman L, Jernigan D, Themba M. *Media Advocacy and Public Health: Power for Prevention*. Newbury Park, CA: Sage Publications, 1993.

Wallston KA, Wallston BS. Health locus of control scales. In *Research with the Locus of Control Construct, Vol. I*, Lefcourt H (ed). New York: Academic Press, 1981.

Ware JE, et al. Choosing measures of health status for individuals in general populations. *Am J Public Health* 71(6): 620-625, 1981.

Warner KE. Financial analysis of workplace health promotion programs. Presented at the annual meeting of the American Journal of Health Promotion, Colorado Springs, CO, February 22-26, 1994.

Warner KE, Luce BR. *Cost-Benefit and Cost-Effectiveness Analysis in Health Care: Principles, Practice, and Potential*. Ann Arbor, MI: Health Administration Press, 1982.

Weiner B. *Human Motivation: Metaphors, Theories, and Research*. Newbury Park, CA: Sage Publications, 1992.

Windsor RA, Baranowski T, Clark N, Cutter G. *Evaluation of Health Promotion, Health Education and Disease Prevention Programs, 2nd Edition*. Mountain View, CA: Mayfield, 1994.

Windsor RA, et al. The effectiveness of smoking cessation methods for smokers in public health maternity clinics: A randomized trial. *Am J Public Health* 75(12): 1389-1392, 1985.

Woods PJ (ed). *Is Psychology the Major for You?* American Psychological Association, 1200 Seventeenth Street, NW, Washington, DC, 1987.

World Health Organization (WHO). *Report of the Working Group on Concepts and Principles of Health Promotion*. Copenhagen, 1984.

World Resources 1988-1989. A Report by the World Resources Institute and the International Institute for Environmental Development. New York: Basic Books, 1988.

Zaltman G, Duncan R. *Strategies for Planned Change*. New York: Wiley, 1977.

Index